THE USE OF CREATIVE THERAPIES WITH SURVIVORS OF DOMESTIC VIOLENCE

THE USE OF THE CREATIVE THERAPIES WITH SURVIVORS OF DOMESTIC VIOLENCE

Edited by

STEPHANIE L. BROOKE, Ph.D., NCC

CHARLES C THOMAS • PUBLISHER, LTD.
Springfield • Illinois • U.S.A.

Published and Distributed Throughout the World by

CHARLES C THOMAS • PUBLISHER, LTD.
2600 South First Street
Springfield, Illinois 62704

ISBN 978-0-398-07818-8 (hard)
ISBN 978-0-398-07819-5 (paper)

Library of Congress Catalog Card Number: 2008012538

With THOMAS BOOKS *careful attention is given to all details of manufacturing and design. It is the Publisher's desire to present books that are satisfactory as to their physical qualities and artistic possibilities and appropriate for their particular use.* THOMAS BOOKS *will be true to those laws of quality that assure a good name and good will.*

Printed in the United States of America
CR-R-3

Library of Congress Cataloging-in-Publication Data

The use of the creative therapies with survivors of domestic violence / edited by Stephanie L. Brooke.
p. ; cm.
Includes bibliographical references and index.
ISBN 978-0-398-07818-8 (hard) -- ISBN 978-0-398-07819-5 (pbk.)
1. Victims of family violence--Mental health. 2. Art therapy. 3. Play therapy. 4. Music therapy. 5. Psychiatry, Transcultural. I. Brooke, Stephanie L.
[DNLM: 1. Domestic Violence--psychology. 2. Sensory Art Therapies--methods. 3. Cross-Cultural Comparison. 4. Stress Disorders, Post-Traumatic--therapy. 5. Survivors--psychology. WM 450 U84 2008]

RC569.5.F3U84 2008
618.92'8582230651--dc22

2008012538

CONTRIBUTORS

I extend my deepest appreciation to the following contributors for sharing their expertise and experience about their work with survivors of domestic violence. Each of these contributors was selected on the basis of his or her experience with respect to clinical issues, diversity in theoretical orientation, or treatment modality. As you read each chapter, it is my hope you will share in my appreciation for the insights contributed by the following individuals:

Liora Abrahams Brosbe, MA

Liza Avetikova, MPS

Brian L. Bethel, MEd, PCC-S, LCDC III

Meredith B. Carleton, MPS, ATR-BC, LCAT, CCLS

Meg Chang, EdD, LCAT, NCC, ADTR

Amy Clarkson, MMT, MT-BC, CP, LCAT

Sandra L. Curtis, Ph.D., MT-BC, MTA

Alexia Electris, MPS, ATR, LCAT

Janice Hnath, MPS, BCSCR, ATR-BC, LCAT

Ellen Horovitz, Ph.D., LCAT, ATR-BC

Fern Leventhal, Ph.D.

Kristin Long, LCAT, RDT/BCT

Athena P. Madan, MA

Dawn Lorraine McBride, Ph.D.

Mary L. McGinnis, MA, LMHC, LMFT, NCC, CLA

Barbara McKechnie, LCAT, RDT, LPC

Charles E. Myers, MA, LPC, LMHC, NCC, RPT-S

Deborah K. Pierce, MA, RDT/BCT

Joshua A. Thomas-Acker, MS, LMHC, LPC, NCC, CAP

Sonali Senroy, BA

PREFACE

The *Use of the Creative Therapies with Survivors of Domestic Violence* is a comprehensive work that examines the use of art, play, music, dance/ movement, drama, and supervision with respect to treatment issues relating to family violence. The author's primary purpose is to examine treatments approaches which cover the broad spectrum of the creative art therapies. The collection of chapters is written by renowned, well-credentialed, and professional creative art therapists in the areas of art, play, music, dance/ movement, and drama. In addition, some of the chapters are complimented with photographs of client art work, diagrams, and tables. The reader is provided with a snapshot of how these various creative art therapies are used to treat male and females suffering from domestic violence. This informative book will be of special interest to educators, students, therapists as well as people struggling with family violence issues.

S.L.B.

CONTENTS

ILLUSTRATIONS

Page

Chapter 1

Chapter 2

Chapter 3

Chapter 4

Chapter 7

Plates

Chapter 11

Chapter 14

Chapter 15

Chapter 16

THE USE OF CREATIVE THERAPIES WITH SURVIVORS OF DOMESTIC VIOLENCE

Chapter 1

INTRODUCTION: ART THERAPY ASSESSMENTS WITH A CHINESE SURVIVOR OF DOMESTIC VIOLENCE

Stephanie L. Brooke

In 2005, I had the opportunity to present on art therapy assessments at the first International Creative Arts Therapy conference in Beijing, China. The conference was designed for professionals who used or were interested in the arts as a method of healing. I was one of two "foreign" friends presenting at the conference. Profession Fucius, the chair of the conference, arranged for the foreign friends to do individual sessions with a client. I had the opportunity to do art therapy assessments with a 41-year-old Chinese woman who presented with the problem of debilitating menstrual pain. This chapter will describe the one session I had with this woman, who we later discovered was a witness to domestic violence. She gave permission to discuss this case and publish her artwork.

Sue, not her real name, started off by discussing the painful periods she had each month. Right off the bat, she related the fact that she had two abortions. In talking about this pain, which she had no explanation for and had been checked by a doctor, she related about the recent breakup with her boyfriend. "Why do I always end up with this sort of man?" she exclaimed. She seemed exasperated. In taking a transactional view, she would often play the parent role and care taker of the man in her life. The parent role forced the boyfriend into the child role and power struggles ensued. This was a repeating pattern in her life. I decided to try a few assessments with her: the Kinetic House-Tree-Person Test (Burns, 1987) and Family Centered Circle Drawings (Burns, 1990). I started off with some baseline exercises such as the affective color chart, which I developed when working with clients, and line drawings representing the emotions (sad, happy, angry, fearful - see Appendix). I will start off with a brief review of the assessment covering the purpose, validity and reliability as determined by the author, desirable features, undesirable features, and overall evaluation. For a more in depth review of the assessments, please see my book, *Tools of the Trade: A Therapist's Guide to Art Therapy Assessments* (Brooke, 2004).

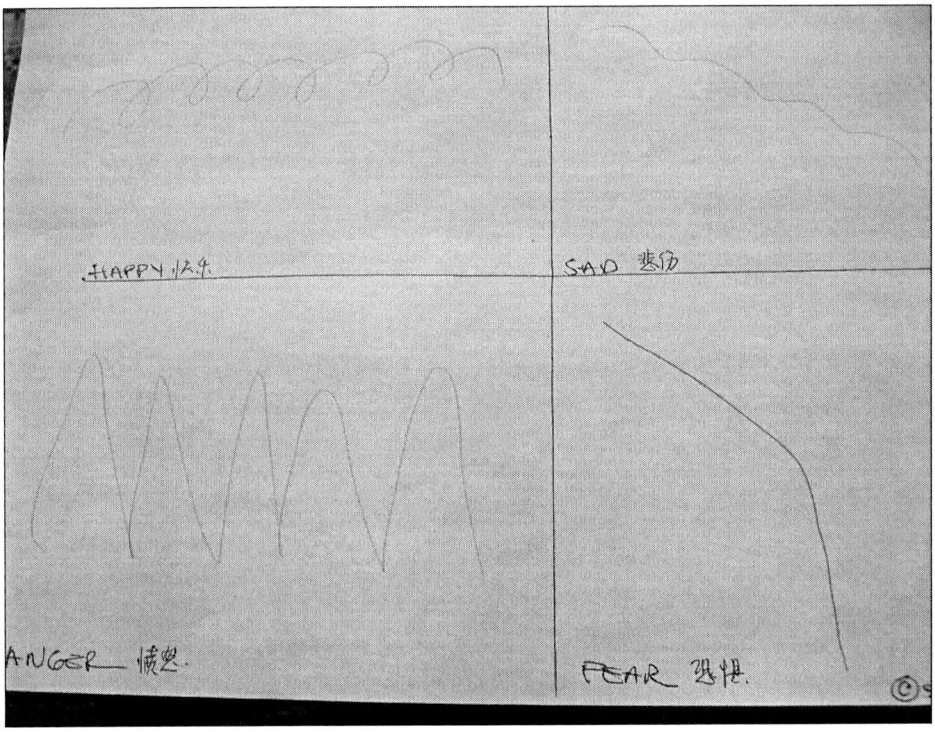

Figure 1. Line Drawings.

Kinetic House-Tree-Person Test

Because of the limitations of the House-Tree-Person Test (HTP) and the Draw a Person Test (DAP), researchers moved toward the development of kinetic assessments. "Projective, non-kinetic techniques are criticized because they restrict the depiction of important family dynamics that provide the greatest insight into a child's feelings and perceptions, and his family's roles, influences, and interactions" (Knoff & Prout, 1985, p. 51). One assessment that incorporated a kinetic component was the Kinetic House-Tree-Person Test (KHTP).

As opposed to the HTP, the KHTP combined all three images, house, tree, and person, on one page. In addition, the drawing introduced physical activity of family members. Despite the clinical value of the HTP, Burns (1987, p. 5) remarked on a few limitations:

1. The HTP was standardized on patients in a psychiatric setting. Literature on the HTP focused on diagnostic labeling such as "Organics, Schizophrenics, etc."

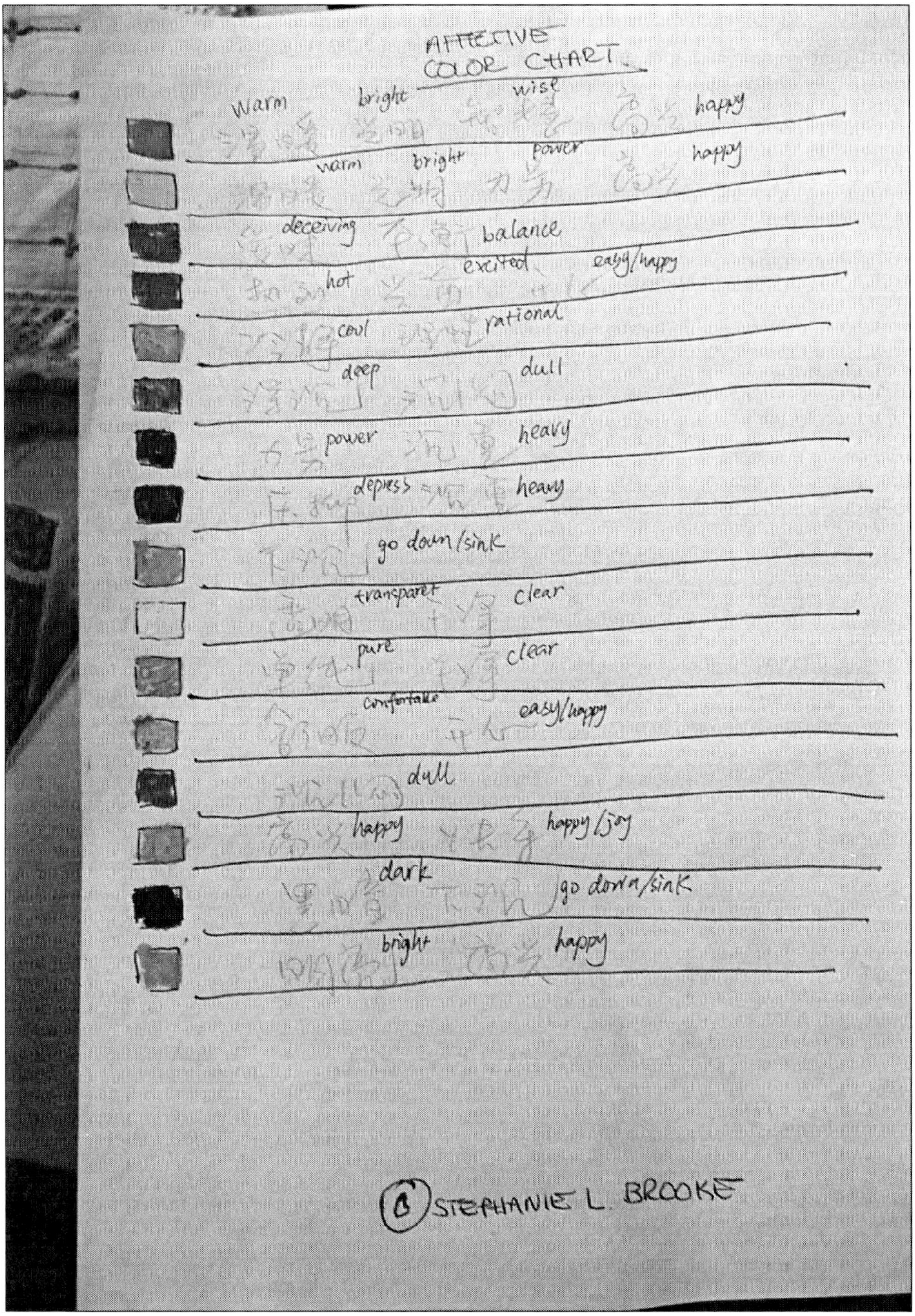

Figure 2. Affective Color Chart (see also Appendix).

2. Placement of the images occurred on separate pieces of paper that did not allow for action or interaction.
3. Interpretation of the HTP was Freudian and reduced all images to fit within this matrix.

The KHTP was developed to surpass some of the limitations presented by the HTP, which resulted in more clinical information about the client.

The purpose of the KHTP was to furnish information on the parameters of a client's perspective that may otherwise remain illusive using some traditional drawing techniques such as the HTP. "The K-H-T-P is useful in understanding the dynamics in many types of clinical situations, thus enhancing the healing process" (Burns, 1987, p. 7). The KHTP assessment was devised to tell a story; to create a visual metaphor about self.

Validity and Reliability as Determined by the Author

Burns (1987) did not incorporate reliability or validity information in his book. He mentioned that kinetic drawings have been reliably scored (Burns & Kaufman, 1972; Knoff & Prout, 1985); yet, he did not provide further information. To date, reliability, and validity for the KHTP has not been examined. Although the KHTP was based on the HTP, it cannot be expected to rely on the research used to support the HTP. Additional research is necessary in order to confirm that the KHTP is a reliable and valid art therapy assessment.

Desirable Features

The test was easy to administer. Further, the manual included several case examples to assist the therapist with interpretation. Adding a kinetic component was a valuable idea. Moving figures will yield more information about personality as compared to static figures. Additionally, combining the house, tree, and person all on one page produces more information than when viewed separately. For instance, when the tree was leaning slightly away from the house, this may indicate growing independence and moving away from family attachments (Burns, 1987). Another possibility was having a person attached to the house. This may suggest a need for nurturing (Burns, 1987). By viewing the interaction of these objects, the therapist was able to glean more information than viewing the house, tree, and person separately.

Not only were attachments and proximity important, but also the order in which the items were drawn may reveal information about the client's personality. When the client draws the tree first, it may reveal that "life energy and growth are most important to the drawer. This was typical of people trying to grow or stay alive" (Burns, 1987, p. 102). If the client draws the house first, it may show a need to belong to the earth (a place to survive), need to belong to the body (body needs or obsessions), a need to belong to society, a home for nurturing, or a home for giving and receiving nurturing (Burns, 1987). If the client draws the person first, it may suggest concern with control of feelings, showing off or hiding the body, showing success, a nurturing person, or a joyful person.

Another desirable feature of the KHTP was the incorporation of Maslow's (1954) theory to create a developmental model for the assessment. Burns (1987) modified Maslow's approach to interpret the items on the KHTP. He came up with the following five levels (p. 54):

Level 1: Belong to Life: Desire for life, survival, safety, rootedness.
Level 2: Belong to body: Acceptance of body, seeking control of body addictions and potential.
Level 3: Belong to society: Search for status, success, respect, and power.
Level 4: Belong to self and not self: Self now defined to include not self as a pregnant woman accepts her child; compassion, nurturing, giving love; meta motivation.
Level 5: Belong to all living things: Giving and accepting love; self actualization; sense of good fortune and luck; creativity; celebration of life.

Burns interpreted each item on the KHTP within this framework. Further, he divided each level into Approachers and Avoiders. Burns (1987) provided a similar breakdown for the developmental levels of the tree and person. In addition, he included several examples of drawings to indicate the various stages of development.

Burns (1987) also presented an appendix that summarized the general characteristics of the images drawn. These were hypotheses used when judging projective drawing techniques: They involved pressure factors, line or stroke characteristics, drawing size, and placement of the drawing. For instance, if a drawing was placed low on the page, it was said to suggest feelings of insecurity (Buck, 1948; Burns & Kaufman, 1972; Jolles, 1964), feelings of inadequacy (Buck, 1948; Burns & Kaufman, 1972; Hammer, 1971; Jolles, 1964), or depressive tendencies (Buck, 1948; Hammer, 1971; Jolles, 1964; Machover, 1949). Burns (1987) also furnished a summary of individual characteristics of the house, tree, and person.

Undesirable Features

The KHTP may be difficult to interpret when a symbol occurs that were not included in the case examples or the summary tables. For instance, I had one client who drew her person in the shape of a mandala, with two legs, and several eyes. It was not clear how to interpret this figure or where to place it within the developmental model presented by Burns (1987).

Although Burns (1987) provided a table for the scoring of attachments, he did not include scoring information when presenting the case examples. These tables were simplified in that they only note the presence of attachments and figures. Their significance was not discussed. For instance, I would have liked more information on clients who included deceased persons or political figures in their drawings. Obviously, these figures were important; yet, Burns (1987) did not present a framework for interpretation.

As Gould (1990) notes, the manual was not organized and is often unclear. The intended use of developmental levels is not made clear in the manual; therefore, interpretation from a Maslowian perspective is difficult.

Overall Evaluation of the KHTP

Many have argued about the universal interpretation of symbols. Whether archetypes or cultural symbols, interpretation without the client's input is not valid. Burns (1987) warned against the over interpretation of drawing symbols; "Interpretation of all symbols depends on the level of consciousness of the producer of the symbol at the time the symbols was produced and the level of consciousness of the interpreter at the time of interpretation. There is obviously room for a great deal of error" (Burns, 1987, p. 143). With this thought in mind, Burns (1987) suggested a procedure for interpreting symbols based on level of consciousness. For example, water can have various meanings depending on the consciousness level (p. 147):

Level 1: Survival, embryonic stage
Level 2: "Juices flowing," hedonistic
Level 3: "Power of sea," water beats rock
Level 4: Nurturing, refreshing, useful
Level 5: Flexible, humble, serene, calm

This breakdown was provided for only a few of the symbols. It was not clear how the therapist would use this breakdown when other symbols were present. This point addressed the main weakness of the manual: The interpretation of symbols or drawing features that were not presented by Burns (1987). Granted, the client was the source for interpreting all symbols but what if the client was nonverbal or was unable to communicate the meaning of the item? Regardless of this weakness, the KHTP yielded some valuable information about the client's perception of self, the environment, and the family. The kinetic component was a valuable addition to the HTP. The interaction of the items as well as the developmental model was a strong improvement over the HTP.

Overall, the test was easy to administer and the case examples were interesting. Additional research information is needed on this assessment, especially the reliability and validity of symbol interpretation. In addition, it would be interesting to have information on the chromatic version of the test. Color choice may reveal additional information about the client. The investigation of possible cultural differences that may be found in the KHTP would be worthwhile.

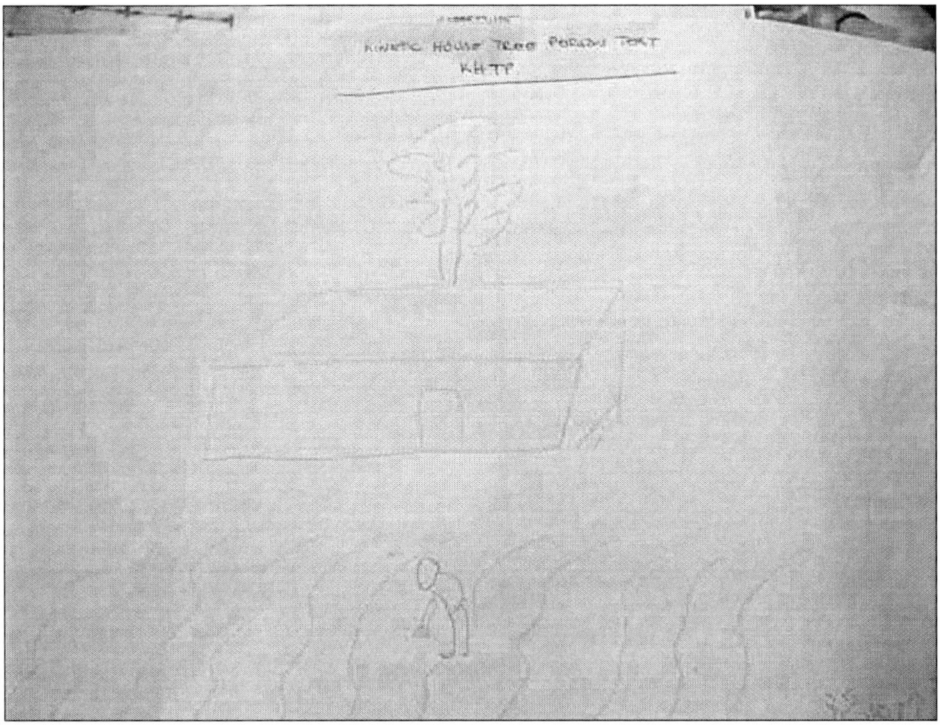

Figure 3. KHTP.

Sue drew the house first, then the person, and last the tree. When the client draws the house first, it may show a need to belong to the earth (a place to survive), need to belong to the body (body needs or obsessions), a need to belong to society, a home for nurturing, or a home for giving and receiving nurturing (Burns, 1987). The drawing is very impoverished and shows a person working in the field, much like she had done when she was growing up. She drew lines associated with happiness in the tree while the field was represented with sad lines. There is no access to the house which possibly indicates lack of interest in establishing environmental contact (Burns, 1987). There are no windows in the house. Additionally, the person would not be able to access the door. This may indicate a person who appears to want people in their space but the really want them out (Burns, 1987). Also, there is no doorknob on the door. This is associated with people who want privacy and do not want their space invaded (Burns, 1987).

The tree is also attached to the house, stemming right out of the center of the house. It has circular lines for the leaves possibility indicating a lack of direction in her spiritual life. According to Burns (1987), attachment of two figures means a "Symbiotic relationship most frequently found where the drawer has two aspects of life intertwined, usually inhibiting growth" (p. 131).

The person is drawn hunched over with no features. Although she was instructed to draw a whole person, it resembles more of a stick figure. Both the tree and the person were created using heavy lines. Burns (1987) suggests that heavy pressure may be due to the following:

1. Extremely tense individuals.
2. Organic conditions, possibly encephalitis or epileptic conditions.
3. Assertive, forceful, ambitious persons.
4. Aggressive and possible acting-out tendencies (p. 181).

The person is the smallest image on the page possibly suggesting feelings of insecurity (Buck, 1948; Burns & Kaufman, 1972), possible depressive tendencies (Machover, 1949), or regressive tendencies (Burns, 1987; Machover, 1949). The assessment was completed in five minutes possibly indicating resistance to the task.

Family-Centered Circle Drawings

The Family-Centered Circle Drawings (FCCD; Burns, 1990) assessment was based on the concept of inner parents and the relationship to the self. Through the creation of symbol systems in drawings, therapists may determine how clients relate to their parents. Specifically, clients' emotions towards their parents and barriers between them were discussed in comparison to the clients' inner parents. Since symbol systems were created by the client, they were unique and served to bring the person closer to center (Burns, 1990).

FCCDs were based partly on Rorschach's findings relating to increased projective material with symmetry. Although standardized inkblot tests were previously used, Rorschach (1942) was the first to apply inkblots to assessment of personality as a whole (Anastasi, 1988). Rorschach (1942) discovered that symmetrical inkblots produced more responses and more unconscious material than asymmetrical inkblots. Burns (1990) incorporated this research by placing individual family members in a centered, symmetrical matrix. By drawing parents and self, the client may begin to see parent-self relationships more clearly and the impact on her own inner parents.

Jung's work with mandalas also contributed to the FCCD. According to Burns (1990), a mandala was a centered symbol in a symmetrical design.

> Psychologically speaking, a mandala image is one that emphasizes the totality of something, usually showing quite clearly a periphery and a center. In its historical sense, the term mandala refers to certain very structured meditation symbols used in Buddhism, often consisting of a four-gated square or circular city with a central image (to be meditated on) and lesser images surrounding it. (Hall, 1983, p.76)

Jung extensively studied mandalas in his search for balance and health (Rubin, 1987). Additionally, Jung was a novice artist who worked through his own conflicts by painting and sculpting: "In fact, Jung's theories can best be understood in the context of the value he attached to the subjective reality of spontaneously generated images" (Rubin, 1987, p. 93). The FCCD combined the use of the mandala with the concept of centering and artistic expression. Burns (1990) perceived that the key to these drawings was centering:

> By centering a symbol and focusing upon it in a symmetrical matrix, one may elicit deep emotional reactions. In the religious world focusing upon centered symbols such as a cross, star, lamb, divine figure, and so on may bring insights and healing. In the projective drawing world, centering upon the self-created images of the parents or of the parents and the self may also bring insights and healing. (Burns, 1990, p. 2)

By placing family figures in the center of the circle, Burns (1990) believed that it would increase projective material. Using this approach, the therapist fostered a dialogue with the client's inner parents in order to determine barriers and emotional conflicts.

The purpose of the FCCD was to gain information about the client's family and relate it to the client's view of self and his/her inner parents. According to Burns (1990), this technique allowed the client to see self more clearly in relationship to each parent. Positive and negative associations were made around the symbols systems that the client created. The FCCD was recommended for those clients who need to get in touch with their inner parents. The objective of Burns' (1990) approach was to furnish counselors with an awareness of the client's visual communication potential. Also, therapists may be able to provide a broader interpretive context that was not heavily dependent on verbal skills.

Validity and Reliability as Determined by the Author

Burns (1990) did not present reliability or validity data on the FCCD. Also, he did not use a population to standardize this assessment. The validity of the items in the Appendix was questionable. The test manual did not include many examples of children's or adolescents' work. Most of the clients were in their thirties and forties. Other demographic characteristics of the clients were not presented. Whether the FCCD was a valid and reliable instrument for children or adults was unclear. It would be interesting to collect data on the interpretations of a variety of practitioners such as art therapists, counselors, and psychologists to see if there was reliable agreement among professionals as to the interpretation of these drawings. To date, no research was available that examined the reliability and validity of this assessment, or research that used the FCCD as a therapeutic tool.

Desirable Features

The FCCD was an interesting assessment in that it provided information about the client with respect to their parents. It was different from the Kinetic Family Drawing (KFD; Burns & Kaufman, 1972) in that the therapist was able to see the client's relationship with one parent at a time and focus in on one particular symbol. When I implemented the FCCD in private practice, the client gained insight from the types of symbols that were drawn in relation to self and to their parents. This assessment seemed to be more helpful in uncovering the barriers in the client's past relationship with their parents as opposed to discovering or getting in touch with their inner parents.

Undesirable Features

Burns (1990) did not outline what types of drawing media the administrator should make available to the client. It was difficult to tell from the drawings included in the book what type of medium was used and if it was consistently used. The addition of color may significantly influence the outcome of the assessment; yet, this was not addressed by Burns (1990).

Interpretation of the FCCD appeared limited. It focused only on the drawing and neglected other aspects of the domain. For instance, observing a client's affect while drawing does yield important information. In addition, the manner in which something was drawn or erased may be significant to the interpretation of the drawing. Some may consider the FCCD a "cookbook" approach (Koppitz, 1968). Burn's (1990) FCCD did not contain a list of symbols that the counselor looks up for interpretation. Much of the interpretation was left up to the client, which has a positive function. Yet, it did follow the cookbook approach to art therapy in that it neglected to observe the manner in which the drawings were completed. Valuable information regarding client affect may be missed if the therapist did not observe the drawing process.

Overall Evaluation

Burns (1990) combined free association, family of origin work, object relations, and Jungian mandala symbolism to create an assessment that helped the client view self in relationship to parents and inner parents. Through a series of centered circle drawings, the client created a visual dialog about his/her relationships with the family. The book contained many examples of each of these drawings.

Although Burns (1990) provided large collection of drawings and explained how to create them, they were in black and white. The colors and media used were not discussed. Thus, the reader lacks a complete visual sense of the drawings. Paint, pastels, inks, and watercolors were some of the materials that clients can manipulate when creating art. Texture of the material was often a reflection of the artist's inner experience or feelings:

> As one avenue to self-definition, we have usually had some choice of art materials, and have on occasion asked that people define themselves by choosing to be an art medium or process, and sharing their reasons. We have found that their choice is intimately related to how they see themselves, i.e., soft or hard, flexible or firm, fragile or strong, colorful or bland, etc. The choice of medium then evolves into a productive activity with that medium, in both cases self-defining and enhancing self-awareness. (Moreno, 1975, p. 113)

Art therapists use the characteristics of art materials for diagnostic purposes. For instance, watercolors involve complex layering. This medium was unpredictable and transparent in nature that allowed the artist spontaneous expression. Since watercolors were hard to control, Robbins (1987) stressed that people who employ this medium were spontaneous individuals who accepted change and relinquished omnipotence. Working with oils was a time consuming process because it entailed layering. People who used this medium were patient, allowed change, and preferred a predetermined challenge (Robbins, 1987). The use of pencil indicated a need for control, structure, and firm boundaries (Robbins, 1987). Finger paint was a direct form of expression. Betensky (1973) described finger paint as an agent of regression that provided an important outlet for stress. These were just a few examples of media as they related to personality characteristics. Although painting may not be an appropriate medium for this assessment, the choice of color would be revealing. For instance, a client may use colored pencils, oil pastels, or crayons to create the FCCD.

Additional information was needed regarding the reliability and validity of the FCCD. It was an interesting approach that revealed information about the client's relationship with self and family; yet, the assessment lacked important data regarding administration requirements, interpretation, and a norm population. Riley (1991) felt that this assessment may be of more interest to mental health professionals as opposed to family therapists as family therapists may be reluctant to ascribe meaning to symbols.

Research on the relationship between the KFD and the FCCD would be beneficial. One advantage of the KFD was that it observed sibling systems. Sibling interactions greatly affect the dynamics of the family system. "There is a high level of interaction among siblings in the home and that the quality of this interaction is rich and varied" (Abramovitch et al., 1979, p. 1003). In my private practice, Burns' (1990) approach was modified to include siblings. This disclosed important information about the client's relationship issues.

Also, it would be helpful to have more information on the use of the FCCD with children and special populations such as learning disabled, hearing impaired, and culturally diverse individuals. Overall, the FCCD had great potential as an art therapy assessment. With additional research information, the FCCD may be a valuable tool when viewing the client's relationship to self and the family.

After the KHTP, Sue completed the Family-Centered Circle Drawings. She used crayons to complete the assessment. The colors she used are related back to her affective chart.

Sue specifically requested to put her brother in the picture. She drew herself closest to her brother. As her KHTP, she drew another impoverished drawing; yet, the colors were revealing. She drew her mother in blue and blue for Sue represented power. The symbol next to mother was an angry lion. Sue recounted stories of how her mother was always angry. It was here that Sue told the story of the time her mother took a knife/razor and cut the scalp of her younger brother. He bled profusely. Sue was only eight years old at the time and felt helpless. The father was not around and she did not know what to do.

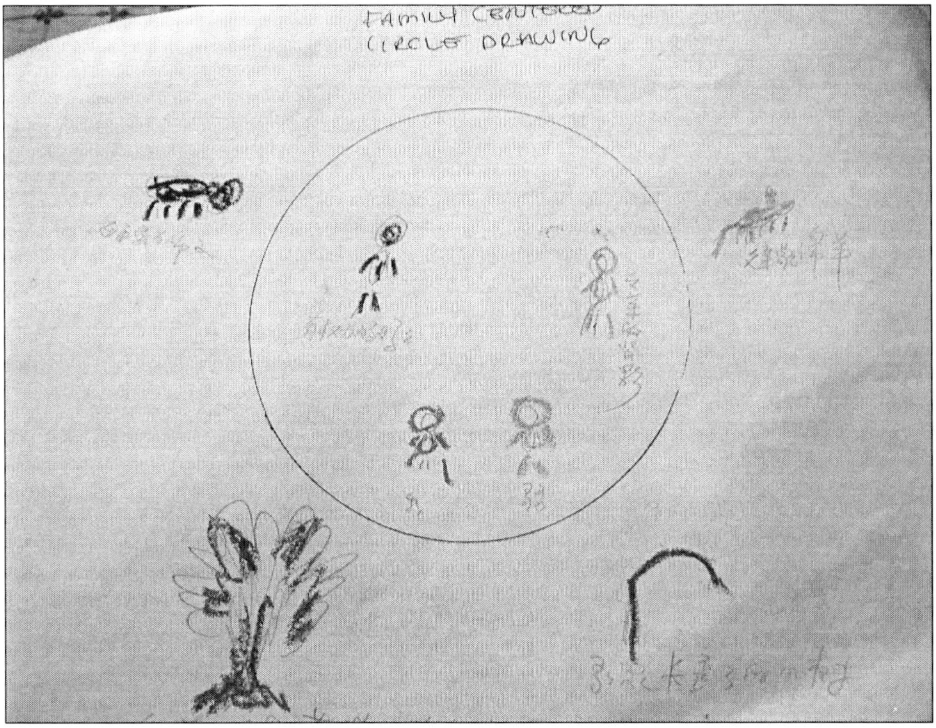

Figure 4. FCCD.

She drew herself in green which represented dullness. She drew a grounded tree next to herself which indicates a strong life force (Burns, 1987). Next to the father, in gold, was a lamb. She described gold as "go down/sink" in her affective color chart. She saw her father as very weak, always giving in to the mother. The brother and self were the smallest figures on the page which may indicate their helplessness when interacting with the mother. There is a great deal of distance between the siblings and the parents indicating possible psychological distance (Burns, 1990). The image next to him was a bending tree and took similar shape to the hunched over figure in her KHTP. It is interesting that there are fear lines in her tree symbol. The father was drawn in grey which represented rational thought.

Father-Centered Circle Drawing

Next, I asked her to put her father in the center of the circle to create a Father-Centered Circle Drawing.

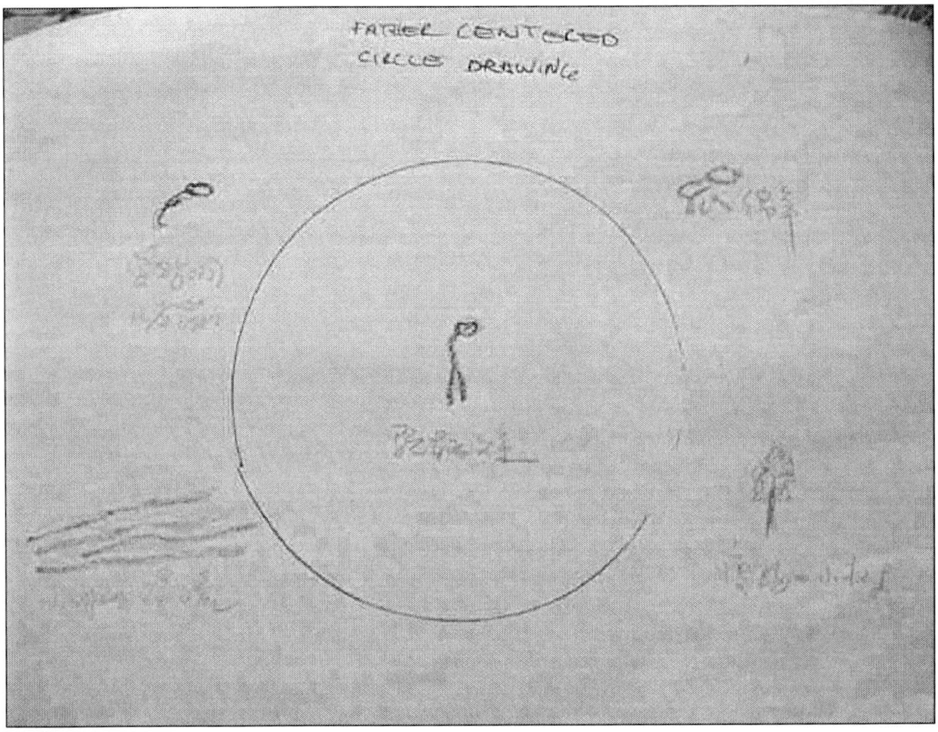

Figure 5. Father-Centered Circle Drawing.

One word that came up repeatedly with this circle drawing was her father was "weak." Sue repeated the word several times. The father was drawn bent over in the shape of fear from her baseline assessment. The figure has no arms which may indicate helplessness. There is a tiny tree drawn next to him which is not grounded. She did not view her father as a very grounded person. The top of the tree is hollow indicating a possible lack of direction in life (Burns, 1987). Next to him is a small brook with lines of possible sadness from her baseline drawing; yet, the color of happiness from her affective chart. She described her father as a "mouse that digs holes"; "always giving in to others." The father was drawn in green which represented dullness. She had a lack of connection with her father and seemed to resent him for not standing up to the mother.

Mother-Centered Circle Drawing

Next, I asked her to draw her mother in the center of the circle. This is when she revealed that her mother used to physically abuse the children.

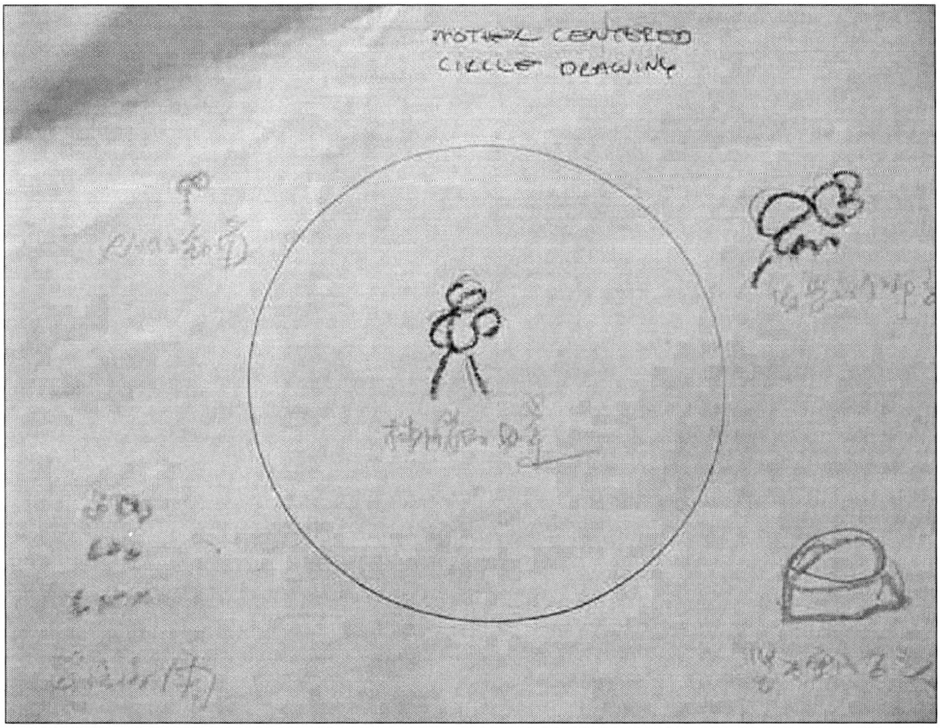

Figure 6. Mother-Centered Circle Drawing.

The mother is drawn with her hands on her hips, as if in an angry posture, in the color of blue which represents power. She drew a grey (rational) rock as one of the symbols next to her mother. Sue drew an angry lion to represent another symbol of her mother. This was a repeated symbol from the FCCD. She drew crying rain and a small sprout which may indicate helplessness.

Self-Centered Circle Drawing

This one Sue seemed kind of stuck on and it took her more time to complete than the other drawings. She described herself as having "muted anger" and Sue questioned this.

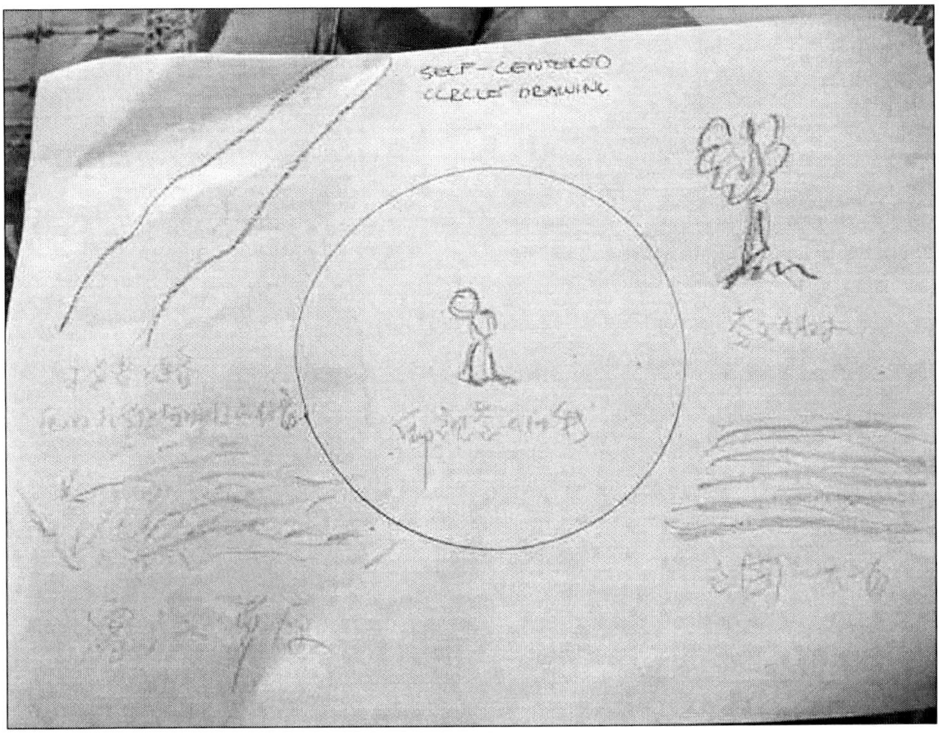

Figure 7. Self-Centered Circle Drawing.

She drew herself in orange (warm, bright, wise, happy–affective color chart) but hunched over in a fear line. Her figure lacks arms which indicates helplessness (Burns, 1987). Also, her figure's feet are backwards in line with the body, a feature I have not yet seen in a client's artwork. I wonder if this indicates that she is stuck. She then said that the figure is actually looking up to the heavens, searching, asking for help. Again, she drew a grounded tree as symbolic of herself. She also drew the sea. Sue said she loves the sea and feels she is the sea. Next, she drew a prairie. Last, she drew a path to represent her search for truth. Sue admitted that she was not very kind to self. She said that she had heart trouble which I understood to be in the emotional context. She concluded by saying she would not love another.

Symbol-Centered Circle Drawing

We concluded the session with the symbol-centered circle drawing. I picked the mother-centered circle drawing and she chose the rock to put in the center of the circle.

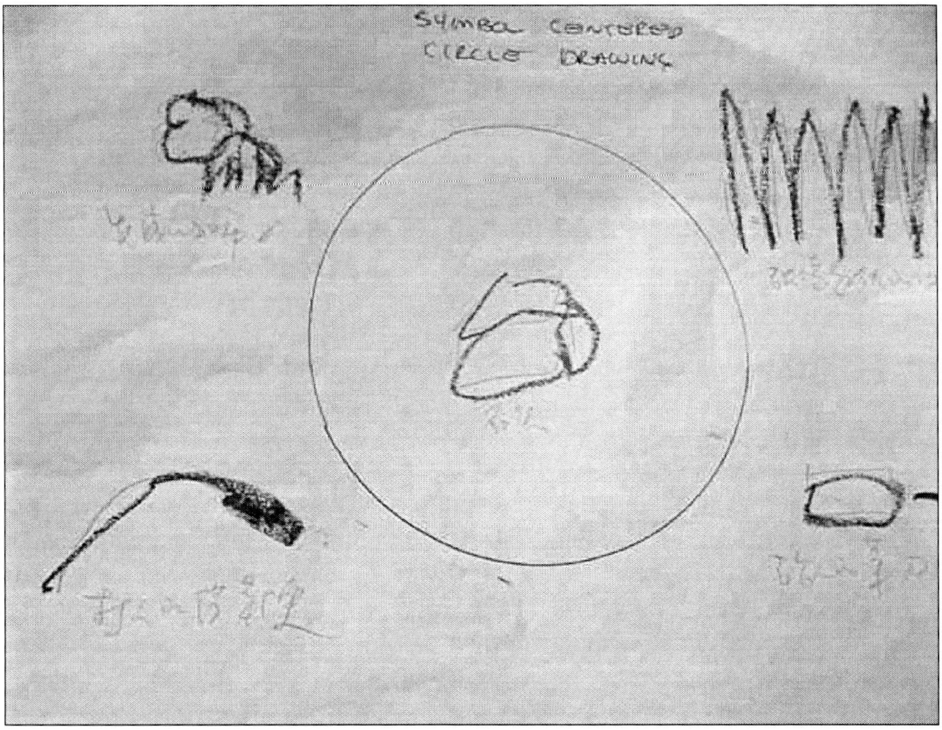

Figure 8. Symbol-Centered Circle Drawing.

The rock is drawn in brown which represented depressed or heavy feelings. She drew the razor first which was used to cut her brother. The razor is drawn in black which represented darkness or a sinking feeling. She also drew the angry lion again to represent how she remembered her mother best. She drew anger lines and used the color of blue (power) as symbolic of her mother. The last symbol was not identified.

I only got a brief view into the life of a survivor of domestic violence. Sue was struggling in relationships in life and that had a lot to do with her growing up as a parentified child. She plays the parent role while the man in her life plays the child role and it results in a struggle for power. Sue is repeating the pattern.

Domestic Violence in China

Family violence strikes nearly one in three families in China, a growing problem which is pushing Beijing to amend its 20-year-old marriage laws (*The Strait Times, 2000*). Serious injuries caused by domestic violence are rising rapidly. One hundred thousand out of the country's 270 million families become broken families each year because of domestic violence. *The South China Morning Post* reported that domestic violence occurred in 30 percent of mainland families, according to surveys conducted by the All-China Women's Federation. Victims include wives and husbands, but are mostly female. According to official figures, domestic assaults resulted in 14 deaths and 240 injuries between 1995 and 1999 (*The Strait Times*, 2000). These are sobering statistics.

This book takes a cross cultural view of domestic violence from the perspective of the victims, primarily women and their children, exploring the issue of family violence in China, U.S., Canada, and India. Chapters 1–4 cover art therapy with survivors of domestic violence, primarily children. Chapters 5, 6, and 7 cover play therapy with children who have witnessed domestic violence. Chapter 8 covers music therapy for abused women. Additionally, Chapter 9 covers music therapy with children who have witnessed domestic violence. Chapter 10 talks about the use of dance/movement therapy with victims of intimate partner and domestic violence, touching on the little discussed issues related to same-sex relationships. Chapter 11 explains family violence with young girls from India–incorporating dramatic play therapy. Chapter 12 covers drama therapy with children on an inpatient psychiatric unit. Chapter 13 discusses the use of drama therapy in domestic violence groups for incarcerated women. Also, Chapter 14 covers the use of drama therapy for women who have survived domestic violence. Chapter 15 explains the use of the creative therapies with mothers and their children. Chapter 16 looks at art and narrative therapy with child survivors of domestic violence. Lastly, Chapter 17 discusses supervision issues in family violence cases.

Appendix

AFFECTIVE COLOR CHART

NAME______________________________DATE:______________________

Directions: For each color, write in the space provided how it makes you feel. Try to move quickly through the colors. There are spaces provided below for you to add colors that you feel were not represented on the chart.

COLOR	FEELING

AFFECTIVE LINE CHART

NAME______________________________DATE:______________________

Directions: For each emotion listed, draw a single line that represents that specific emotion. Try to move quickly through the emotions.

Happy	Sad
Angry	Fear
Surprise	Discomfort

References

Abramovitch, R., Corter, C., & Lando, B. (1979). Sibling interaction in the home. *Child Development, 50*, 997-1003.
Anastasi, A. (1988). *Psychological testing* (6th ed.). New York: Macmillan.
Betensky, M. (1973). *Self-discovery through self-expression: Use of art in psychotherapy.* Springfield, IL: Charles C Thomas, Publisher, Ltd.
Brooke, S. L. (2004). *Tools of the trade: A therapist's guide to art therapy assessments.* Springfield, IL: Charles C Thomas, Publisher, Ltd.
Buck, J. N. (1948). *The House-Tree-Person Technique.* Los Angeles, CA: Western Psychological Services.
Burns, R. C. (1990). *A guide to family centered circle drawings.* New York: Brunner/Mazel.
Burns, R. C. (1987). *Kinetic House-Tree-Person-Drawings: An interpretive manual.* New York: Brunner/Mazel.
Burns, R. C., & Kaufman, S. H. (1972). *Actions, styles and symbols in kinetic family drawings (K-F-D): An interpretative manual.* New York: Brunner/Mazel.
Gould, P. (1990). Book reviews. *American Journal of Art Therapy, 28*(4), 118-120.
Hall, J.A. (1983). *Jungian dream interpretation: A handbook of theory and practice.* Toronto, Canada: Inner City Books.
Hammer, E. F. (1971). *The clinical application of projective drawings.* Springfield, IL: Charles C Thomas, Publisher, Ltd.
Jolles, I. (1964). *A catalog for the qualitative interpretation of the House-Tree-Person (H-T-P).* Los Angeles, CA: Western Psychological Services.
Knoff, H. M., & Prout, H. T. (1985). The kinetic drawing system: A review and integration of the Kinetic Family and School Drawing techniques. *Psychology in the Schools, 22* (January), 50-59.
Koppitz, E.M. (1968). *Psychological evaluation of children's human figure drawings.* New York: Grune & Stratton.
Machover, K. (1949). *Personality projection in the drawing of the human figure.* Springfield, IL: Charles C Thomas, Publisher, Ltd.
Maslow, A. H. (1954). *Motivation and personality.* New York: Harper and Row.
Moreno, Z. T. (1975). *Group psychotherapy and psychodrama.* New York: Beacon House Inc.
Riley, S. (1991). Book reviews. *American Journal of Art Therapy, 29*(4), 119-121.
Robbins, A. (1987). *The artist as therapist.* New York: Human Sciences Press.
Rorschach, H. (1942). *Psychodiagnostics.* Berne: Verlag Has Huber.
Rubin, J. A. (1987). *Approaches to art therapy.* New York: Brunner/Mazel.
The Stait Times. (2000, July 26). Domestic violence pushes China to vary marriage law. Retrieved January 13, 2008 from http://www.hartford-hwp.com/archives/55/354.html

Biography

Stephanie L. Brooke, Ph.D., NCC, teaches sociology and psychology working with Excelsior College, University of Maryland, and Capella University. She also has written books on art therapy and edits books on the use of the creative therapies: *Tools of the Trade: A therapist's guide to art therapy assessments; Art therapy with sexual abuse survivors; The creative therapy manual; The use of the creative therapies with sexual abuse survivors; The creative therapies and eating disorders.* In October 2006, she was the chief consultant for the first Creative Art Therapy Conference in Tokyo, Japan. Doctor Brooke continues to write and publish in her field. Further, Doctor Brooke serves on the editorial boards of PSYCCritiques and the *International Journal of Teaching and Learning in Higher Education.* She is Vice Chairper- son for ARIA (Awareness of Rape and Incest through Art). For more information about Doctor Brooke, please visit her web site: http://www.stephanielbrooke.com

Chapter 2

A STRUCTURAL FAMILY ART THERAPY APPROACH TO DOMESTIC VIOLENCE

Ellen G. Horovitz

INTRODUCTION

While numerous researchers have examined the theoretical construct of utilizing family systems theoretical framework for explaining family and/or domestic violence (Gelles, 1979, 1980, 1982, 1985; Gelles & Maynard, 1987; Gil, 1971; Straus, 1973), few (Horovitz, 1999, 2004, 2005; Horovitz-Darby, 1992; Kozlowska, 2001; Linesch, 1993; Malchiodi, 1997) have discussed the clinical literature, bridged the gap between research and art therapy practice, as well as provided a useful model for clinical intervention. This chapter proposes to model such application using structured family art therapy when working with an oppositional defiant disordered adolescent and his family.

Background and Reason for Referral

A school psychologist, who recognized Paul's propensity for drawing and thought his problems would best be resolved via art therapy, referred him to art therapy. The statement of concern from his sixth grade teachers was "Paul's nervousness, excitability, short attention span, moods, hostility, and poor attitude result in behavior that is disruptive in the classroom and to his own learning. This behavior is not constant but is variable with his mood cycle." As a result he was given the following batteries, which will be reported in the discussion:

- Wechsler Intelligence Scale for Children (WISC-R)
- Bender Gestalt

- House Tree Person Test (Achromatic only)
- Kinetic Family Drawing (KFD)
- Silver Drawing Test for Cognitive and Creative Abilities (SDT)
- Cognitive Art Therapy Assessment (CATA)

Developmental Milestones and Psychosocial Information

At referral, Paul, a white Caucasian eleven-year-old boy, was the younger of two siblings. He had a sister two years his senior named Debra. Biological mother, Cindy, reported that pregnancy, labor, and delivery were all normal. Paul was reported to be a good-natured child and all developmental milestones were reached within normal limits. Cindy reported that the period of time when both her children were babies was a happy and contented one for the entire family. Paul had a pleasant experience through the first grade but by his second grade, it was reported that there had been a "personality conflict" between the child and the teacher. (Apparently, Paul flew into a rage and kicked his teacher in the stomach; she was reportedly pregnant at the time.) As well, it was during this year, that Cindy and her husband, Paul, Sr., separated after several months of marital discord. The mother described herself as having a volatile temper, which easily erupted. Mother presented the father as emotionally "flat." Apparently, their differences were too vast, a divorce ensued, and father remarried one year later; at Paul's age 8 (third grade). While both children were reported to visit their father every Sunday, they harbored negative feelings towards the stepmother, Linda. Paul, however, was much more vocal about his dislike for the stepmother, which was communicated frequently in art therapy session artwork (see Figure 1 for family genogram).

Prior to family art therapy intervention (via this writer), the mother had sought appropriate parent and limit setting from a social worker. While the divorce had adverse effects on both children, the mother indicated that it was the father's lack of involvement and interest that compounded the children's difficulties. (While the mother presently reported having a boyfriend, at intake, she presented the relationship between Paul and her boyfriend as "amicable.")

Mother admitted that she easily lost her temper, had difficulty controlling arguments between Paul and Debra, and swore constantly at the children and that she was "edgy" and suffered from thyroid regulatory problems. At the referral, mother reported missing some jewelry (although Paul denied any wrongdoing) as well as an altercation between Paul and a neighborhood boy that required the other child to receive stitches at a local hospital.

Upon interview, Paul presented as amicable, anxious to please, and admitted that he feared he would be deemed "mental" and have to be institution-

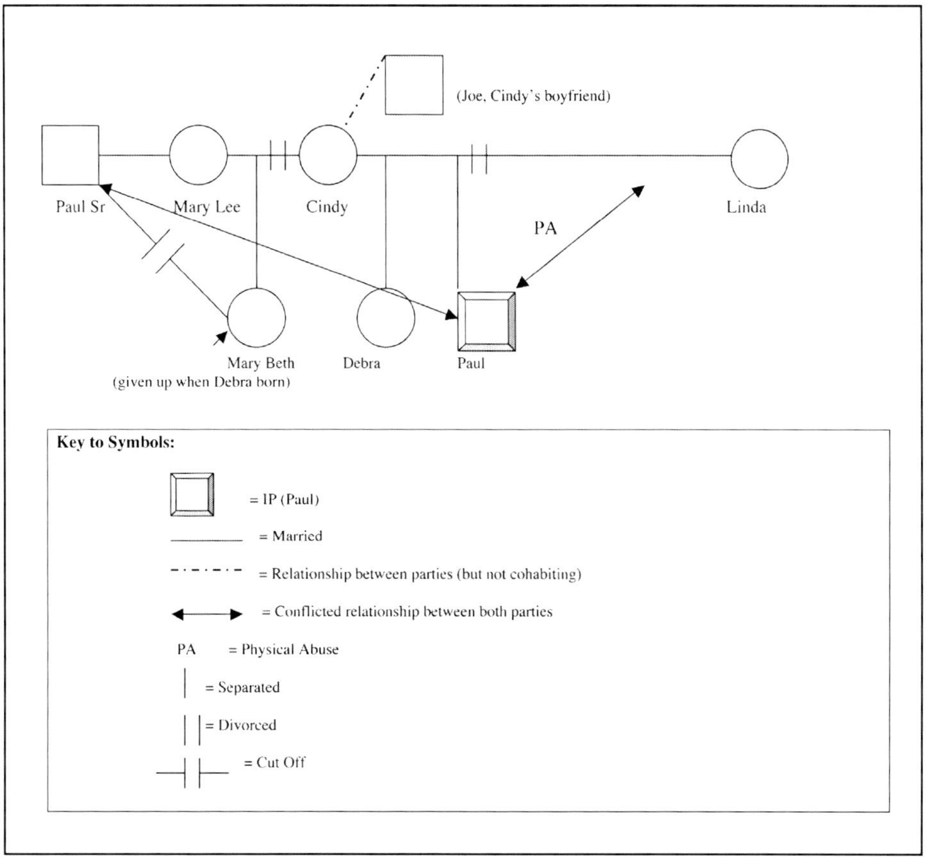

Figure 1. Genogram.

alized. The most notable element was Paul's apparent mastery of professional lingo related to his negative attention seeking behavior: he assumed complete responsibility for his behavior and even noted the reasoning behind his actions. He further explained that visiting his father and stepmother (whom he only referred to as his "father's wife") caused hyperactivity in his behavior on the following day at school. He also made mention of his mother's physical illness and need to try and control his behavior, lest he exacerbate her medical condition.

(*N.B.: Author's Note:* No information about Mary Lee or Mary Beth, father's first wife and child (respectively) that father had begotten, age 18 (Mary Lee's age 15) nor his lack of contact with this family upon Debra's birth with his second wife, Cindy was available on intake. This information came out in the first family session with father and his third wife, Linda.) To boot, in this same interview, Linda expressed her anger with both Paul Sr. as well as Cindy because Paul Sr., underwent a vasectomy while he was married to Cindy. (According to Linda's report Cindy was "screwing around" when Paul Sr. agreed to the operation. She felt "shortchanged" having to care for other's progeny (namely Debra, Paul (Jr.) and Mary Beth (with whom Linda restored relations). While adoption was discussed as a viable option, Paul Sr. steadfastly refused to consider this since he felt neither physically or emotionally equipped to deal with any more children. At this meeting the father admitted to his regret regarding his previous unsuccessful marriages and fear that Linda would also leave him. Despite their mutual disdain on the issue of more children, they seemed to display genuine affection for each other in the interview.)

Results of Art Therapy Evaluation, Psychological Batteries, and Diagnosis

Test Results:

Wechsler Intelligence Scale for Children- Revised

Verbal tests	**Performance tests**
Information 10	Picture Completion 9
Similarities 10	Picture Arrangement 14
Arithmetic 8	Block Design 9
Vocabulary10	Object Assembly 9
Comprehension 9	Coding10
(Digit Span)(10)	

Verbal Scale (VS)IQ 96
Performance Scale (PS) IQ 101
Full Scale (FS) IQ 98

Bender Gestalt:

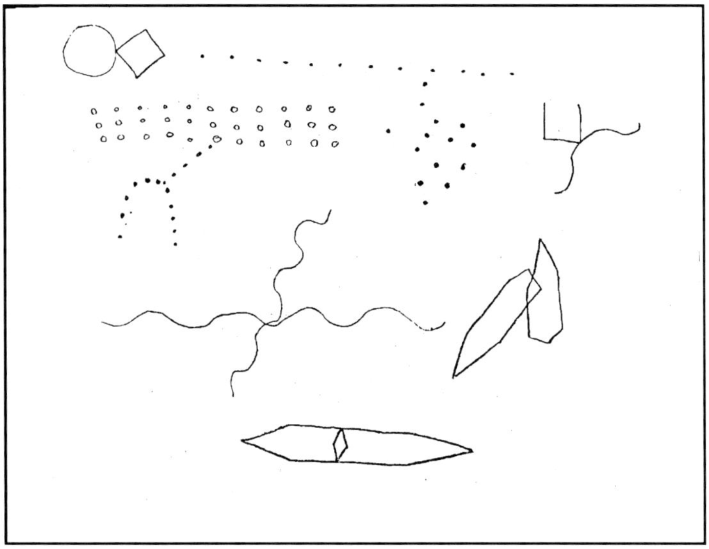

Figure 2. Bender Gestalt.

(N.B.: Since this was conducted prior to the revised Bender Gestalt II, it was reviewed via Koppitz's work (1963) and received a raw score of 1 with a developmental age of 10–0 at his chronological age (CA) of 11–5 (at time of testing).)

House-Tree-Person Test (Achromatic Only)

Most notable was the inordinate amount of time spent on the roof area of the House subtest, suggesting a propensity for both rigidity (need to control impulsivity and aggressive tendencies) with a concomitant desire to release his feelings into fantasy. Order was apparent as Paul requested a ruler to complete his shingling of the rooftop. Of interest, was the Person subtest (combined with Tree response); he illustrated himself flying above the ground via a propelled rocket underfoot. Again this underscored Paul's need for retreat into fantasy and simultaneous aggressive stance (rocket feet) (Hammer, 1980).

Kinetic Family Drawing

Paul drew (left to right) his sister, mother, and father each involved in an independent, physical sport. He then queried, "Do you want me to draw me?" His self representation was one third to one quarter the size of the other figures, illustrating himself making a bed and stating, "Why me?"(Figure 3, KFD). (Regarding the actual grid analysis of the figures, distance from each other and key elements see KFD sheet analysis at addendum - Burns & Kaufman, 1972). The analysis of this test portrayed mother with aggressive cleats on her feet, suggesting perceived power and hostile impulsivity issues, father engaged in weight lifting, implying expected strength and resilience, and sister, Debra, engaged in an enjoyable outlet, foretelling freedom from mundane tasks; yet, he created himself in Cinderella mode (e.g., making his bed, and the only family member differentiated by not engaging in physical activity). (Of interest is father's dumbbell, directly positioned over Paul's head. This may imply Paul's perceived simultaneous identification with the victim / aggressor-role. Moreover, the family system appears to float on the paper, further suggesting instability within the family system. The fact that all members are in isolated activity speaks to the need for communal reparation and shared activity in order to mend this system); Burns & Kaufman (1972); Hammer (1980); Horovitz (2005); Oster and Crone (2004).

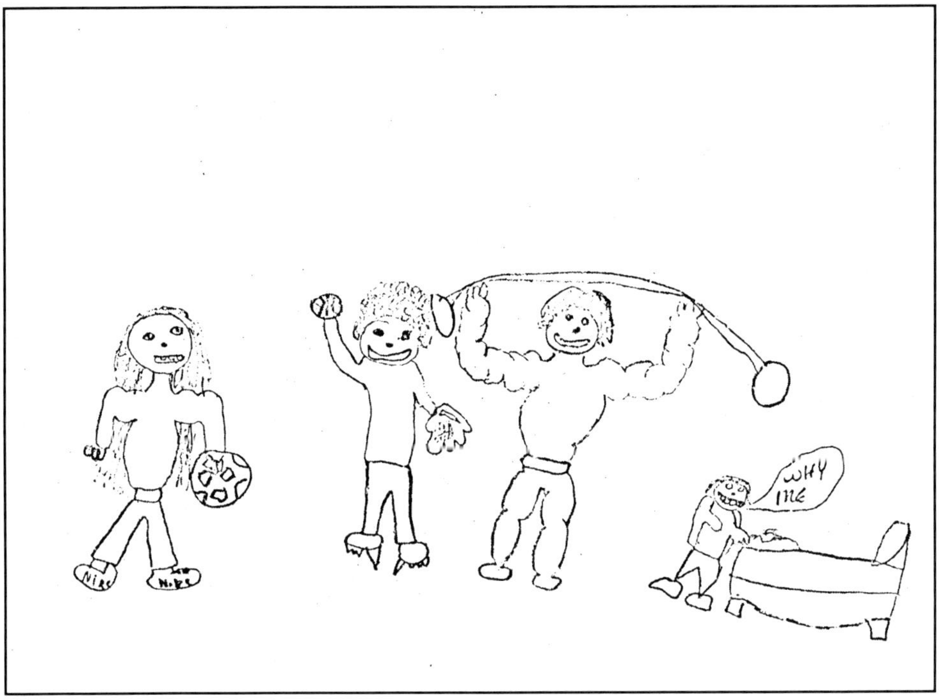

Figure 3. KFD.

Silver Drawing Test

When given the SDT he placed in the 89 percent with a t score conversion of 62.39. Most admirable was his ability in the Drawing from

Observation subtest, where he received a perfect score, thus underscoring his artistic potential. Nevertheless, his impulsivity was clear in his inability to stay within the confine of the page in the Drawing from Imagination subtest, where he drew a dog's tail overlapping onto the preceding page of the Drawing from Observation subtest (Silver, 2002).

Cognitive Art Therapy Assessment (CATA)

The result of Paul's drawing subtest was comparable to the achromatic version of the HTP House subtest: once again, he used a ruler to articulate a rocket, complete with a drill-like nosed protrusion, which he stated could be used to "drill into the enemy." When this writer asked him if he knew who the enemy was, he had no response for the query but became introspective and guarded. The painting subtest, a large street lamp told a different story: here, Paul fabricated an interesting tale of its components: He stated that his father represented the tall streetlamp, the arc-shaped ground below the streetlamp was portrayed to be Linda, a wide open flower (coming from the left section of the ground) was a stand-in for his sister, Debra ("because she can't keep her mouth shut"), the smaller closed flower (emerging from the right section of ground) was deemed himself ("because I keep my feelings to myself") and the sky (air) was his mother, Cindy. When this therapist inquired as to why Linda was the earth from which the children sprung and not his biological mother, he quickly reversed their roles, realizing his error. Nevertheless, his verbal associate to the work produced revealed his Zeitgeist of the current family system and his confusion around loyalty to his mother, father, and stepmother. The final clay subtest, a flat, two-dimensional cat, revealed his need for regression following the painting subtest. Overall, Paul placed in the lower end of Pseudo-Naturalistic Stage of Development, age 12-14 years, according to Lowenfeld and Brittain (1985).

CATA Results:

Drawing Subtest: Gang Age, Age 9–12 years

Painting Subtest: Pseudo-Naturalistic Stage of Development, age 12–14 years

Clay Subtest: Gang Age, Age 9–12 years

Overall Score: Lower end of the Pseudo-Naturalistic Stage of Development, age 12

Recommendations:

Diagnostically, Paul's psychiatric diagnosis fell into the following category:

AXIS I – Oppositional Disorder – 313.81
Attention Deficit Disorder without Hyperactivity – 314.00
AXIS II – No Diagnosis – V71.09

Academically, Paul's performance on standardized tests indicated average capabilities. Comprehension skills varied depending on Paul's level of anxiety and investment in the task (both of which affect his attention and concentration). In general impulsiveness and performance anxiety seemed to be adversely effecting Paul's achievement. Moreover, emotional factors were prohibiting Paul from realizing his intellectual and academic potential.

What was clear after both intakes and the battery of assessments was that biological mother's physical and verbal abuse towards the children would need to be addressed in a manner that was both palatable and life changing. Otherwise, Paul's aggressive tendencies (transitional learned behavior from mother) would be in full throttle as he moved toward late adolescence and onset of adulthood. Paul's ability to utilize intellect to control his behavior was only partially successful. Using fantasy as a means of sublimating impulsive expression, aggression, and power were evident. Indeed he was an obviously distressed child, masked much of his own suffering and censored his behavior as a defense. Among his strengths were a sense of hope, normal intellectual development, good social skills, talent for self-expression through artistic media and a desire for therapeutic intervention to help him navigate his feelings and actions.

Theoretical Research and Intervention Strategies with Familial Domestic Violence

Historical Underpinnings of Domestic Violence

Had it not been for Kempe and colleagues (1962), domestic violence might not have been identified, even though it clearly has persisted amongst humankind for centuries. By the 1990s, family therapists began to scour the literature for the dark underpinnings of family interactions. That time gave rise to literature reviews of sexual abuse and battering (Goldner, Penn, Sheinberg & Walker, 1990). According to Nichols (2007), "The systemic view, now under attack, was that violence was the outcome of cycles of mutual provocation, an escalation, albeit unacceptable of the emotionally destructive behavior that characterizes most marriages" (p. 218). In this writer's opinion, while this may bear some truth, pinpointing domestic violence to simple wife beating was not the answer. If one looks to transitional factors handed down from generation to generation, a more precise model can be established for each familial system, thus giving rise to the need for a structural intervention. Nevertheless, most researchers agree that a systems approach to domestic violence is only effective in mild to moderate violent offenders. It is clearly inappropriate to use conjoint or systems interventions when working with severe, life-threatening violent offenders (Bagarozi & Giddings, 1983; Gelles & Maynard, 1987; Taylor, 1984).

Structural Systems Thinking and Art Therapy

Thus, it seems more fitting to turn to the literature of structural family systems in order to work effectively with the chaos and aftermath of domestic violence. Salvador Minuchin (1974), the kingpin of structural family therapy, theorized that families could be categorized into two distinct patterns: "enmeshed" (chaotically intertwined) and "disengaged" (isolated and ostensibly unrelated). Yet, according to Minuchin and Nichols (1993), enmeshment and engagement tend to be reciprocal. Indeed, structural family therapy gave rise to mapping out the chaotic interactions of the family system in order to more visually delineate interactions and the objectives and goals for the family (art) therapist. So for example in this family system, conflict between the mother and Paul could be represented by the symbol below.

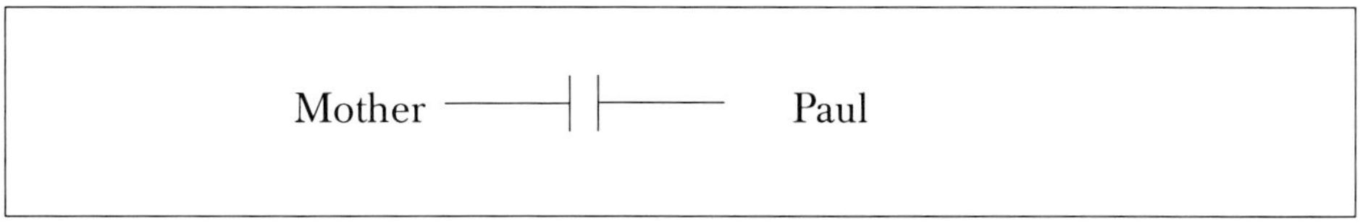

As well, both children's failure to accept stepmother, Linda, could be represented with the "diffuse boundary" of a dotted line between the mother and both children and then a straight line between the father/stepparent so that one can actually visualize the cutoffs such as below.

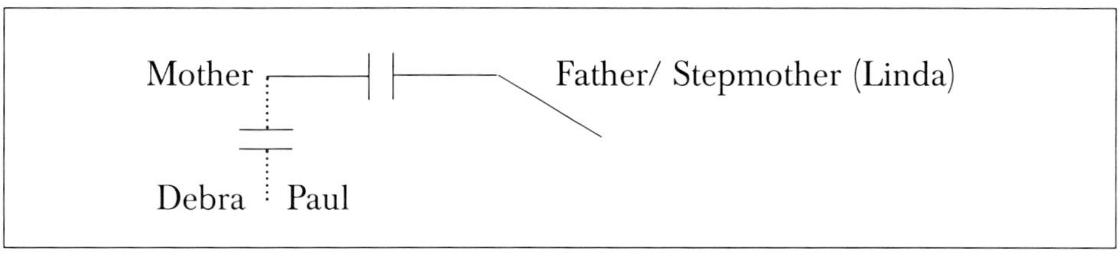

This allows the therapist to visualize both cutoffs and conflicts within the family system. As well, it offers the therapist a visual map from which to operate. For more on the symbols of family structure and explication see Minuchin (1974) and Nichols (2007). Thus after conducting an intake and generating a family genogram the formula below can aptly aid the therapist in working with domestic violence (Nichols, 2007, pp. 135–141):

- Joining and Accommodating (Getting the therapist into the system)
- Enactment (Positioning and creating awareness amongst members)
- Structural Mapping (Accounting for problems and dynamics)
- Highlighting and Modifying Interactions (Focusing on process not content)
- Boundary Making (Realigning relationships between subsystems)
- Unbalancing (Changing relationships within subsystems)
- Challenging Unproductive Assumptions (Relating and viewing the system differently)

(*Author's Note:* It is these last two areas (unbalancing and challenging unproductive assumptions) where the therapist needs to be seasoned and /or under supervision of a more senior family therapist in order to make inroads with families of domestic violence. This cannot be underscored enough. Working with violent families is problematical in itself, but changing the homeostasis of these families (who prefer to remain in these static "sick" systems) can be excruciatingly taxing for even the most seasoned therapist. Ongoing supervision of such casework is highly recommended.) Indeed, Straus (1973) viewed family violence as a "goal-seeking adaptive system"; that is rather than viewing the violence as an aberration, it was viewed as a system product or output, thus contributing to the homeostasis of a "sick" system.)

Moreover, according to Gelles and Maynard (1987), there are three main questions that also need to be considered when working with domestic violence: (a) the extent of the violence, (b) factors related to the violence (e.g., which family members are at risk), and (c) the cause of the violence. Indeed causes appear to be multidimensional and researchers have consistently found the following factors:

1. The cycle of violence – the intergenerational transmission of violence.
2. Low, socioeconomic status.
3. Social and structural issues.
4. Social Isolation.
5. Personality problems and psychopathology. (p. 270)

In sum, reform, engagement, and action lead to new experiences, insight, understanding, and reshuffled structures. By challenging the familial pattern of homeostasis and interaction, members are forced to bypass the symptomatology (domestic violence in this case), examine the clandestine arrangement governing the family's transactional configuration and finally change. In art therapy, this is concretized by familial artwork. The artifacts created sustain, act, and create a visual reminder that results in continuity from session to session. Unlike verbal association, the artwork has the added presence of playing co-therapist and forces the issue ever so gently, just through its presence alone (Horovitz, 1999, 2004, 2005). Indeed, both Kozlowska (2001) and Linesch (1993) highlighted the ability of artwork to (a) facilitate and the exposure to traumatic cues (in a less direct manner), (b) aid children in labeling and articulating affective states, and finally (c) lead to positive family changes and coping behavior.

Family Art Therapy

Objectives and Goals

Initially, it was imperative to establish trust with Paul and his family system. The beginning work was months of individual art therapy with Paul: domestic violence between Paul and his mother had to be quashed and Paul had to learn proactive behavior and quell his aggressive acting out behavior.

While this served to create cooperative behavior and success in the school system, it was clear that the real work would need to be realigning the relationships and subsystems within this family (boundary making). This could not occur without firmly laying the groundwork for Paul to trust the family art therapist with his issues and those of his family. As a result, two sessions with Paul Sr. and his new wife, Linda occurred and five family sessions with Paul and his biological mother, Cindy, transpired to reestablish parental alignment and eliminate diffuse boundaries. Then afterwards, the real work needed to take place with the children, father, and stepmother in order to achieve acceptance of Linda into this family system. As a result, the case will be summarized presenting only the bulk of the work leading up to the eight family sessions that occurred. There were 47 sessions in total.

Thematically, Paul always presented a consistent pattern of ambivalence, the light and dark sides of himself and his inability to regulate these Dr. Jekyll/Mr. Hyde emotions that raged unchecked. While he was able to articulate this to his mother within the family dyads, it did not quell his anger and/or resentment towards mother or her boyfriend, Joe. Yet, in one family art therapy session, Paul and Cindy were able to work conjointly on a large pastel drawing of fruit, wine and vegetables (see Figure 4).

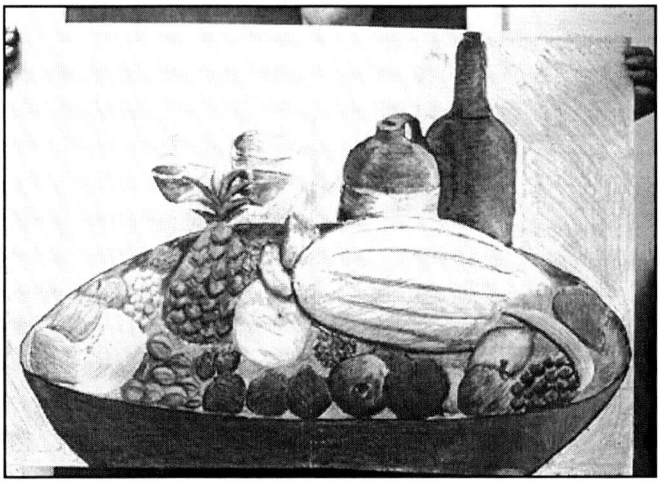

Figure 4. Mother/child dyadic family session.

The drawing (proudly held by Paul for the picture) was a testament to his ability to work cooperatively on a family art therapy task and sublimate his need for unconditional nurturance and acceptance. The large bowl holding the bounty was a direct stand-in for Paul's need for absolute regard and sustenance. While this led to a honeymoon period, one evening, Paul snuck into the mother's bedroom while she and her boyfriend, Joe, slept. He fished $300 out of Joe's pocket and left the bedroom. When this was discovered the next day, Cindy flew into a rage and literally hit Paul over the head with a frying pan. While not hard enough to cause stitches or need for hospitalization, mother had the good sense to call this writer and make an emergency appointment. (Naturally, this writer reported the incident to CPS (Child Protective Services); CPS's response was a verbal discussion with the mother and file of a written report. Intercession generally occurs only when there is a life-threatening situation. This is due to the mass of domestic violence cases.)

When Paul finally admitted to the theft and his concomitant anger towards mother and her boyfriend, he was able to confess the reason he had stolen the money: apparently his bicycle had been stolen the day before and his mother refused to replace it. He was planning to use the money to buy himself a new bicycle. This author requested that both work in clay in order to enact and challenge unproductive actions toward each other. Paul first created a bicycle and then a question mark (which he later painted light blue and dark blue, once again representing the ambivalent, light/darks sides of his personality). The he fashioned a crying and sad face. Mother created herself as Medusa and asked for forgiveness (see Figure 5).

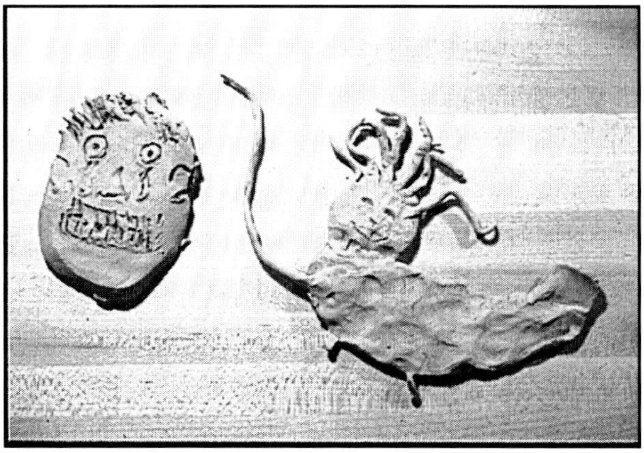

Figure 5. Sad face and Medusa.

The artwork allowed for a medicinal uptake: Cindy was able to witness herself and her untoward reaction toward her son. This insight was in and of itself cathartic for the mother. From that point on, she was able to check her violent behavior just by looking at that sculpture repeatedly. Here the artifact took on the form of shamanistic talisman and curtailed fractious behavior from this point forward. While Paul's violent behavior decreased, he still had difficulty with self-expression and several more family art therapy sessions led to further resolve. Some led to artwork where Paul was able to articulate his anger towards mother as well as Linda. The artwork below (see Figure 6) aptly spells out his unchecked rage: "I feel like a time bom (sic) about to explode."

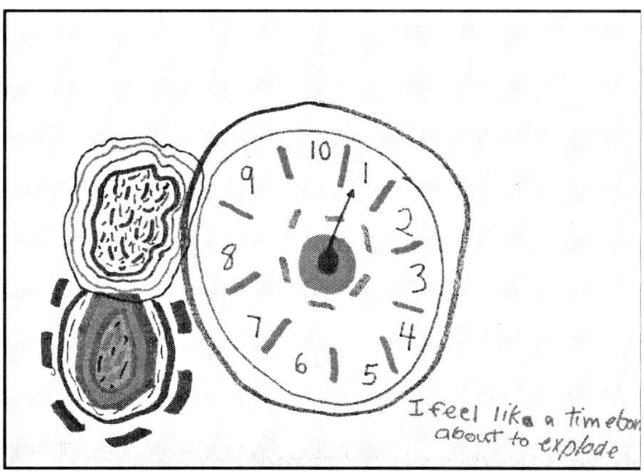

Figure 6. Time bomb.

Family sessions with both children, the father, and stepmother, Linda, next sealed the fissure. Everyone was asked to create him or her self and family members out of clay. Who complained vehemently about wanting to "strangle someone" because of her anger toward Cindy and her husband. (Apparently, she felt that Paul Sr. spent too much money on the children and she was angry with her husband for dispensing these resources on his ex-wife's children as opposed to her.) Paul began to cry and ran out of the therapy room. The author went to comfort him and later enlisted the father to join her.

After this ensued, Linda created a pig, which she directly related to this writer: she blamed the therapist for "squealing" (that is getting family members to release their feelings outwardly). Quietly, Debra worked and fashioned Linda and her father, both were snowmen and without legs or arms, thus suggesting lack of mobility and inability to reach out toward others. (Yet, Linda was serving brownies, thus suggesting Debra's positive connection towards her.) The father was able to create himself, albeit smaller than Linda, suggesting feelings of incompetence and low self-esteem. Both children were created (one smiling, Debra and the other not, Paul). None of the family members had feet again concretizing lack of mobility and inaccessibility (Burns & Kaufman, 1972; Hammer, 1980; Oster & Crone, 2004). Finally, Paul created only "Linda and (his father) connected on a platform" thus suggesting his inability to view them as disparate parts. The fact that they were all head also suggests his view of them as intellectualized and unfeeling toward himself (Burns & Kaufman, 1972; Hammer, 1980; Oster & Crone, 2004). Below are all the images after being fired and painted (from left to right: Debra's father and stepmother; father's family; Linda's pig and Paul's connected platform rendering of Linda and father).

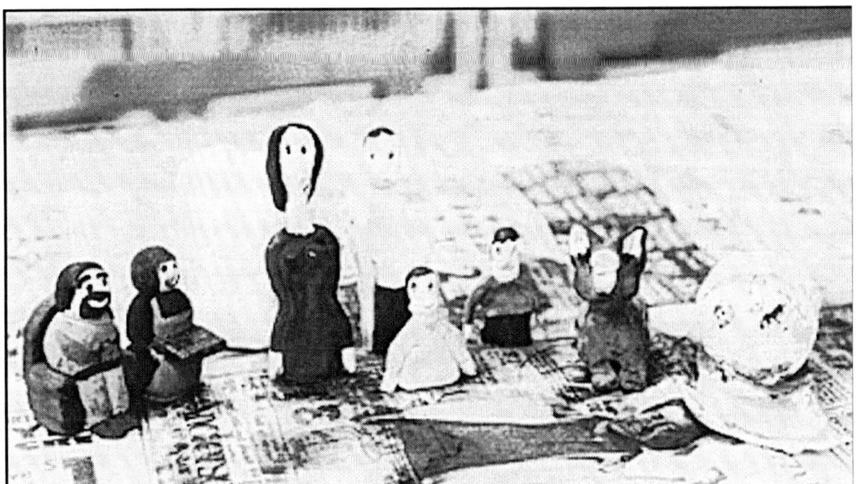

Figure 7. Family portraits.

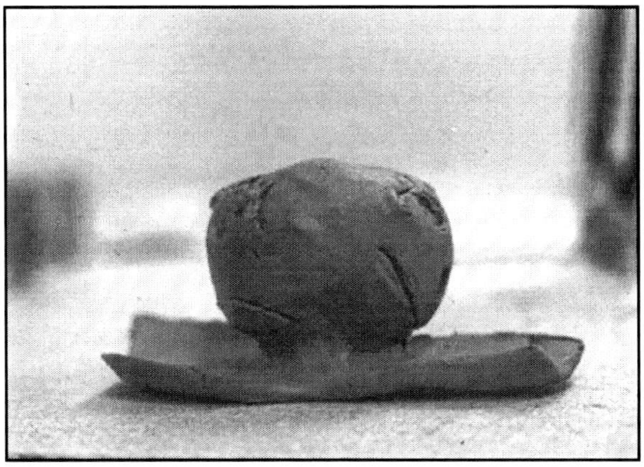

Figure 8. Paul's platform person of father (left) and Linda (right).

Despite the tumultuous session, both Linda and the father thanked the art therapist for the session and agreed to return. Because Paul was doing so well, the family decided to terminate treatment but three months later, the father called demanding a family session for himself, Linda, and Paul, Jr.: the reason was that they were convinced that Paul had stolen some of Linda's jewelry. All were asked to do a drawing together. Primarily, Linda sat at the table and refused to participate. Paul and his father settled on the creation of a "universe of planets," revealing considering the issues of distance, space and an atmospheric temperature that is cold. Yet, their planets brewed with heat spots and fire rings, foretelling the unexpressed emotion beneath the sublimated drafting. Fortunately, in between sessions, the father called to reveal that the "robber had been caught" and Paul was cleared of the suspected thievery. While the damage had been done, Paul had learned from previous challenging unproductive assumptions (Nichols, 2007) and did not take this to heart. He neither raged against his subsystems nor retaliated and instead quietly forgave his father and Linda as he completed the drawing with his father (see Figure 9).

Conclusion and Follow-Up

Family art therapy coupled with a structural family systems approach had allowed for substantial restructuring. Violent behavior had been quelled, new communication patterns were observable, parental subsystems were strengthened and sibling subsystems had been appropriately regulated. A six-month follow-up indicated that positive restructuring changes had been maintained. At the session's end, Paul gifted this worker with a card and hugged her upon departure. (Below is the interior image of the card, Figure

10.) His words, "Bye, Bye, Ellen, Keep on Trukin" (sic) suggest that Paul finally could see the road ahead and had the perspective and ability to traverse his course.

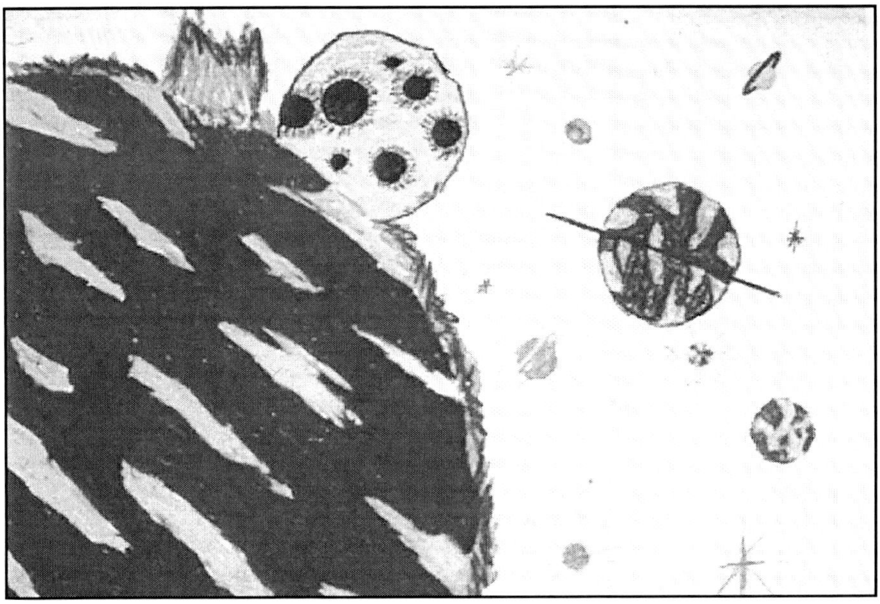

Figure 9. Universe.

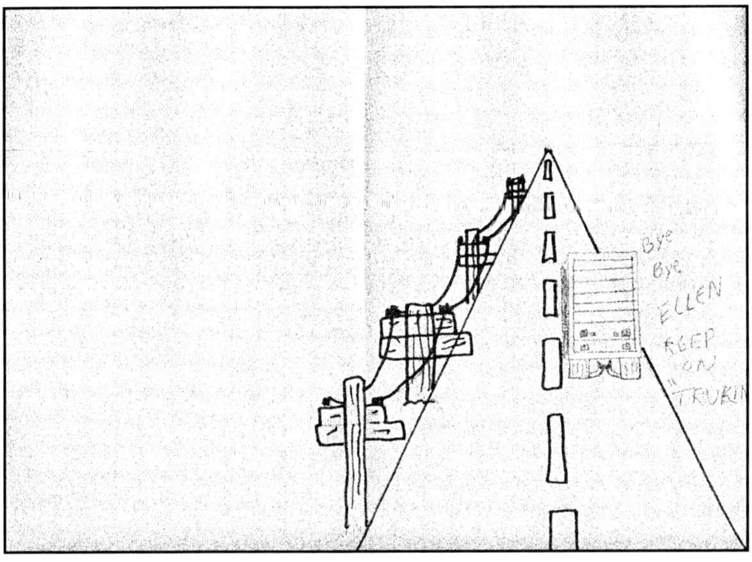

Figure 10. Goodbye card.

(Rare Follow-up: Of interest was that ten years later, Debra showed up to a presentation by this writer and after the session, she revealed herself. She had so changed that she was unrecognizable to this author.) Debra had blossomed into a beautiful young woman, who was currently practicing as a special education therapist. She thanked this writer for all her work and revealed that Paul was now in college and working towards completion of his baccalaureate degree.

Structure does aid those that are in chaos and clearly this particular approach of using structural family art therapy when working with an oppositional defiant disorder adolescent and his family was just the right ticket to enact a reorganized, robust family system, based on health and newfound communication.

Domestic Violence Terms

Low, socioeconomic background: A leading cause of domestic violence.

Social Isolation: Leads to violence

Transitional Conflicts: Intergenerational psychosocial acts learned from previous generations

Structural Family Therapy Terms

Boundary Making: Realigning relationships between subsystems

Challenging Unproductive Assumptions: Relating and viewing the system differently

Disengaged: Isolated and ostensibly unrelated

Enmeshed: Chaotically intertwined

Enactment: Positioning and creating awareness amongst members

Highlighting and Modifying Interactions: Focusing on process not content

Homeostasis: Systems that do not change

Joining and Accommodating: Getting the therapist into the system

Structural Mapping: Accounting for problems and dynamics

Unbalancing: Changing relationships within subsystems

Appendix

K-F-D ANALYSIS SHEET

K-F-D ANALYSIS SHEET

Name: ______________________ **Age:** _____ **Date of Birth:** ___/___/___ **Sex:** __________

I. STYLE(S) (Circle)

A. Compartmentalization
B. Edging
C. Encapsulation
D. Folded Compartmentalization
E. Lining on the Bottom
F. Lining on the Top
G. Underling individual figures

II. SYMBOL(S)

A. ____________ D. ____________
B. ____________ E. ____________
C. ____________ F. ____________

III. (A) ACTIONS OF INDIVIDUAL FIGURES

Figure	Action
1. Self	____________
2. Mother	____________
3. Father	____________
4. Older Brother	____________
5. Older Sister	____________
6. Younger Brother	____________
7. Younger Sister	____________
8. Other (Specify)	____________
____________	____________

(B) ACTIONS BETWEEN INDIVIDUAL FIGURES

Figure	Action	Recipient
1. Self	____________	____________
2. Mother	____________	____________
3. Father	____________	____________
4. O.B.	____________	____________
5. O.S.	____________	____________
6. Y.B.	____________	____________
7. Y.S.	____________	____________
8. Other	____________	____________

IV. CHARACTERISTICS OF K-F-D FIGURES

A. Arm Extensions
1. Self 5. O.S.
2. Mother 6. Y.B.
3. Father 7. Y.S.
4. O.B. 8. Other

B. Elevated Figures
1. Self 5. O.S.
2. Mother 6. Y.B.
3. Father 7. Y.S.
4. O.B. 8. Other

C. Erasures
1. Self 5. O.S.
2. Mother 6. Y.B.
3. Father 7. Y.S.
4. O.B. 8. Other

D. Figures on Back
1. Self 5. O.S.
2. Mother 6. Y.B.
3. Father 7. Y.S.

E. Hanging
1. Self 5. O.S.
2. Mother 6. Y.B.
3. Father 7. Y.S.
4. O.B. 8. Other

F. Omission of Body Parts
1. Self 5. O.S.
2. Mother 6. Y.B.
3. Father 7. Y.S.
4. O.B. 8. Other

G. Omission of Figures
1. Self 5. O.S.
2. Mother 6. Y.B.
3. Father 7. Y.S.
4. O.B. 8. Other

H. Picasso Eyes
1. Self 5. O.S.
2. Mother 6. Y.B.
3. Father 7. Y.S.
4. O.B. 8. Other

I. Rotated Figures
1. Self 5. O.S.
2. Mother 6. Y.B.
3. Father 7. Y.S.
4. O.B. 8. Other

V. K-F-D Grid

A. Height
1. Self_____5.O.S._____
2. M._____6. Y.B._____
3. F._____7. Y.S._____
4. O.B._____8. Other____

B. Location of Self

____

C. Distance of Self From:

Mother____________ Brother____________
Father____________ Sister____________
Other (Specify)____________

References

Bagarozzi, G. A., & Giddings, C. W. (1983). Conjugal violence: A critical review of current research and clinical practices. *The American Journal of Family Therapy, 11*(1), 3-12.

Burns, R. C., & Kaufman S. H (1972). *Action styles and symbols in kinetic family drawings (KFD).* New York: Brunner/Mazel.

Gelles, R. J. (1979). *Family violence.* Beverly Hills, CA: Sage Publications.

Gelles, R. J. (1980).Violence in the family. A review of the research in the seventies. *Journal of Marriage and the Family, 42,* 873-885.

Gelles, R. J. (1982). Domestic criminal violence. In M. E. Wolfgang & N. A. Weiner (Eds.), *Criminal violence* (pp. 210-235). Beverly Hills, CA: Sage Publications.

Gelles, R. J. (1985). Family violence. In R. Turner (Ed.), *Annual review of sociology, 11*: 347-367. Palo Alto, CA: Annual Reviews, Inc.

Gelles, R. J., & Maynard, P. E. (1987: July). A structural family systems approach to intervention in cases of family violence. *Family Relations. 36,* 270-275.

Gil, D. (1971).Violence against children. *Journal of Marriage and the Family. 33,* 637-648.

Goldner, V., Penn, P., Sheinberg, M., & Walker, G. (1990). Love and violence: Gender paradoxes in volatile attachments. *Family Process. 29,* 343-364

Hammer, E. (1980). *Clinical applications of projective drawing techniques.* Springfield, IL: Charles C Thomas, Publisher, Ltd.

Horovitz, E. G. (1999). *A leap of faith: The call to art.* Springfield, IL: Charles C Thomas, Publisher, Ltd.

Horovitz, E. G. (2005). *Art therapy as witness: A sacred guide.* Springfield, IL: Charles C Thomas, Publisher, Ltd.

Horovitz, E. G. (2004). *Spiritual art therapy: An alternate path* (2nd ed.) Springfield, IL: Charles C Thomas, Publisher, Ltd.

Horovitz-Darby, E. G. (1992). Countertransference: Implications in treatment and post treatment. *Arts in Psychotherapy, 19,* 379-389.

Kempe, C. H., Silverman, F., Steele, B. F., Droegemeuller, W., & Silver, H/K (1962). The battered child syndrome. *Journal of American Medical Association, 181*(4), 107-112.

Koppitz, E. (1963). *Bender Gestalt Test for Young Children: Research and Application.* New York: Grune & Stratton.

Kozlowska, K. (2001). An art therapy group for children traumatized by parental violence and separation. *Clinical Child Psychology and Psychiatry, 6*(1), 49-78.

Linesch, D. (1993). *Art therapy with families in crisis.* New York: Brunner/Mazel.

Lowenfeld, V., & Brittain, W. L. (1985) *Creative & mental growth* (6th ed.). New York: Macmillan.

Malchiodi, C. A. (1997). *Breaking the silence: Art therapy with children from violent homes* (2nd ed.). Philadelphia: Brunner/Mazel.

Minuchin, S. (1974). *Families and family therapy.* Cambridge, MA: Harvard University.

Minuchin, S., & Nichols, M. P. (1993). *Family healing: Tales of hope and renewal from family therapy.* New York: The Free Press.

Nichols, M. P. (with Swartz, R. C.). (YEAR?). *The essentials of family therapy* (3rd ed.). Boston, MA: Pearson, Allyn & Bacon.

Oster, G. D., & Crone, P. (2004). *Using drawings in assessment and therapy* (2nd ed.). New York: Brunner/Mazel Publishers.

Silver, R. (2002). *Three art assessments.* New York: Brunner-Routledge Publishers.

Straus, M. A. (1973). A general systems theory approach to a theory of violence between family members. *Social Science Information. 12*(6), 105-125.

Taylor, J. W. (1984). Structured conjoint therapy for spouse abuse cases. *Social Casework, 63,* 11-18.

Biography

Ellen G. Horovitz, Ph.D., LCAT, ATR-BC is Chair of the Creative Arts Therapy Depart- ment, Professor/Director of Graduate Art Therapy and the Art Therapy Clinic at Nazareth College of Rochester, New York. She has had over thirty years of experience with myriad patient populations and specializes in family art therapy with the deaf. Doctor Horovitz currently is in private practice. Doctor Horovitz is the author of numerous articles, book chapters and the following books: *Spiritual Art Therapy: An Alternate Path, A Leap of Faith: The Call to Art, Art Therapy As Witness: A Sacred Guide* and *Visually Speaking: Art Therapy and the Deaf.* As well, Doctor Horovitz has directed and produced ten films available in DVD format. (Doctor Horovitz's films are available through www.arttxfilms.com.) Doctor Horovitz is past President Elect of the American Art Therapy Association (AATA). For additional information contact: Doctor Ellen G. Horovitz, ATR-BC, Director of Graduate Art Therapy/Nazareth College, 4245 East Avenue/ Rochester, NY 14618. E-mail: ehorovi4@naz.edu, ehorovi4@naz.edu

Chapter 3

HEALING THROUGH CLAY: A CASE STUDY OF A CHILD WITNESS OF DOMESTIC VIOLENCE

LIZA AVETIKOVA

Introduction

It is estimated that 70 percent of school-age children from low socioeconomic areas have witnessed assaults, arrests, drug deals, gang violence, shootings, and domestic violence (Skybo, 2005, p. 263). Studies on domestic violence have explored its proposed causes, outcomes, and effects. While most of the earlier literature has discussed only women as the victims of violence, studies in the last few years have emerged focusing on children as domestic violence victims as well (Fantuzzo & Mohr, 1999; Hill, 2002).

Researchers are taking various angles in looking at the problem of domestic violence and its effects on children. Wolfe and colleagues (2003) talk about exploring different populations and familial situations, such as parental conflict and/or divorce by conducting retrospective studies of exposure experienced by adults as children, simulated conflict studies, and studies of children exposed to domestic violence in their homes (p. 173). Other researchers are looking at the influence of the environment on the frequency of occurrences of domestic violence (e.g., Saxe, Ellis, Fogler, Hansen, & Sorkin 2005). Saxe and colleagues see domestic violence as all part of the poor environment, in addition to drug and alcohol abuse, poverty, inadequate schools, community crime, and racism. Researchers found that such factors contribute to the perpetuation of violence in homes and, in turn, to trauma in children.

Studies (English et al., 2003; Osofsky, 1999) conducted on school-age children and adolescents have found that domestic violence can affect children on emotional, cognitive, and behavioral levels, as well as be the cause for physical health problems, laying the foundation for negative externalized and internalized behaviors (English et al., 2003; Ornduff & Monahan, 1999; Wolfe et al., 2003). Negative externalized behaviors include various acting-out behaviors, such as aggression and delinquency, poor academic performances, reduced social competencies, anger, and physical violence towards others (McAlister Groves, 1999; Ornduff & Monahan, 1999; Refvem, 2000; Wolfe et al., 2003). Internalized behaviors include depression, low self-esteem, and anxiety (McAlister Groves, 1999; Ornduff & Monahan, 1999; Refvem, 2000; Wolfe et al., 2003).

More important, for the purposes of therapy, are feelings that underlie the emotional responses to the violence and terror. Reaching beyond the manifested behaviors, McAlister Groves (1999) discusses those feelings. She lists the fears of death and loss, feelings of rage, guilt, and responsibility for the violence.

Moreover, children are believed to erase the traumatic events from their conscious memories and disassociate words and feelings due to the fear of re-experiencing the event (Ornduff & Monahan, 1999; Johnson, 1987). Johnson (1987) explains this phenomenon through neurological processes. He refers to two ways in which memory is encoded in the brain. Through photographic memory, a more primitive process, the events are recorded precisely the way they happened and are recalled only when triggered by similar stimuli. The other, more mature way of memory recording, is through association. An event is recorded and reconstructed through various parts of the memory. With severe psychological trauma, events seem to be recorded in a more primitive photographic form. When a similar stimulus triggers a memory it is recalled in vivid detail. This precise recollection is referred to as flashbacks. However, unless there is a concrete stimulus, the event is absent from the conscious memory of the individual and access to it or, for the purposes of this chapter, to feelings associated with it is closed through means of verbal intervention. Because one's childhood experiences are encoded through photographic memory it is logical to assume that such traumatic experience as parental abuse or witnessing thereof would be unavailable for verbal processing (p. 9).

Role of Art in the Treatment of Trauma

Conventional psychotherapy relies on verbal means of communication to access and work through the issues. While that might be a substantial enough intervention for an adult, children require more interactive and creative modalities, such as art therapy. Art therapy is the therapeutic intervention that not only allows one to express oneself nonverbally, but also helps one channel his or her negative feelings into an outside object through a creative activity in the safety of a therapist-client relationship. As mentioned above, Johnson (1987) stresses that victims of psychological trauma are often unable to express their experience adequately through words. Through art, an individual has a chance to externalize his or her feelings, as well as formulate a creative visual representation of his or her experiences. This process directs internalized feelings, such as aggression, into an object outside of oneself and controls externalized behaviors, such as acting out. Having one's feelings represented in this way, gives a client the opportunity to process his or her feelings, reflect on them, and accept them so he or she can learn to eventually let go and move on (pp. 9–10). Malchiodi (1990) and Johnson (1987) talk about art as a way to distance the traumatic experience from the self, providing safety from it, and thereby, helping to release built up tension and anxiety. A victim can discuss his or her feelings from the point of view of his or her creation, instead of speaking in the first person. This safe and controlled externalization of the experience facilitates verbal therapy.

Malchiodi (1990) lists four areas of intervention for a child victim or witness of domestic violence that can be facilitated through the use of art. The first is communication of feelings, as children from homes that have been influenced by parental aggression have been taught to not express their feelings regarding the situation at home. In art therapy, such feelings can be safely expressed and channeled through art materials. Another area of intervention is reducing the parentification of the child. Often, in households where there is parental aggression, children are caught between the fighting adults. Because of the chaos and confusion at home, a child may be forced to take on more responsibilities than the average child. Particularly with the presence of younger children, an older sibling may find him or herself in a parental role, having to take care of younger brothers or sisters. Art, furthermore, becomes a container for the stresses in a child's life. A sense of control is essential to a child's ability to deal with stresses in his or her life. By making choices about the execution of an art piece, a child maintains control over his or her experience. Finally, a positive self-image constantly needs to be encouraged in a child from a violent home. The above-mentioned areas of art intervention provide an art therapist with the needed avenues to help address and develop healthy self-images of these children.

Case Study–Tommy

This chapter explores how the above mentioned four areas of intervention with a witness of domestic violence can be addressed with the use of art therapy and, particularly, how they can be addressed more efficiently with the use of clay as the primary medium. The study was done at an agency in New

York City that services victims of domestic violence. The subject of the study was a 9-year-old boy who had witnessed parental violence. The presenting problem was Tommy's reported inability to concentrate on tasks, persisting anxiety about wanting something but not knowing what it was, and difficulty making friends at school. Within the first two sessions, it became clear that Malchiodi's (1990) four areas of intervention – expression of feelings, un-parentification, giving back control and promoting a positive self-image – were to become central to my work with Tommy. In working through these areas, many of the behaviors and feelings discussed above, such as anxiety, acting out, poor academic performance, feelings of guilt, responsibility, and anger were addressed.

Four major themes were present in my work with Tommy, which had to be explored and developed in order to facilitate Tommy's growth in the above mentioned areas. Of course, in the actual sessions the themes were not, and could not be, as clearly delineated; however, it is helpful to outline them when discussing the work. The development of trust was essential before Tommy could feel comfortable enough in the relationship to verbalize his feelings. The themes of protection and nurturance led to the exploration of Tommy's role in the family and the beginning of his letting go of the parental role. Additionally, destructive and constructive feelings had to be explored with enough flexibility and acceptance on the part of the therapist to give back to Tommy a sense of control. Finally, working on Tommy's feelings of competence and supporting his individualization was important for the growth of a new positive self-image.

Building Trust

Trust is an essential aspect of any therapeutic relationship and was particularly important in this study. Already in the second session, Tommy asked me if there was anyone else I was talking to about what happened in sessions. Receiving a reassuring answer, and with the help of art materials, Tommy told me of a traumatic incident that happened when he was five, when his mother called the police and his father was taken away. Though Tommy felt safe enough with me early in the relationship to tell me about the trauma of what had happened, once he verbalized the experience, he closed up. The re-experiencing of the events had triggered defense mechanisms that, according to his mother, were in effect four years ago. In conversation with me, Tommy's mother reported that around the time of the divorce that followed shortly after the recalled incident, Tommy had stopped talking and became quiet and withdrawn. Similarly, after recalling the traumatic incident in the session, Tommy withdrew, shut down, and would not go back to talking about his feeling about what had happened. In an attempt to re-establish a sense of trust, I suggested we do a dual drawing (see Figure 1 and Plate 1) as a way to nonverbally clarify each other's boundaries. Through his images and body language, Tommy made it clear that he needed his space and time and that I had to allow him both.

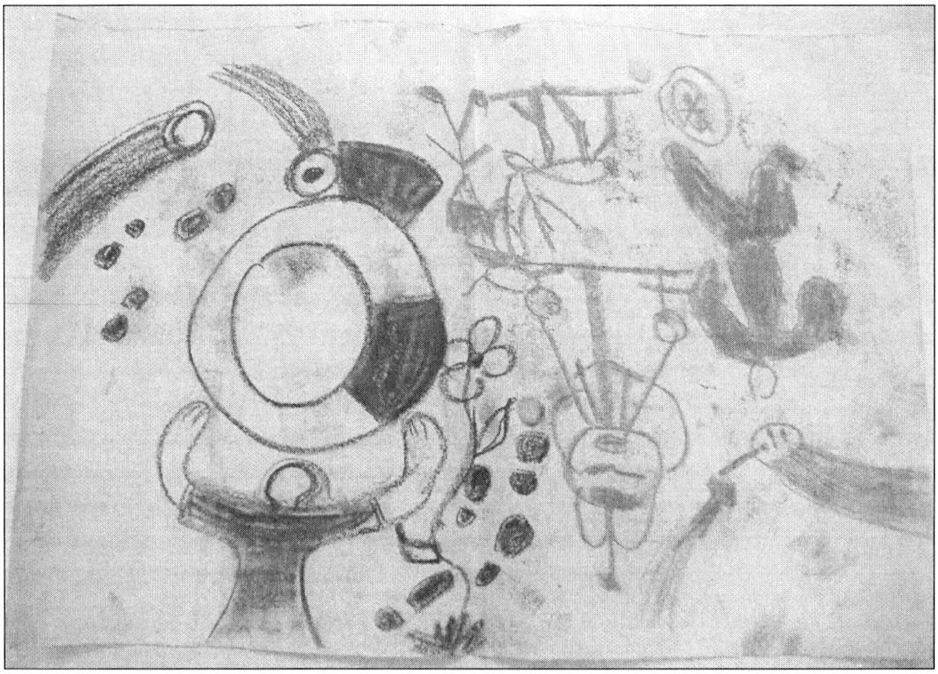

Figure 1. Dual drawing (see also Plate 1 in color).

A shift in the relationship happened in the next session with the introduction of clay. As clay absorbed Tommy's frustration and anxiety and provided a visceral sensory experience, Tommy began to open up. Clay, by nature, offered numerous metaphors with which to process Tommy's feelings. Molding, shaping, re-shaping, bending, supporting, assisting, attaching, connecting, letting be, were all terms that Tommy could emotionally relate to.

In working with the Bird Monster (see Figure 2 and Plate 2) and, later, with the horn lizard (see Figure 3 and Plate 3), Tommy began to process his feelings metaphorically, as he spoke about the creatures and the art process, rather than himself. Clay gave Tommy an opportunity to process concepts in a non-threatening way, contributing to his sense of trust towards me as the therapist.

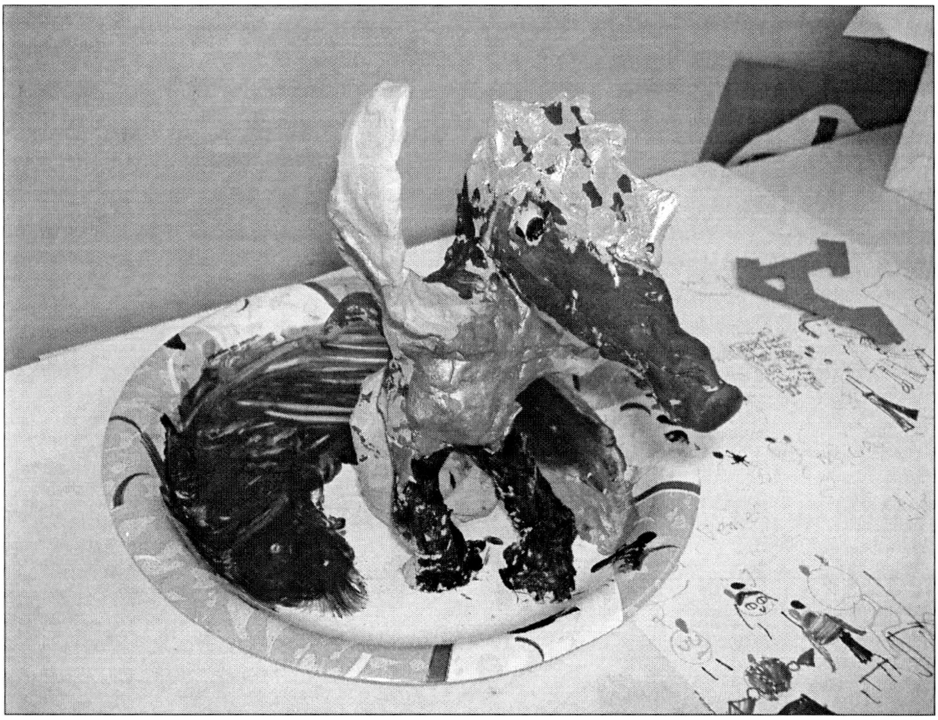

Figure 2. Bird Monster (see also Plate 2 in color).

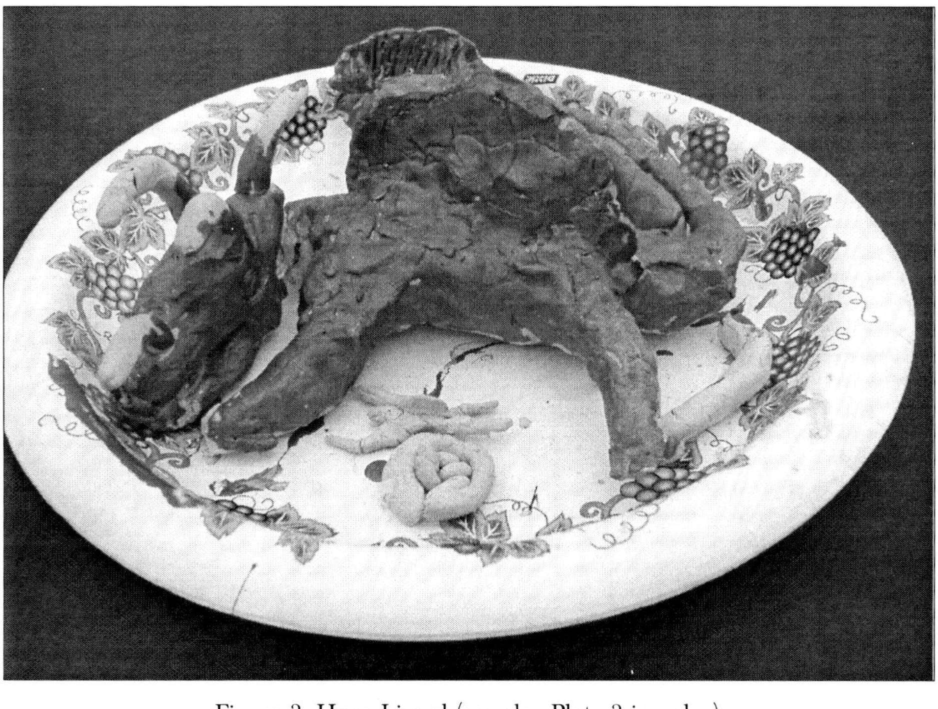

Figure 3. Horn Lizard (see also Plate 3 in color).

Additionally, the three-dimensionality of the figures made them more life-like and contributed to Tommy's treatment as he viewed them almost as his pets. He took care of them, made up families for them, and took great pains to fix parts of them that would break off. Because both figures were left at the agency between sessions, Tommy began to see me as the "other protector" of his creatures; and thus worthy of being trusted to take care of them in his absence, and by extension, worthy of being trusted to take care of Tommy himself.

Making Sense of Protection and Nurturance

Themes of protection and nurturance came up in the first session and remained a big part of Tommy's treatment. Tommy explored those themes through his clay characters and by looking directly at his relationship with his parents and his sisters. In both cases, the roles of the protected and the protectors continuously interchanged, reflecting Tommy's conflicting feelings of needing to be the child and feeling responsible for the situation at home. Tommy's protectors persistently needed to be protected and the nurturers needed to be nurtured. For example, in the first session, Tommy used markers to make a picture of a Million-Dollar-Robot (see Figure 4), describing the character as someone who would protect Tommy. In the same session, Tommy said that he also wanted to have a smaller robot that he, Tommy, would protect. Similarly, at home, Tommy naturally felt the need to be watched over and cared for; however, as a child-witness of domestic violence, he also felt that it was up to him to protect and provide support for his family.

Skybo (2005) offers a possible explanation for the phenomenon. She points out that children's egocentric thinking contributes to their sense of responsibility for the violence at home. They see themselves as the cause of all things, and it is only natural that they see themselves as the cause of parental aggression as well. The element of fantastical thinking also leads to their sense of omnipotence and fantasies of fixing the situation at home. As long as the violence goes on or parents stay separated, the child thinks that it is up to him or her find new ways to resolve the situation. In fact, Tommy often talked about his wish to bring his parents back together.

Though Tommy brought up themes of protection and nurturance in relation to the drawing of the robot (see Figure 4), it was with the introduction of clay that he was able to really play out and explore their meaning. In contrast to the robot, Tommy's treatment of the Bird Monster (see Figure 2 and Plate 2) reflected a sense of deeper-seated concern for the figure's well-being. He became upset when a part of the Bird Monster would break, and laughed

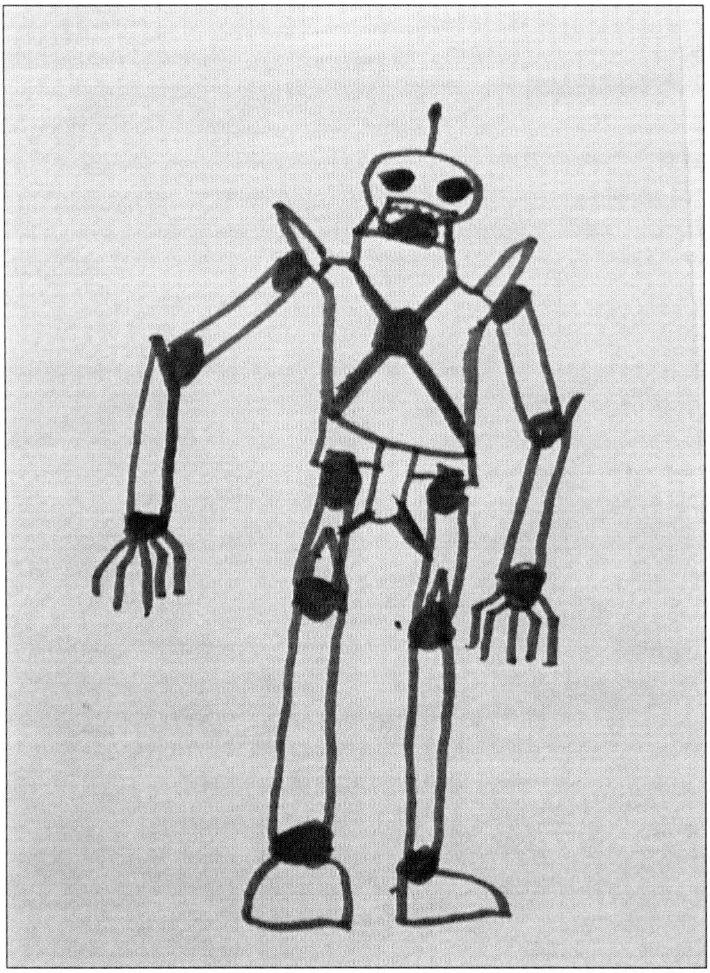

Figure 4. Million-Dollar Robot.

when a section would come out the way he planned it. Tommy took on the role of the care-taker in working on the Bird Monster as he asked for the researcher's assistance to find a way to support the figure's head in the beginning of sculpting and continued to care for it by strengthening its legs in the following sessions.

While the Bird Monster (see Figure 2 and Plate 2) seemed to require Tommy's protection, Tommy's next creature, the Horn Lizard (see Figure 3 and Plate 3) was entirely self-sufficient. Tommy described the Horn Lizard as shooting blood out of its eyes to fight the enemies and attacking them with its horn. Tommy solved the problem of weak legs by sculpting the Horn Lizard lying on its stomach. Of course, with that decision, Tommy eliminated the possibility of mobility for the creature. He seemed to have compensated for this limitation by endowing it with the ability to protect itself another way.

As vicious as Tommy made the Horn Lizard (see Figure 3 and Plate 3) sound, a nurturing quality soon emerged in the process. In one of the sessions, as Tommy was absentmindedly rolling a small piece of clay between two fingers, he suddenly remarked that it looked like an egg and proceeded to make a nest with five eggs, reportedly, for the Horn Lizard to protect. Interestingly, there were five people in Tommy's immediate family. For the duration of that session, Tommy was fully involved with the making of the nest.

In our further explorations of the imagery, Tommy struggled to reconcile the two seemingly opposite sides of the horn lizard–the attacker and the protector. After a number of sessions in which we discussed various aspects of the creature, Tommy finally verbalized this twofold quality when he said that even scary animals protected their eggs. The Horn Lizard's aggressive nurturance was likely reflecting Tommy's view of his parents', and particularly, mom's relationship to himself and his twin-sisters. There was a lot of anger in Tommy's tone when he spoke about the time that his mother called the police, which Tommy saw as the cause for the parents' separation.

Tommy's need to be the adult came out in the protective tone and affect when he talked about his younger twin sisters. In the second session, after Tommy drew the picture depicting the incidence with the police, I asked Tommy why he did not include his two sisters in the drawing. Tommy replied that they were too young to know what was happening and he never told them. Not only was he shielding them form the violence by excluding them from the picture, it sounded like Tommy thought that it was his responsibility to tell his sisters why their parents were not together. After some consideration, he drew the sisters into the picture. Tommy's feelings of responsibility became further apparent when Tommy considered telling them what happened, saying: "Maybe *I* need to tell them, because maybe they should know."

Tommy did not bring up the concept of siblings again until a few sessions later when Tommy was working with clay and made a clay nest for the Horn Lizard (see Figure 3 and Plate 3). As he was making the nest, Tommy specified that there will be five eggs that the lizard would protect. Tommy continuously brought up the idea of the lizard protecting its eggs, as well as the idea of protection by attacking.

The idea of attacking to protect paralleled Tommy's discussion of the safe people in his life. Tommy associated the ability to protect with physical strength as he reported that his father and his Karate instructor made him feel safe because they knew Tae Kwan Doe and Karate, respectively. To

Tommy, protecting, invariably meant attacking. Before Tommy would be able to begin to equate protection and nurturance with less aggressive actions, such as shielding, he needed to explore those concepts as he understood them and talk about what protection and nurturance meant to *him.* The making of the Horn Lizard (see Figure 3 and Plate 3) aided this process as Tommy kept coming back to the thought that even though the Horn Lizard attacked its enemies in a seemingly vicious manner by squirting blood out of its eyes and attacking them with its horn, it was doing so to protect the nest with its eggs.

Destructive and Constructive Feelings

Giving Tommy a sense of control, and at the same time, instilling in him an understanding that his familial situation was not up to him to fix became another focus of the treatment. As mentioned above, children from violent homes are stuck in the vicious cycle of feeling responsible for the situations in their homes and not being able to "fix" it. Constant failure to bring about peace contributes to a sense of loss of control and low self-esteem, resulting in declining behavior. One area in which a therapist can help a child feel in control is his or her fantasy. In fact, Hoffman (2003) states that children's aggressive behaviors are due to their inability to contain those behaviors in their fantasies (p. 547). Once a child is given the space to freely fantasize, the need to act out those fantasies in reality decreases. In the case of Tommy, clay facilitated the exploration of fantasy in two ways. Firstly–as a structured, but not rigid material, clay allowed Tommy to change his mind regarding design and relatively easily fix mistakes. Secondly–clay absorbed much of Tommy's negative feelings and helped Tommy safely project his emotions onto the figures, which in turn, helped him process those emotions.

The medium had to be malleable enough for Tommy to manipulate and control it, but firm enough to provide structure and guidance for the times when words and/or emotions became too overwhelming and therefore, difficult to manage. In other words, Tommy needed something more visceral to reach through his defenses into the inner self, but something that would also provide enough structure to contain his affect. Markers, used to draw the robot (see Figure 4), were too structured; the image did not hold Tommy's interest into the next session. On the other hand, paints were too freeing. Tommy used watercolor paints once to depict what was merely a copy of a house that he drew in the session prior (see Figure 5 and Plate 4) as a response to my directive of drawing a house. There was no emotional connection to the painted house, neither in the detached manner of painting, nor in the attempted discussion. Though chalk pastels that were used in the fol-

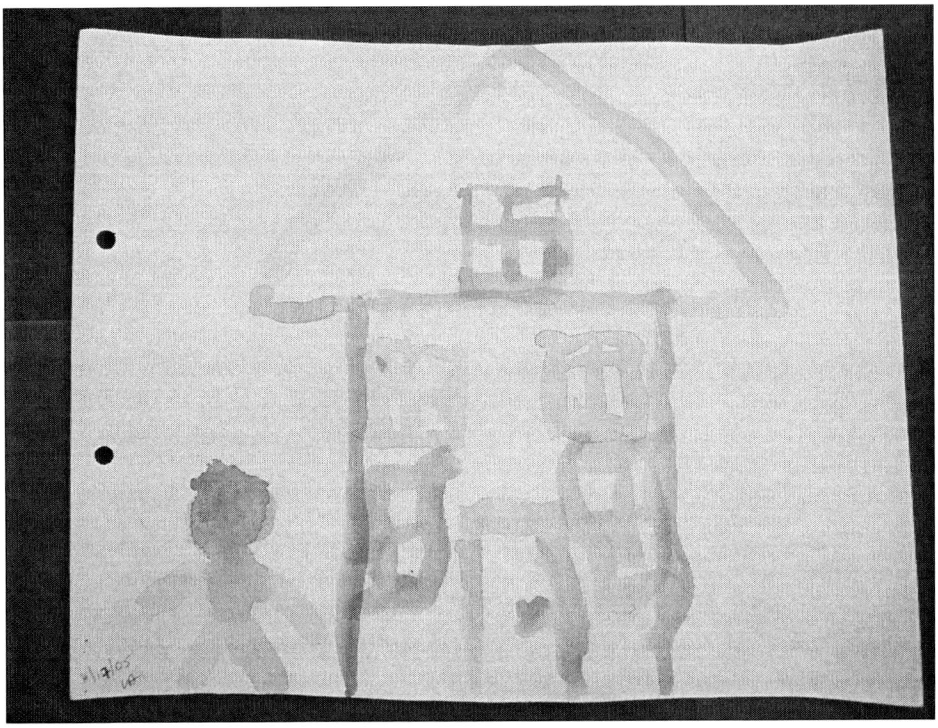

Figure 5. Watercolor House (see also Plate 4 in color).

lowing session to make a dual drawing (see Figure 1 and Plate 1) had a simultaneously loose; yet, structured quality, they were too dry to engage Tommy for the duration of the drawing.

One possibility I would like to suggest for the difference in response to the two media is that an instrument of two-dimensional media serves merely as the conductor of artistic expression, leaving a distance between the maker of art and the art itself. In that distance, there are pastels, pencils, paints, brushes, markers, and other tools, with the help of which, one creates. In contrast, clay *becomes* the artistic expression. Clay tools used in the work with clay are there only to assist the artistic experience, not serve as the main means for creation. When working with clay, there is nothing between the maker and the art. Unlike working with two-dimensional media, where a client either requires another object to manipulate materials such as paints or collage, or uses materials such as pastels or markers to depict an image, in work with clay, the *material* becomes the image, receiving the impact of the affect directly. As the result of molding clay in the client's hands, the product that comes out becomes, almost literally, a physical extension of the client's inner self in the moment.

In Tommy's case, what came out were figures that he called Bird Monster (see Figure 2 and Plate 2) and Horn Lizard (see Figure 3 and Plate 3). A monster was representative of the destructive side of Tommy and his view of that figure was reflective of his view of himself, as was supported by the session in which Tommy only took Bird Monster home after he made sure that it was strong enough to stand on its own. Horn Lizard represented Tommy's need to be protected, as well as his conviction that it was up to him to protect his family.

Henley (1991) talks about his choice of clay in the work with children due to the medium's propensity to encourage sensory stimulation and absorb and redirect the discharge of aggression. Clay absorbed Tommy's aggression and anger, allowing for the emergence of more positive forces, such as victory over enemies. Unlike destructive elements in the dual drawing (see Figure 1 and Plate 1), that were simply a "monster roller coaster," an "evil man," or a "rocket that was destroying a meteor," forces that were destructive without a flip positive side to them–the Bird Monster (see Figure 2 and Plate 2), though a monster, was destroying the evil.

Using a pencil at the beginning of treatment to depict the traumatic incident at home was easier at the time because it is a dry, minimally engaging medium that permitted Tommy to keep a safe distance from the experience. Using a pencil helped Tommy to relate what had happened, however, the medium was not involving enough to penetrate through the defenses to be able to process Tommy's feelings about the matter. Clay, with its visceral, sensual quality, accessed the self under the surface as well as absorbed some of the aggressive energy, making it easier for Tommy to express his anger verbally. Clay contained Tommy's aggression, making it unnecessary for Tommy's defenses to hide the true emotion.

Using archetypes, such as monsters, protectors, destroyers, evil man, old man, roller coaster, weak legs, lost head, twins, parents, and others he related to the various parts of himself and of people around him, and began to reconcile the "good parts" of the self with the "bad." By projecting the weak and destructive aspects of himself onto the Bird Monster (see Figure 2 and Plate 2) and the Horn Lizard (see Figure 3 and Plate 3), respectively, Tommy was able to process, accept, and begin to understand the possibility of coexistence of weakness and strength, and nurture and aggression.

Developing Competency and Establishing Individuality

As mentioned above, children witnesses of domestic violence see themselves as directly influencing and responsible for the violence (Skybo, 2005). Children try to control or fix events around them, but their failure, as they inevitably fail, results in their poor view of themselves, and, consequently, difficulty regulating their emotions and/or behaviors (Hoffman, 2003). Furthermore, Winnicott (1971) and Wolfe and colleagues (2003) talk about a child's loss of self as a result of their futile attempts to resolve the situation at home.

In work with Tommy, it became very important to validate and develop his sense of self. By teaching him certain skills for clay work and mirroring back Tommy's feelings as they were projected in his artwork, the researcher was able to begin to explore and develop Tommy's sense of competency and begin to establish and solidify his sense of individuality. The actual mastering of clay building techniques greatly contributed to Tommy's developing sense of self. Though Tommy had used clay before, he gained additional skills necessary to improve the quality of his figures throughout the duration of our work. When making the Bird Monster (see Figure 2 and Plate 2), Tommy learned one way to create supports for individual parts of the piece and how to reinforce the weaker elements. Making the Horn Lizard (see Figure 3 and Plate 3), Tommy learned how to score and slip - a technique to join two pieces of clay that have been left out to dry–and, in combination with what he had already learned in making the Bird Monster, was able to complete the Horn Lizard almost entirely on his own.

As Tommy's figures began to reflect closer Tommy's expectations for them, a change in Tommy's affect happened as it shifted from concentrated and serious to more relaxed and playful. When he saw that the Bird Monster's (see Figure 2 and Plate 2) legs remained strong after he had fixed them, as he excitedly exclaimed: "I told you it'd stick!" Tommy displayed the same excitement in the second session of working on the horn lizard when he saw that it did not crack: "Look! It's still together!"

The process of strengthening of the legs took much of the time and became a noteworthy part of Tommy's reconciliation of his role in the family that would not have been possible had he been using two-dimensional media. As if mirroring Tommy's uncertain position at home, the Bird Monster (see Figure 2 and Plate 2), though seemingly strong, would not stand on its own. The body and the head were too heavy for the weak legs. This aspect offered a rich context for metaphorical exploration of Tommy's feelings and coping mechanisms. Tommy constructed the head and the body relatively quickly, but the art process slowed down when he began making the creature's legs. Despite Tommy's struggles to make the figure stand up, the legs were coming out too thin to hold the body up. Eventually, I suggested Tommy add more clay to the legs. Tommy seemed to like the suggestion; however, as he was adding clay to the legs, he kept taking pieces of clay away and stretching out the legs, making them thin again. Just like Tommy was struggling to carry the weight of the feelings inside him, the Bird Monster was struggling to support the weight of its body. With much emotional and technical support from me, Tommy got the Bird Monster to stand on its own by the end of the session.

However, once the Bird Monster (see Figure 2 and Plate 2) was painted, Tommy said that he wanted to leave it at the agency. Tommy was excited about the figure in prior sessions and I attempted to explore Tommy's sudden indifference to it. As Tommy was reaching for a fresh piece of clay that was on the table, I drew his attention back to the Bird Monster and asked whether he liked making him. Tommy said he did. We talked about the process of making the figure, discussed how creative Tommy has been in making him, how it was difficult to get the figure to stand and how we finally got him to stand on his own. As we spoke, Tommy picked up the Bird Monster and held him in his hands. One of the legs was shaky. Tommy picked up a piece of clay and began to repair the leg with an effortless and familiar; yet, deliberate gesture. We continued to talk about the Bird Monster. Tommy said that he liked making the Bird Monster's head, but not the rest of it. He, again, expressed that he wanted to work on a different figure and leave the Bird Monster at the agency; however, he continued to repair the leg.

When the leg seemed to hold up better, Tommy said that maybe he would take it home. I commented that it seemed that Tommy did not want to take the Bird Monster (see Figure 2 and Plate 2) with him only if the leg was shaky. Tommy agreed that now that the leg was strong enough he wanted to take him home. By the end of the session, the leg was reinforced and the Bird Monster was standing strong. Tommy seemed pleased and said he wanted to give the Bird Monster to his mother. As Tommy held the Bird Monster in his hands to carry him out of the room, he accidentally dropped the figure on the table. When the tail and part of a wing fell off, Tommy seemed disappointed, but said that he would fix it himself at home. He proudly carried the Bird Monster out and presented it to his mother.

This change in affect and attitude can be explained in terms of Winnicott's (1971) discussion on projection in creative play. According to Winnicott, in creative play, a child manipulates external phenomena in the service of fantasy and invests that external object with fantasy meaning and feeling. In other words, a child projects his or her feelings onto the object of choice. Projection plays a tremendous role in the therapeutic work. Clay, as three-dimensional medium, makes working with projection that much easier. When a client's characters are looked at as representations of him or herself, the language with which those characters are discussed becomes a way to metaphorically process the client's experiences and feelings, strengths and weaknesses, accomplishments, and insecurities. Karkou and Glasman (2004) cite Refvem who stresses the importance of verbally processing the artistic experience. Talking about the experience of making art allows for the development of metaphors that can be applied to various aspects of the client's life.

As long as Tommy saw the Bird Monster (see Figure 2 and Plate 2) as himself, he needed to see the creature as stable and self-sufficient. As long as the Bird Monster's legs kept cracking and the figure kept falling, there was no room for it at home, since Tommy saw himself as the figure that held his family together. The acceptance of the Bird Monster was a two-step process. First, Tommy had to allow me, as an outsider, to enter his space and help him with the construction of the figure. Second, Tommy needed to make the figure strong and balanced enough to stand on its own. Once the figure was standing, it did not matter that other parts of it fell off. The tail or the wings were not the essence of the creature.

At the end of our time, Tommy was expressing with more ease his feelings and thoughts about his family situation. He was also more readily expressing his wants and needs, and asking for assistance when needed. Acting out behaviors at school decreased, and Tommy was able to concentrate better on his school work. Finally, though Tommy's fantasy of bringing his parents back together never completely disappeared, Tommy began to talk about his parents being together more in terms of his wish for it to be true, and less in terms of it being his responsibility.

In working with victims of domestic violence, it has already been recognized that art is a helpful modality in accessing, processing, and re-shaping of the traumatic experiences of the victims (Malchiodi, 1990; Johnson, 1987). However, clay, literally and figuratively, adds another dimension to the therapeutic work, facilitating a more efficient and deeper connection to the feelings underlying the behaviors. Clay, by nature, requires molding, shaping, and re-shaping by the client; it allows for movement, destruction, and rebuilding–all aspects that are important in dealing with one's anger. It requires a physical investment more so than two dimensional media. A witness of domestic violence has to reconstruct the view of his- or herself, of the world around them and re-evaluate how much influence they actually have on the situation. Clay allows for manipulation that lends itself to all the right metaphors to accomplish those changes, at the same time, respecting the necessary distance (Henley, 1991). Tommy had remarked in on of the sessions: "A sponge is a tool. . . . Water can be a tool. . . . Anything can be a tool." Though it is unlikely that Tommy was consciously aware of the powerful implications of his statement, on the unconscious level, he was learning a new coping mechanism in which, rather than shutting down and becoming emotionally distant, one can use the available resources as "tools" to improve one's situation.

Malchiodi (1990, p. 101) stresses the importance of allowing for spontaneous artistic expression arguing that to be more authentic and, therefore, more meaningful to the individual than art work that arises from a particular directive. Henley (1991) also considers spontaneity important in working with victims of domestic violence, as it creates a sense of control of which they were deprived and so desperately need to feel. He points out that because of the earthy, grounding qualities of clay, it triggers an impulse in a client to manipulate it, to mold it and shape it, which, in turn, promotes spontaneous expression. In such spontaneous manner, a Bird Monster (see Figure 2 and Plate 2) emerged, which proved to be invaluable for Tommy's development of individuality. When Tommy began to build the Bird Monster, he preferred to work by himself, without much input from the researcher. As the sessions progressed, Tommy developed enough ego-strength to not only accept the researcher's suggestions, but ask for help when he needed assistance.

Such heavily traumatic experience as domestic violence is difficult to process for even an adult who has developed adequate defenses and coping mechanisms. For a child who functions using primary defenses and is still figuring out which coping strategies work for him or her and which do not, the task of reconciling and making sense of the trauma is too much to handle on a conscious, reality-based level. Children revert to fantasy to help them figure out their situation (Ornduff & Monahan, 1999). Clay offers a balance between play and reality. It triggers our early memories of tactile experiences (Henley, 2002) facilitating therapeutic regression, which in turn, allows the client to reach affective states associated with the trauma. On the other hand, clay has its natural boundaries, through which it stimulates integration and self-control keeping the artist grounded in reality.

Using the Bird Monster (see Figure 2 and Plate 2) and the Horn Lizard (see Figure 3 and Plate 3), Tommy explored numerous themes that reflected his developmental stage as well as his familial situation. Tommy cultivated a stronger sense of self and built up confidence, developing individuality. He played with the idea of destructive and constructive forces as energies that could co-exist. Tommy continually worked out ideas of protection and nurturance as related to him and his family and friends. With this last theme, came the theme of responsibility; responsibility for all those that relied on him for protection. With time, through metaphor and play, Tommy developed enough trust within the therapeutic relationship to give over some of that role to the researcher as he allowed the researcher to assist in the execution of and care for his figures.

Clay required for direct contact with the material as well as assistance from the researcher leading to the development and building of trust between the researcher and Tommy that is so vital in the therapeutic work. Once a deeper trust was established, I was able to address Tommy's sense of competency and begin to establish individuality through the exploration of his fantasy, through improving his skills in working with clay, and through projecting his feelings onto the clay creatures.

The use of clay also helped Tommy's understanding and making sense of the ideas of protection and nurturance by absorbing some of the anxiety associated with the traumatic experience and making Tommy's feelings more manageable. Tommy was able to direct his anxiety into clay and explore protection and nurturance through his clay characters.

Finally, clay was instrumental for allowing Tommy a sense of control by facilitating decision making with the possibility of changing his mind. Tommy struggled to reconcile destructive and constructive forces within himself, as clay absorbed aggressive and destructive energies. Once aggression was channeled into clay, Tommy explored the seemingly conflicting parts of his personality by assigning various qualities to his clay characters, eventually exploring the same themes by looking at his relationship with family and friends.

Terms

Art Therapy – Art therapy is the use of art making process, within a therapeutic, professional relationship, by people who experience illness or trauma, or by people who seek personal growth.
Association – Process of recalling past experiences by relating similar events.
Parentification – A situation, in which a child assumes, or is given adult responsibilities due to various unfortunate situations at home.
Photographic memory – Process, in which past experiences are recorded in the brain in the form of images.
Score and slip technique – A method, which allows to join two pieces of clay, minimizing the possibility of breakage.

References

English D., Marshall, D., & Stewart, A. (2003). Effects of family violence on child behavior and health during early childhood. *Journal of Family Violence, 18*, 43-57.

Fantuzzo, J. W., & Mohr, W. K. (1999, Winter). Prevalence and effects of child exposure to domestic violence. *The Future of Children, 9*, 21-32.

Henley, D. (1991). Facilitating the development of object relations through the use of clay in art therapy. *American Journal of Art Therapy, 29*, 69-76.

Henley, D. (2002). *Clayworks in art therapy.* London: Jessica Kingsley Publishers.

Hill, A. (2002). *The impact of domestic violence on children's psychological well-being.* Unpublished doctoral dissertation, Biola University, La Miranda, CA.

Hoffman, L. (2003). A psychoanalytically oriented approach as primary and secondary prevention: Discussion of Joy Osofsky's "psychoanalytically based treatment for traumatized children and families." *Psychoanalytic Inquiry, 23*, 544-552.

Johnson, D. R. (1987). The role of the creative arts therapies in the diagnosis and treatment of psychological trauma. *Arts in Psychotherapy, 14*, 7-13.
Karkou, V., & Glasman J. (2004). Arts, education and society: The role of the arts in promoting the emotional wellbeing and social inclusion of young people. *Support for Learning, 19*, 57-64.
Malchiodi, C. (1990). *Breaking the silence: Art therapy with children from violent homes.* New York: Brunner/Mazel.
McAlister Groves, B. (1999). Mental health services for children who witness domestic violence. *The Future of Children, 9*, 122-132.
Orduff, S., & Monahan, K. (1999). Children's understanding of parental violence. *Child and Youth Care Forum, 28*, 351-364.
Osofsky, J. D. (1999, Winter). The impact of violence on children. *The Future of Children, 9*, 33-49.
Refvem, J. (2000, March). *The witnesses walk your halls: The school counselor and student victims of domestic violence.* Paper presented at the meeting of the American Counseling Association, Washington, DC.
Saxe, G. N., Ellis, B. H., Fogler, J., Hansen, S., & Sorkin, B. (2005). Comprehensive care for traumatized children. *Psychiatric Annals, 35*, 443-448.
Skybo, T. (2005). Witnessing violence: Biopsychosocial impact on children. *Pediatric Nursing, 31*, 263-270.
Winnicott, D. W. (1971). *Playing and reality.* London: Routledge Classics.
Wolfe, D. A., Crooks, C. V., Lee, V., McIntyre-Smith, A., & Jaffe, P. G. (2003). The effects of children's exposure to domestic violence: A meta-analysis and critique. *Clinical Child and Family Psychology Review, 6*, 171-187.

Biography

Liza Avetikova, M.P.S. is an art therapist for Psychological Trauma Center in Los Angeles, California, working in an intercity elementary school. She received her M. P. S. in art therapy and creativity development from Pratt Institute, Brooklyn, NY. This present chapter is based on her experience as a primary therapist for children affected by domestic violence during her second year internship at a New York agency designed to offer services and resources to children and families affected by domestic violence.

Chapter 4

FINDING PEACE THROUGH ART: ART THERAPY WITH CHILD SURVIVORS OF DOMESTIC VIOLENCE

MEREDITH B. CARLETON

Introduction

"Our fantasy is over." Four simple words speak volumes, inscribed with conviction at the bottom of a child's painting. The eleven-year-old appears simultaneously buoyant and defeated as he fills his paper with opulent color, an image of a sailboat on a tranquil sea. A black sphere looms in the corner of the paper, emphasized by streaks of motion that threaten the tiny boat with a grim promise. "Our fantasy is over," he explains in reference to his family: the fighting, the bruises, the pain. He contemplates the whereabouts of his father, whom he concurrently fears and longs for. He cries for his siblings and his mother, trying desperately to pick up the pieces of their fragmented lives and move on. And yet, when this boy leaves my office, he does so with an air of freedom and innocence. He joins the group of his peers playing UNOÆ in the playroom, laughing greedily at his stack of cards, as if life had not dealt him such an unfortunate hand.

It is this quality that amazes me about children; this extraordinary ability to laugh, to find joy amongst sadness; the resilience to look hopefully towards the future, despite never seeing evidence that what lay ahead will promise anything but more pain. Art therapy provides a creative outlet for emotional exploration, and in my work with child survivors of domestic violence, I have learned just how powerful tool creativity can be in bringing the cycle of family violence to a halt.

There was a time not long ago when parents and professionals alike believed that mere witness to domestic violence was not significant enough to cause lasting damage or trauma in a child's life. As long as the child was

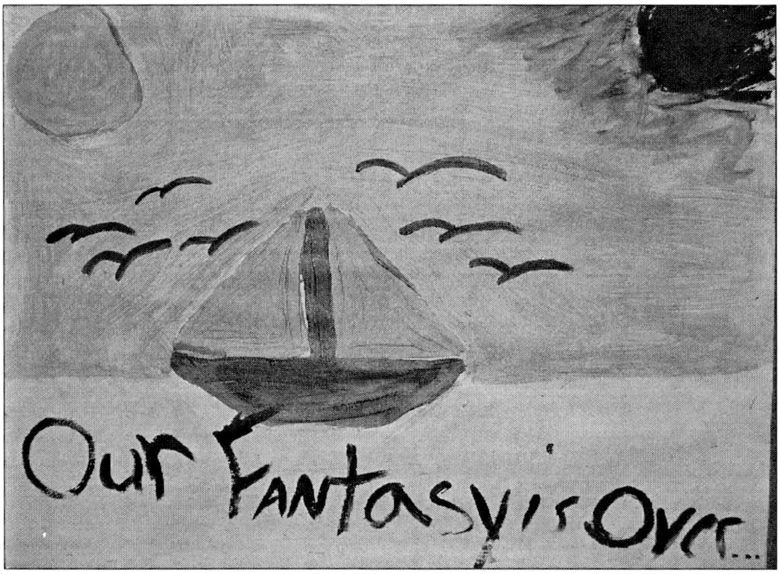

Figure 1. Painting created by 11-year-old boy in PALS program (see also Plate 5 in color).

not physically abused, there was little focus on the long or even short-term ramifications of witnessing inter-parental violence. In more recent studies, however, such as an in-depth literature review conducted by Rossman, Hughes and Rosenberg, (2000), it has been suggested that both behavioral and emotional problems are significantly higher in children that come from homes plagued with domestic violence. Additional research conducted by Carlson and Strauss concludes that between 2.3 and 10 million children witness violence between their parents in the United States each year (as cited in Rossman, Hughes & Rosenberg, 2000). Furthermore, it has been estimated that as many as 15 percent of children are exposed to physical and/or verbal aggression between their parents (Rossman, Hughes, & Rosenberg, 2000). With staggering statistics on childhood exposure to domestic violence being published in recent years, it is no wonder the psychological and emotional well-being of these young survivors are finally being considered and addressed.

Special Population

The PALS program (Peace: A Learned Solution) was designed to serve children between the ages of 4 and 12 who have been victim of or witness to domestic violence, as well as provide emotional support for the non-offending parent and the family unit as a whole. Families come to our program in various stages of the healing process, though for the most part, the acute trauma has likely past. During the six-month program cycle, most of the families we serve are in the process of moving on in their quest for a peaceful home, often after a separation or divorce has occurred. With the abusive parent no longer in the home, the remaining family members can begin to emerge from the traumatic cycle of violence, and begin the long journey towards self-expression and acceptance.

One might wonder what happens to those children still living in an abusive environment; do they not need an arena for safe, creative expression, too? As a therapist, my goal is to equip children with tools for healing, and to empower them to embrace their emotions, foster familial communication, and build self-esteem; all issues that can be dangerous if the source of the abuse is still a prominent fixture in their lives. To teach a child to access and embrace his/her pain and emotions in an unsafe environment can be far more detrimental than maintaining the survival-mode mentality. And so with heavy hearts we often have to turn these families away. Without passing judgment, we refer them to the 24-hour domestic violence hotline, counseling and psycho-educational programming, and invite them to reach out to us again in the future.

Once the intake process is completed, children are matched with a therapist for individual work, as well as enrolled in a group comprised of children homogeneous in age and sex. Whenever possible, children are offered a combination of modalities, such as individual art therapy and group music therapy, to provide multiple opportunities for connection with a therapist and with their own individual creativity. Children go through an initial assessment period in each modality that involves pre-testing, mandated by DYFS (Division of Youth and Family Services), as well as a creative assessment. In an effort to establish basic trust and assess a child's artistic development and skill level, I engage each child in a simple progression of drawing, painting, and sculpting, allowing the child the freedom to choose their subject matter. There is much to be learned from these initial pieces of artwork beyond the child's level of ability, including a basic understanding of personality, self-esteem, current/presenting issues, and level of trauma and repression of that trauma. While preliminary in nature, art assessments can provide a jumping off point for further creative endeavors, as well as a solid basis for comparison with later works.

Based on the initial assessments, the multi-disciplinary treatment team designates goals for each child, chosen from a bank of various milestones and objectives (see Appendix). The progress and regression with regards to these goals are continually addressed and documented each week by the child's therapists. The child's progress is closely monitored and reviewed by the treatment team on a monthly basis, to ensure the utmost level of therapeutic service for each child.

Recent research has suggested that one feature distinguishing child survivors of domestic violence from victims of other traumatic experiences, is that the child is robbed psychologically of both his/her parents. With one parent acting as a terrorizing abuser, the other parent is focused on fear and survival, thus the child is often left without nurturing parental refuge (McAlister Groves, 2002). Because of this devastating circumstance, while child participants in the PALS program, they are engaged in their respective creative arts therapy sessions, the non-offending parent is involved in our parenting support group. This group is designated for parents to discuss issues they face in the wake of their domestic violence experiences, such as custodial concerns and behavioral challenges in their children, etc. All families are also offered family therapy, to support their journey in healing the family as a unit. Creative arts therapies are integrated into the parenting groups and family work whenever possible, to provide some insight into the creative process, as well as provide insight into conflict and communication issues that might otherwise go unexpressed in traditional talk therapy.

Creative Approach

Art therapists utilize a multitude of materials to foster creativity and make a connection with their clients. Within the PALS program, the therapists address the following basic psychosocial components: safety/trust, emotions, relationships, communication/conflict resolution, and self-esteem. Though these topics are overlapping, and by no means exhaustive, they provide a basic framework for healing and, at the very least, a solid foundation for growth. During a six month period of therapy, all of these goals may be addressed, or in the case of many children whose lives have been more profoundly damaged by domestic violence, often only a few of these areas are addressed in depth. Also, it should be noted that while the following cases are all illustrated by examples that use a directive art therapy approach, some of the greatest and most significant strides I have witnessed are achieved through an open studio approach, where the child is given the time, space, materials, and freedom to create without agenda.

Stage 1: Safety/Trust

Therapeutic Intervention: Cooperative Drawing

In the forming stages of any therapeutic relationship, it is essential to establish a sense of trust between the client and the therapist. With a child who has been a victim of domestic violence, this initial period is of utmost importance, particularly as their sense of trust has been compromised by a lack of safety in their home life. They have been taught to care for and rely on themselves rather than their caregivers, as their abusive parent has proven too dangerous, and the non-offending parent has most likely existed in survival mode, unable to attend their child's basic needs for stability and expression. Often, the result is a premature loss of childhood innocence.

Peter

Peter was five years old when he joined the PALS program. In his young life, he had witnessed much discord in his parents' marriage, culminating in a divorce that left Peter and his sister in deep emotional turmoil. Peter's mother, who is visually impaired, endured great emotional and verbal abuse from Peter's father, and her disability contributed to this already skewed balance of power. Peter and his older sister relied solely on their mother for emotional support, though had to depend on themselves for other needs, due to their mother's physical limitations and their father's abusive, often neglectful behavior. Once the divorce was in process, Peter and his mother and sister moved from their home in Florida all the way to New Jersey, leaving the abuse behind but carrying with them the memories, the trauma, and a whole new set of challenges that would come with living on their own.

Like most children whose lives have been touched by domestic violence, Peter still loved and admired his father, wanted very much to see him and was devastated by his absence. Unfortunately, however, Peter's father had alternate intentions. Once living in New Jersey, their contact with Peter's father dwindled. He did not fight for custodial rights, and nor did he take advantage of the visitation rights granted to him. Not only had Peter and his sister been mistreated by their father, they had now been abandoned him also, compromising Peter's ability to trust and feel safe, even in the presence of those whom were closest to him. The results of the trauma Peter experienced were manifest in bouts of extreme separation anxiety when mom was absent, fluctuation between emotional extremes, temper tantrums, and a general lack of positive attitude and affect.

Peter's mother reported that he was an extremely talented young artist, though he was initially quite timid, and reluctant to participate and communicate with me. In order to help ease the transition into the therapeutic relationship, I employed a cooperative drawing technique, a simple yet effective method of engagement. By taking turns adding to a drawing on a shared page, it becomes possible to establish trust between therapist and client through collaborative art-making, and therefore symbolically bond in the shared therapeutic space. While facilitating a cooperative drawing session, emphasis is also place on respect of one another's boundaries, process over product, and last but not least, having fun!

Initiating a mutual drawing with even the most basic line or shape serves as an invitation into the shared space, and in Peter's case, was extremely successful in helping to begin an artistic dialogue. A curvy line would become a vast sea with mermaids and sharks, while a circle would be transformed into face as part of a family portrait. Sometimes the mood of the drawing would be silly and abstract, while others would be more reality based, but all helped in some way to provide a sense of trust and commonality, and a foundation for later independent expression.

Stage 2: Emotions

Therapeutic Intervention: Clay Sculpture Journey

The definition of domestic violence has broadened to include spurning, terrorizing, denial of emotional responsiveness, isolating, corrupting/exploiting, and mental, physical and emotional neglect (Rossman, Hughes & Rosenberg, 2000), thus the resulting trauma experiences by victims of such atrocities encompass a plethora of emotional and behavioral difficulties. Only after a basic sense of trust has been established can we begin to explore such emotions. For some children, this means developing a basic emotional vocabulary, and most importantly, granting them permission to feel. When a home is wrought with domestic violence, feelings become dangerous. Anger and sadness need to be masked with joy so as not to disturb the delicate balance of a volatile relationship. Thus, it is essential to support each child in rediscovering their emotional self, validating their fears, their anger and their anxieties, and ultimately help them to alleviate the guilt that inevitably develops while allowing themselves to feel.

Mark

Mark is the oldest of three children, and from an outsider's perspective, would appear to be a perfectly healthy, well-rounded kid, and in many respects this is true. What one would not expect at first introduction to Mark, is that this eleven year old boy came from an explosive home, and was plagued with anger and manipulation. His father is a successful, well-respected man, who to the rest of the world seemed to have it all. Behind closed doors, however, he was often controlling and demeaning to his wife and children, and was prone to bouts of property destruction and terroristic threats.

When Mark came to PALS, he had perfected the act of the being the ideal child; straight A's in school, a star on the local soccer team, creative, musical, and popular amongst his peers. Mark's mother described a boy who was determined to be perfect, to show the world, and his father, that he was worthy of love. In these efforts, however, Mark swallowed his feelings, pushed his fears and insecurities deep down inside, denied his emotions, and put on a happy face. After all, everyone loves a happy, successful kid.

When Mark first started attending art therapy, he was content creating perfect pictures with a pencil and ruler, and organized mosaics created symmetrically to look like geometric puzzles. He was open to trying about anything, as long as he could make it pretty and keep the process cerebral and non-threatening. And yet, Mark was never satisfied with anything he made, as his creations could never possibly live up to his impossible standards for perfection. The more I encouraged Mark to explore his feelings artistically, the more his insecurities shone through, as he created perfect, calculated, frame-worthy art. Likewise, his style of communication was equally calculated and free of emotion, as our discussions tended to be somewhat superficial.

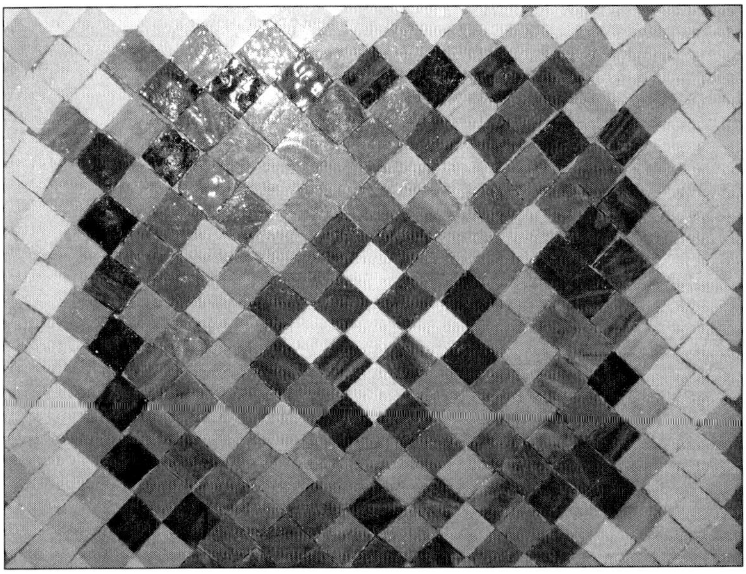

Figure 2. Mosaic created by 11-year-old boy in PALS program (see also Plate 6 in color).

Once initial trust and safety had been established, I decided to challenge Mark with a directive that undoubtedly had the potential to be emotionally charged. It was at this point that we began working with clay, which, by nature, is messier, less controllable and requires more physical and emotional investment than the pencil drawings he had been so content creating. But the real challenge went beyond the material itself. To instill a sense of control, I encouraged Mark to manipulate the atmosphere in the art room, in order to create a soothing and comfortable environment. He accomplished this by dimming the harsh, fluorescent lights and selected some familiar music to play in the background. I then provided Mark with a mound of clay, and invited him to close his eyes, and create a sculpture that felt good in his hands. By completely removing the emphasis and pressure of creating something that *looked* good, it allowed Mark the opportunity to create something that *felt* good.

Mark was resistant to this process at first, trying to open his eyes, and then attempting to create a recognizable object despite the fact that he could not see what he was doing. With some encouragement and perseverance, however, there was a shift in Mark's demeanor. While it was understandably difficult for him to surrender himself in this manner, to concentrate on feeling rather than appearance, he was clearly liberated by the experience. The regressive, muddy nature of the material combined with the freedom of creating without agenda resulted in a breakthrough for Mark; as he molded the clay, he shared a story about a mud fight he once had with his father and brother on a camping trip in early childhood, which he recalled as being the most fun they had ever had together.

By shifting Mark's creating process from his head to his hands, he was able to create a piece of art that was more emotionally derived. The process resulted in the first creation for which he had no prior expectation, thus Mark was finally satisfied with the product. His hands had been his only tools, and as such, the product was a true extension of himself. Mark expressed for the first time feeling content with his creation, and seemed at peace to have shared such an intimate, poignant memory of his father in the process.

Stage 3: Relationships

Therapeutic Intervention: Puppet Making

A family that is plagued with domestic violence often perpetuates a cycle of guilt and self-reliance. Healthy relationships are replaced with dysfunctional ones, as children become caretakers for younger siblings, even for their own parents. Residual effects often include Post Traumatic Stress Disorder (PTSD) resulting in extreme fear of being vulnerable to others, thus making healthy relationships almost impossible without some type of intervention. In fact, studies have shown that of the two factors most accurately predicting PTSD, sexual abuse and witnessing chronic domestic violence, the latter actually seems to be more harmful overall when compared with children whom are direct victims of child abuse (McAlister Groves, 2002). Furthermore, children who have been witness to prolonged domestic violence and abuse often end up victimizing one another, or even victimizing their non-offending parent much as they have witnessed.

Elisa

Seven-year-old Elisa spent her entire young life as a helpless witness to her family's demise. As the youngest member of a large family, Elisa was accustomed to chaos and tumult from birth. Her father had been abusive towards her mother for nearly two decades, his actions so manipulative that he was capable of turning the entire family against their mother. Utilizing control and deception, Elisa's father convinced his eldest children that their mother was trying to destroy the family. He fabricated tales of his wife's adultery and substance abuse, until the older children became convinced that their mother was a villain, and began replicating the abusive behavior they had witnessed. Elisa became a casualty of the situation, as she watched her mother flee the family home to seek safe shelter, leaving Elisa to be cared for by adolescent siblings whom had become perpetrators themselves, and were engaging in self-destructive behaviors.

By the time Elisa's mom had won the vicious custody battle over Elisa and her nine-year-old sister, their teenaged siblings, who were old enough to choose their custodial parent, had already been acting as young girls' caretakers. Their father's continued neglect only served to reinforce the teenagers' rebellious and unhealthy behaviors, and Elisa was witness to dangerous and harmful acts, including harassment of her own mother.

As Elisa's mother attempted to salvage what remained of her relationship with her two youngest daughters, it became apparent just how much trauma Elisa had experienced in the preceding months. The dysfunctional environment in which she had been living promoted vulgar, disrespectful language and behaviors, which Elisa ultimately replicated towards her mother. Elisa's emotional and physical health had been neglected during her mother's four-month absence from the family home, as there was no responsible, nurturing caretaker to tend to these basic needs. Thus, when Elisa joined the PALS program, she was completely shut down emotionally. She viewed her mother as a peer rather than a parental figure, and spoke to her as such. In her mother's presence, Elisa would tantrum and scream obscenities, while in her absence she more closely resembled a typical seven-year-old girl.

Elisa's behavior was a clear indicator of Post Traumatic Stress Disorder, as the combination of her mother's abandonment, her father's neglect and her dysfunctional home life proved extremely damaging. In response to these harrowing circumstances, Elisa shut down emotionally in order to protect herself from further pain, and was displaying great anger and resentment towards her mother. When I attempted to address any feelings of pain or sadness with Elisa directly, she would disassociate, and completely shut down. With this in mind, understanding just how fragile Elisa's emotional state was, I offered her the opportunity to create a puppet, onto which she could project any feelings that felt unsafe for her to own and express herself.

Puppet making is a favorite in the PALS program, and is executed utilizing methods that range in cost, level of difficulty, and varying time commitments. In order to make Elisa's puppet, we layered wet plaster-coated cotton strips onto a partially inflated balloon. Once dry, the balloon could be popped and retrieved from a small hole in the plaster, where a stick was inserted to serve as the puppets body/handle. Elisa was given the choice to create an animal or human, and then provided the materials necessary to decorate her puppet any way she desired.

Elisa chose to make her puppet a girl, which she described as being the youngest sibling of a large family. Her completed puppet served as a nonthreatening figure to be used in dramatic play. Though she was reluctant to play out scenarios specific to her own life experiences, I was able to play and communicate with her puppet using other puppets, demonstrating healthy examples of communicating one's thoughts and feelings through metaphor. Elisa responded well to this process, as she enjoyed the creation process and the playful interaction between puppets, and was even able to extract meaning relevant to her own life on occasion. For example, when her puppet witnessed an argument between two other adult-figure puppets, her puppet cried and hid beneath the table, noting that it frightened her to see mommy and daddy fight.

Given the immense trauma Elisa endured, it is understandable and even expected that her progress throughout the PALS program would be very gradual, and interspersed with periods of regression. By engaging her in artistic endeavors and dramatic play, however, the emotions that have been overwhelming, and therefore repressed, were now somewhat accessible when channeled through safe, productive means.

Stage 4: Communication/Conflict Resolution

Therapeutic Intervention: Creating a Game

Communication in families where domestic violence is prevalent is often severely compromised. Children witness volatile arguments, and often try to become a mediator or peacemaker. There is little if any respect present in

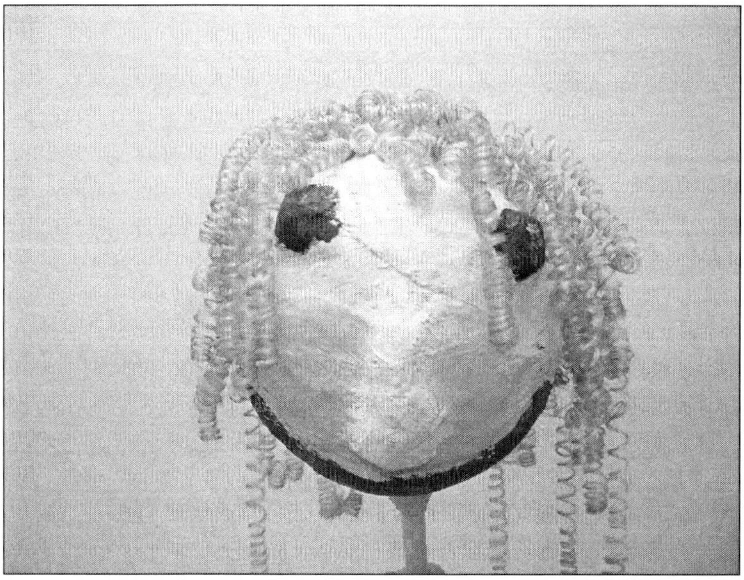

Figure 3. Puppet created by 7-year-old girl in PALS program (see also Plate 7 in color).

much of family communication, and children repeat patterns that are modeled for them by their caregivers. Also, living in fear of the next event of domestic violence, these children often suppress their own needs, and stop genuinely communicating altogether. It is imperative that these children learn methods for effective communication, and gain tools to utilize when challenges inevitably arise.

John

John is another example of a child survivor of domestic violence that suffers in silence. To the world, he appears to be a healthy, outgoing ten-year-old boy, whose life would likely be an extension of his parents' perfect marriage. But John has endured a great deal of pain and trauma, having witnessed his father attack his mother's body and character with increasing regularity over the recent years.

John is the middle child who, as stereotype might suggest, often gets lost in the shuffle. Upon his parents' divorce, John's older brother took on the role of the "man of the house," and became their mother's confidant, while his younger sister received constant attention for her emotional outbursts and simply for being the youngest child. John, on the other hand, was relatively easy-going, smart and athletic, and did not actively seek out attention or support from his family.

For John, the most troublesome aspect of his parents' divorce was the loss of his father, with whom he shared some truly meaningful memories as a young child. Because he was not the oldest child, he was spared some of his father's harsh criticism. Since he was not the youngest, he was not seen as a nuisance because of frequent temper tantrums. In fact, when compared with his siblings, John actually had a healthy relationship with his father, making his feelings of loss and abandonment that much stronger when his father finally moved out. Nevertheless, John witnessed much discord between his parents, and was the victim of his father's dramatic mood swings and severe discipline tactics; yet, in his absence he idealized his father, and longed for a relationship with him.

Some of John's fondest childhood memories are of hours spent playing chess with his father. Neither of his siblings had ever taken much interest in the game, thus it was a pastime only he and his father shared. During their scheduled visitation time, John looks forward to opportunities to play chess, as it seems the game provides and arena for communication and father-son bonding not otherwise available in his life. In light of this, I suggested that John might create a special chess set for he and his father to use together. John was immediately taken with this idea, and enthusiastically set out to create this unique symbol of their relationship.

John created a chess set using a canvas board, painted with care using metallic gold, silver and copper paint. To create the chess pieces, John glued stacks of colored mosaic tiles, topped with as assortment of trinkets and seashells to designate the king, queen, pawns, etc. As John worked on his masterpiece, he spoke with nostalgia about his experiences playing with his father, emphasizing it as a highlight amongst the day-to-day tumult of their troubled home. While he may never be able to communicate with his father the pain and longing and sadness he feels, when playing the chess game he created, they would be able to meet on safe, common ground.

Part of the healing process for victims of domestic violence is often coming to terms with the limitations of others, specifically the abusive parent. By supporting a child in creating a game, one can emphasize peaceful coexistence as well as verbal and artistic communication. In creating his chess set, John was able to begin to gain acceptance of his situation, create opportunities for positive interactions with his father, while celebrating his creativity and self-expression with each round of chess.

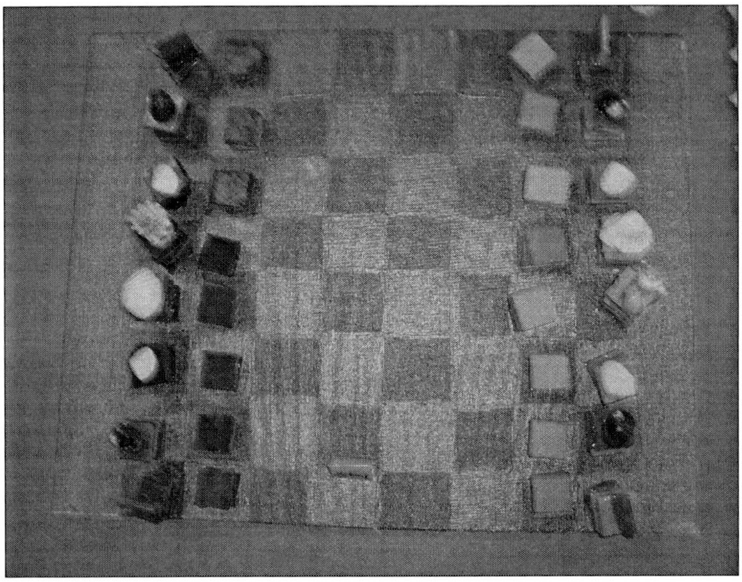

Figure 4. Chess set created by 10-year-old boy in PALS program (see also Plate 8 in color).

Stage 5: Self-Esteem

Therapeutic Intervention: Art to Share

Perhaps one of the most detrimental effects of domestic violence on children is low self-esteem. These children are constantly disrespected and disregarded by the abusive parent, causing them to feel devalued. This can lead to a constant struggle to be the best at everything in order to win approval, or to completely withdraw for fear they will never measure up. Furthermore, harboring guilt about one's own responsibility for the domestic violence or parents' separation can lead to plummeting self-image.

Kate

Kate never quite felt like she fit in, even within her family. She had very few friends, and gravitated towards younger children that she could care for, avoiding connections with children her own age. At eight years old, she was her mother's only child, and her father's youngest child by nearly twenty years. From early childhood, she never seemed to be able to live up to her father's expectations, and lived in the shadows of her much older siblings. Her mother is extremely loving and attentive to Kate as a rule, though when circumstance turned violent and unsafe at home, nothing could sooth Kate, for the memories of the most frightening events continue to occur over and over again in her mind.

Kate shared her recollections of the last confrontation between her parents, when her mother came home later than expected to find her father enraged. Kate remembered vividly how it felt to see her bicycle thrown down a flight of stairs in anger, and remembers clearly how terrified she felt to see her father, an alcoholic, scream and threaten her mother. This was the most physically violent moment that Kate can recall witnessing, though the stories of verbal and emotional abuse are plentiful. Kate expressed feeling that she had never and would never be good enough to please her father, and after months of therapy was able to express her anger over this rejection.

In response to feeling devalued, Kate developed a fascinating coping mechanism, that resulted in vast fluctuations in behavior. One moment, Kate would he speaking in a very juvenile, babyish voice, crawling around on the floor, impersonating an infant, and in the next moment would be speaking poetically about growing older, becoming a teenager, and gaining the freedom she so longed for. For Kate, the present was just too painful to bear, while the past and the future seemed ideal. Kate spent the first several weeks of treatment wanting only to finger-paint, telling stories about her friends at after-school-care, all of whom were far younger than she. She explained that the finger-painting made her feel "like a kid again," and she seemed content regressing to a childlike demeanor.

When Kate was not imitating the mannerisms and speech of a toddler, she was fixated on adolescence, even when given the directive to create a portrait of herself as she is. In response to this prompt, Kate chose to create a life-sized self-portrait by tracing her body and then painting and embellishing it to look like herself. Despite the directive, however, the finished portrait was not an illustration of her present self, but rather a vision of a thirteen-year-old Kate, titled "The Me I Want to be When I'm 13." She accompanied her portrait with a narrative that mentioned a part-time job, lots of friends, and most memorably, a girl who is never sad.

It is difficult to isolate a specific turning point for Kate, as with each passing month she seemed to shift into a more confident little girl. Over time, the fluctuations in the personas she presented dwindled, until she seemed content just being herself. Due to an extension granted by DYFS, I was fortunate enough to see Kate in therapy for full year, during which time she underwent tremendous growth. When a new group of peers joined the program in the second six-month cycle, Kate seemed to have an air of confidence I had not seen before, as she was proud to share her knowledge and experience with the new kids, and take on a leadership role. Suddenly, in stark contrast to the role she had been locked into with her family, Kate could now feel like she had something to offer her peers, rather than embody the role of the youngest daughter that would never quite measure up, always feeling like she was a thousand steps behind.

Part of every child's graduation from the PALS program includes participation in an Arts Festival, wherein each child has the opportunity to share any artwork or musical explorations, should they feel compelled to do so. In addition, the children contribute a favorite song to a community CD. Each family receives a copy of the music compilation, to serve as a symbol of their growth throughout the program, and a transitional object to help them cope with the separation. In addition to welcoming the children's contributions to the festival gallery, I offer children the opportunity to contribute a piece of artwork to be used as the cover of the CD, and Kate was happy to accept this challenge. She put a great deal of thought into her design, wanting it to convey the feelings of peace and joy she has felt along her journey. Her completed image contained a tree, flowers, and sunshine, and the words "PALS" and "Friends." The image was simple but joyful, and the immense pride and satisfaction she felt in sharing her artwork with the rest of the community was truly inspired.

As a witness to the demise of her parents' marriage, and victim of eight years of her father's demeaning, controlling behavior, Kate's self-esteem was suffering. She was so conscious of her limitations, and of her place in her family and in the world, that her day-to-day life seemed almost unworthy of recognition or celebration. Through art therapy, Kate was able to reflect on her longing for the past and the future, and rejoice in all that is beautiful and rewarding about being an eight-year-old girl in the present, perhaps for the very first time.

Conclusion

In her book, *Children Who See Too Much*, Betsey McAlister Groves (2002) states that "Domestic violence, violence that occurs between adult caregivers in the home, seems to be the most toxic form of exposure to violence for children" (p. 50). Long gone is the time when professional and common beliefs suggested that children witness to domestic violence emerged unscathed. We now understand that there are many lasting effects on children that, if left untreated, further perpetuate the cycle of violence.

Art therapy is a tremendously healing vehicle, through which child survivors of domestic violence can begin to find and create peace. By uniting creative interventions with comprehensive treatments goals, art therapists can support these children in increasing their self-esteem as well as begin to build healthier communication and relationships, while rediscovering the joy and innocence of simply being a child.

Appendix

PALS THERAPEUTIC GOALS

PALS Therapeutic Goals

1. Learn and practice self-soothing strategies.
2. Remain grounded and focused for task completion.
3. Strengthen impulse control and self-regulation abilities.
4. Maintain appropriate personal boundaries.
5. Develop a healthy sense of autonomy.
6. Demonstrate respect for adults and peers.
7. Achieve greater awareness of feelings.
8. Learn to express and to contain expression of feelings in healthy ways.
9. Show compassion for the feelings of others.
10. Find and develop one's voice.
11. Relate to peers in a cooperative and peaceful manner.
12. Communicate in an assertive and effective manner.
13. Demonstrate good listening skills.
14. Demonstrate empathy for others.
15. Learn peaceful strategies for resolving disagreements.
16. Develop problem-solving skills.
17. Increase understanding of how domestic violence has affected one's life.
18. Communicate feelings and needs to parents.
19. Build healthy relationships with siblings.
20. Identify/develop a support network.
21. Develop positive peer relationships.
22. Increase self-esteem.
23. Identify one's areas of strength.
24. Identify one's core hurts and recognize one's core value.
25. Broaden sense of self to include new roles and capabilities.
26. Increase spontaneity and creativity.
27. Identify hopes, dreams and goals for the future.
28. Express feelings regarding changes that have occurred and anticipated changes.
29. Increase acceptance of losses/changes which have occurred.

Terms

Art Therapy: Art therapy is the therapeutic use of art making, within a professional relationship, by people who experience illness, trauma, or challenges in living, and by people who seek personal development. Through creating art and reflecting on the art products and processes, people can increase awareness of self and others, cope with symptoms, stress, and traumatic experiences; enhance cognitive abilities; and enjoy the life-affirming pleasures of making art. Source: www.arttherapy.org
Domestic Violence: Any hurtful or unwanted behavior perpetrated upon an individual by an intimate or prior intimate. Includes physical, psychological, and emotional abuse. Primarily a learned behavior whose effects, without intervention, become more destructive over time. Source: www.turnaroundinc.org
Post Traumatic Stress Disorder (PTSD): Post Traumatic Stress Disorder (PTSD) is the result of a severe and extraordinary stressor in the person's life that may be environmental (a large fire, hurricane), war, or violent crime (armed robbery, child abuse, rape), or the witnessing of violent incidents. Source: www.psychologytoday.com
Self-Esteem: A realistic respect for or favorable impression of oneself; self-respect. Source: www.dictionary.com

References

McAlister Groves, B. (2002). *Children who see too much.* Boston: Beacon Press.
Rossman, B. B. R., Hughes, H. M., & Rosenberg, M. S. (2000). *Children and interparental violence: The impact of exposure.* Philadelphia: Brunner/Mazel.

Biography

Meredith B. Carleton, M.P.S., A.T.R.-B.C., L.C.A.T., C.C.L.S, earned her BA in psychology from Lehigh University, and her MPS in Art Therapy and Creativity Development from Pratt Institute. In addition to earning her board certification from the American Art Therapy Association, and her LCAT (Licensed Creative Arts Therapist) in New York, Meredith is also a Certified Child Life Specialist (CCLS). Meredith has dedicated her work thus far to serving children, be they survivors of domestic violence and sexual assault, or plagued with terminal illness. She has spent nearly three years working with the PALS (Peace: A Learned Solution) program, at SAFE in Hunterdon, formerly Women's Crisis Services of Hunterdon County, NJ, both as the program Art Therapist and as Coordinator of Children's Services and Child Advocacy. Meredith also facilitates Art Therapy groups in the Morris County Juvenile Detention Center and Morris County Youth Shelter, as a part of Creative Heartwork, Inc.

Chapter 5

THE ROYAL ROAD: USING PLAY TO HEAL CHILDREN WHO HAVE EXPERIENCED DOMESTIC VIOLENCE

Charles E. Myers

Introduction

A six-year-old Hispanic girl plays in the dollhouse. She places the girl doll in the bedroom and "locks" the door. Next, she moves the parent dolls outside the bedroom door. The mother slaps the father and screams, "Don't ever touch my daughter again!" The child's play is so intense that she is not conscious of the therapist, still in the room.

A five-year-old African-American boy takes an adult tiger and a tiger cub. He has the mother caring for the cub. Then the mother bites the cub. The cub cries out in pain as the mother continues to hurt him. This play is repeated with elephants, snakes, and other animals throughout the session.

A four-year-old African-American boy picks up two Barbie-style dolls, a male and female. He methodically undresses them. He places the dolls together. The child has the dolls kiss, then moves them against each other in a clearly sexual manner. Then suddenly they stop, the male strikes the female repeatedly, finally, throwing her across the room. Through the entire play session the child's affect is completely flat.

Domestic Violence

Since the 1970s, domestic violence has emerged from behind closed doors. Prior to this time, the tendency was to think that domestic violence did not happen, or at least it never happened to anyone in your family, your friends, your neighborhood. And if it did happen in your family, the attitude was 'what happens at home stays at home' (Carlson, 1984). Nationally, people are increasingly willing to acknowledge the existence of domestic violence and its impact on it has on our society and our children (Kot et al., 1995). Domestic violence is now recognized as a family legacy that crosses social class, education, and income levels (Lloyd, 1990). In a survey by Straus and Gelles (1990), more than 25 percent of couples reported at least one incident of physical aggression occurring in their relationship.

Domestic violence's impact on children is invasive and pervasive. The family environment of homes in which domestic violence occurs is chaotic (Tyndall-Lind, et al 1999), and jeopardize a child's physical and emotional well-being, safety, and development. Moore, Pepler, Mae, and Kates (1989) identified the following characteristics of homes with domestic violence: a lack of stability and consistency, poor problem-solving skills of the parents, salient models of aggressively responding to social problems, and apparent acceptance of the use of violence to resolve conflicts.

Edleson (1999) found child witnesses of domestic violence experience increased difficulties, as compared with child non-witnesses of domestic violence, with: (1) behavioral and emotional functioning, (2) cognitive functioning and attitudes, and (3) long-term developmental problems. Behavioral and emotional problems included higher levels of aggression, anger, and hostility; fear, anxiety, withdrawal, depression, and low self-esteem. Cognitive functioning and attitudes encompassed lower cognitive functioning, poor school performance, lack of conflict resolution skills, pro-violence attitudes, and limited problem-solving skills. Long-term developmental effects included increased levels of adult depression, trauma-related symptoms, and low self-esteem.

Carlson (1984) reported children who have experienced domestic violence often experience the sudden loss of a parent or caregiver. Domestic violence may result in the breakup of the relationship, incarceration, Child Protective Services removal of the child from the home, and/or physical or emotional abandonment by the parent(s) or caregiver(s). Developmentally, young children are egocentric, believing they cause the events that happen in the world around them. It is common for children to misunderstand the domestic violence occurring around them and the resulting situations following the violence (Huth-Bocks, Schettini, & Shebroe, 2001). Children are likely to internalize what is happening around them and experience guilt and shame.

Importance of Play

Rousseau wrote in the 1700s of play as being essential to the healthy development of children (Bratton, Ray, Rhine, & Jones, 2005). Play is the central activity of childhood and the single most important means by which they learn about themselves, others, the world around them and their place in that world (Landreth, 2002). The importance of play in the lives of children is evident in its pervasiveness in childhood. The United Nations proclaimed play as a universal and inalienable right of childhood, emphasizing the importance of play to the development and wholeness of children. Through play, children learn to respect themselves, to control their feelings responsibly, and to be creative in confronting problems. Children can imagine and test new possibilities and ways of being.

Children use play to explore their inner world and to express their true self, which is full of needs, wishes, and wants. Children use play to organize their experiences and personal worlds, to resolve conflicts, and to communicate their feelings (Landreth, 2002). Through play, children develop their capacity to be creative in confronting problems and finding solutions. Play has a reality of its own as an activity in which children explore their identities in relation to others (Cattanach, 1992).

Play and activity are the natural mediums of communication for children (Axline, 1964; Ginott, 1959; Landreth, 2002). Play is also the young child's primary mode of emotional expression (Hall, 1997). Through play, children can communicate what they are unable to say in words. Children can use toys to express emotions about their self-perceptions, about others, and about significant events they have experienced (Ater, 2001).

Play is the most natural and healing process in childhood. Erikson (1963) believed children have the capacity to find recreation and to self-cure when engaging in play. Play is particularly useful with traumatized children, such as those children who have experienced domestic violence, as they are more likely in general to express their innermost feelings and fantasies much more readily through play than verbalization (Mann & McDermott, 1983). The recognition of the importance of children's play in their healing and growth is paramount, and its value of to children and to the therapeutic process with children is crucial (Caplan & Caplan, 1974).

Developmentally, children lack the cognitive, verbal facility to express how they feel, and emotionally are unable to focus on the intensity of what they feel in a manner adequately expressible in a verbal exchange (Landreth, 2002). Children use the symbolic language of play to express their inner worlds and experiences. Piaget (1962) stated play bridges the gap between a child's concrete experience and abstract thought. The symbolic function of play is central to the manner in which children communicate. Children use symbolic play to create a special world, a safe place, set in their own time and space aside from "ordinary" life. Children have a clear understanding of the boundaries of play and signal their intention to begin and to end play in ways which keep the boundaries clear (Cattanach, 1992).

Play is the child's means of self-expression, an opportunity for a child to "play out" feelings, thoughts, and experiences as an adult might "talk out" difficulties (Mader, 2000). Landreth (2002) stated, "Children's play can be more fully appreciated when recognized as their natural medium of communication. Children express themselves more fully and more directly through self-initiated spontaneous play than they do verbally because they are more comfortable with play. For children to 'play out' their experiences and feelings is the most natural dynamic and self-healing process in which children can engage" (p. 14).

Play Therapy

Garry Landreth (2002) described play therapy is a "dynamic interpersonal relationship between a child (or person of any age) and a therapist trained in play therapy procedures who provides selected play materials and facilities the development of a safe relationship for the child (or person of any age) to fully express and explore self (feelings, thoughts, experiences, and behaviors) through play, the child's natural medium of communication, for optimal growth and development" (p. 16).

When working with a child, it is important for a therapist to consider the developmental level of the child when deciding what approach to utilize. Children behave and think differently from adults, and the therapist's approach to working with them must reflect this difference (Ater, 2001; Webb, 2002). Children are able to use the healing and growth process of play naturally and independently, except when trauma has significantly interrupted these processes (*Cochran, 1996*).

Play is the natural treatment approach for working with children. Play allows children the ability to externalize trauma and to work through the trauma at their own pace (Allan & Lawton-Speert, 1989). Play therapy is a primary, and usually the most appropriate, intervention for children. It is therapeutic approach based on the understanding that play is the child's natural medium of self-expression (Homeyer, 1999). Play therapy naturally undertakes the hard work of child psychotherapy in the appealing guise of play. Play therapy has been adapted to accommodate the world of childhood, using the medium of play as the means of communicating symbolically with the child (Webb, 2002).

Play has been used by child therapists with children since the 1920s. Anna Freud (1926/1982) used games and toys as a way to build a relationship with her child patients, while another child analyst, Melanie Klein (1932), used the child's play as the basis for interpretations to the child. Another play therapy pioneer is David Levy (1938), who helped children recreate traumatic events through a structured play format. Other innovators included Fredrick Allen (1942), Clark Moustakas (1959), Virginia Axline (1947), and Landreth

(2002), all of whom emphasized the natural growth process of children as key to helping the child individuate and develop basic self-esteem (positive regard). Achievement of these goals in play therapy occurs through recognition of the child's feelings as expressed in the play and through the therapist's belief in the child's strengths and potential for growth and change (Webb, 2002).

The purpose of play therapy is to help children through the medium of play in the context of a therapeutic relationship. Play therapy incorporates the unique meaning of play to children and the importance of understanding the symbolism of the child's play language (Webb, 2002). Therapists who understand the importance of play in the lives of children, and that children naturally communicate through play, are well on their way to understanding the world of children. Conversely, therapists who employ adult-style talk counseling with children send a very clear message to child clients: "I am unwilling to enter your world of communication; therefore if this process is going to work, you have to leave that world and come into my adult world, which includes my level of thinking and communication" (Sweeney & Homeyer, 1999). The responsible therapist goes to a child's level and communicates with children through the medium with which they are comfortable (Landreth, 2002).

Rationale for Play Therapy

Ray, Armstrong, Warren, and Balkin (2005) stated play therapy is based on the developmental understanding of children based on Piaget's (1962) theory of cognitive development. Piaget recognized children and adults differ in how they understand and process information. Sweeney (1997) stated adult therapy depends heavily on the formal operations of Piagetian development. Adult communication by its very nature is abstract and sophisticated, whereas the communication of children is concrete and simple.

Children (Ray, Armstrong, Warren, & Balkin, 2005) in the "Preoperational Stage" (2–7 years of ages) are "acquiring the skill of language in which symbols are used to mentally represent objects" (p. 360). These children are in the process of developing understanding and knowledge internally, but lack the ability to communicate their experiences to the world around them. Preoperational children use play as a primary way to communicate their internal awareness of self and others. Children in the "Concrete Operations Stage" (8–11 years of age) grow "in personal ability to reason logically and organize thoughts coherently" (p. 360). These children are able to manipulate ideas and accept societal rules, but are limited in their ability think abstractly. With play, Concrete Operation children are able to gap the bridge between concrete experience and abstract thought.

The nature of child's play and play therapy are both fundamentally preoperational. Play and language are contrasting forms of representation of an individual's thoughts, feelings, and experiences. When a therapist insists a child communicate cognitively and verbally, in essence the therapist is asking the child to translate symbolic thoughts into the therapist's accepted medium of communication of talk. Play and fantasy do not carry this limitation. Children are able to create without the restriction of translating their creation verbally. Therefore, children and play do not lend themselves to the Formal Operationalism of abstract thought and verbal communications, as they are in fact preoperational. The therapist must approach and understand children from a developmental perspective (Landreth, 2002).

Through play, a sense of connection, of understanding develops between the child and the therapist quickly and smoothly (Kottman, 2001). The therapist's willingness to and ability to "speak" in the child's language conveys a respect for the child that the child may have never experienced previously. By being present with the child, watching how the child plays, the toys the child chooses, and when the child switches from one activity to another, the therapist is able to enter and learn much of the child's world.

An important role of the play therapist is to provide children with opportunities to prove to themselves that they have the potential to be successful. Play therapists provide a safe and accepting environment in which children use play to learn about themselves and the world around them (Landreth, 1987). Engaging children through play therapy allows the children to share their stories and experiences, and provides the therapist the opportunity to understand the child's phenomenological world (Axline, 1969; Ginott, 1959; Landreth, 2002; Moustakas, 1953; Mullen, 2002). By engaging in the process of play, children attempt to reduce overwhelming experiences in their lives into manageable situations through symbolic representation, thereby creating an opportunity for self-expression (Johnston, 1997). Children are able to use symbolic materials in play to create the necessary therapeutic distancing from the traumatic experiences (Mann & McDermott, 1983) to engage in growth and healing. Play therapy provides children with a safe and protected space where they can enact, ingest, and assimilate traumatic experiences slowly over time. The child is able to divide overwhelming experiences and emotions into small quantities, manageable components, and handle those experiences through play. Children can then become empowered and able to express their feelings and master their environment through play (Allan & Lawton-Speert, 1989).

Child-Centered Play Therapy

Child-centered play therapy gives voice to the child. Through child-centered play therapy, children are able to express their inner experiences. The child-centered play therapy philosophy considers play as essential to the healthy development of children. Play gives concrete form and expression to a child's inner world. Children are able to give meaningful symbolic expression to emotionally significant experiences through play. Children are able to transform, through play, what may be unmanageable in reality to manageable situations through symbolic representation, providing children with opportunities for learning to cope by engaging in self-directed exploration (Landreth, 2002).

Child-centered play therapy is based on a philosophy resulting in attitudes and behaviors for living one's life in relationships with children. It is both a basic philosophy and an attitude of deep and abiding belief in the ability of children to constructively self-direct their play in ways that are healing and significant to them (Landreth & Sweeney, 1997). The child-centered play therapist believes deeply in and trusts implicitly the inner person and direction of the child. The play therapist's objective in a play therapy session is to relate to the child in ways that will release the child's inner directional, constructive, forward-moving, creative, self-healing power. When children genuinely experience this philosophical belief within the playroom, they are empowered and their developmental capabilities are released for self-exploration and self-discovery, resulting in constructive change (Landreth & Sweeney, 1997).

Axline (1969) clarified the nature of the interaction between the therapist and child in the child-centered approach in her eight basic principles that serve as a guide for therapeutic contact with the child (Landreth, 2002):

1. The therapist is genuinely interested in the child and develops a warm, caring relationship.
2. The therapist experiences unqualified acceptance of the child and does not wish that the child were different in some way.
3. The therapist creates a feeling of safety and permissiveness in the relationship so the child feels free to explore and express self completely.
4. The therapist is always sensitive to the child's feelings and gently reflects those feelings in such a manner that the child develops self-understanding.
5. The therapist believes deeply in the child's capacity to act responsibly, unwaveringly respects the child's ability to solve personal problems and allows the child to do so.
6. The therapist trusts the child's inner direction, allows the child to lead in all areas of the relationship and resists any urge to direct the child's play or conversation.
7. The therapist appreciates the gradual nature of the therapeutic process and does not attempt to hurry the process.
8. The therapist establishes only those therapeutic limits that help the child accept personal and appropriate relationship responsibility.

Play Therapy and Domestic Violence

The treatment of children who have experienced or witnessed domestic violence is difficult. These children have experienced a parent or caregiver, a person normally associated with protection and nurturance, as being harmful, either directly to the child, or to someone significant to them. Play therapy addresses the needs of these children through a developmentally appropriate approach.

The lives of children are sometimes intruded upon in very traumatic ways and are so often outside their own control (Sweeney & Homeyer, 1999). Children who have experienced domestic violence often feel powerless and vulnerable (Tydall-Lind et al., 1999). Therapeutic interventions, therefore, should not only be nonintrusive, but also provide high level of safety for children. Play therapy provides children a safe place in which they can naturally express their experiences, feelings, and desires (Kot et al., 1995). Through the use of play, play therapists can address trauma-related issues effectively, while providing an emotionally safe environment for the process of healing to occur (Gallo-Lopez, 2000).

Cattanach (1992) identified four basic concepts of play. First, play is central to the child's way of understanding the world. Second, play is a developmental process and in therapy, the child moves back and forth along a developmental continuum as a way of discovering individuation and separation. Third, play is a symbolic process through which the child can experiment with imaginative choices appropriately distanced from the consequences of those choices in "real" life. Finally, play happens in a therapeutic space, where the child's creative life starts and the child experiences for the first time the psychological significance of art.

Play therapy frees the child, allowing the child to emote without the need to translate emotions into verbal expressions. Play provides children with courage, empowering them to heal what is hurting (Homeyer, 1994) The play experience generates a feeling of relief and mastery for the child, promoting healing, and growth (Hall, 1997). Healing can only occur within safe boundaries; this is especially true for sexually abused children who have experienced a traumatic violation of their boundaries (Brooke, 2007). Through play therapy, children come to an acceptance of what has happened to them and learn new ways of coping to protect themselves from further abuse (Ater, 2001; Cattanach, 1992).

Play Therapy Skills

Play therapists (Landreth, 2002) utilize a number of therapeutic skills that communicate to the child four basic messages: "I am here," "I hear you," "I understand," and "I care." The basic play therapist skills include (Kottman, 2001): (a) tracking behavior to establish a relationship with the child, (b) restating content to build rapport, (c) reflecting feelings to help the child to feel understood, (d) limit setting, (e) returning responsibility to the child, and (f) dealing with questions.

It is important for the therapist to allow the child to decide when to deal with issues. The play therapist appreciates the gradual nature of the therapeutic process and does not attempt to hurry the process (Axline, 1969; Landreth, 2002). Given a safe therapeutic environment and relationship, children will deal with those issues in the order most important to them (Homeyer, 1999).

Limit setting is important in play therapy (Landreth, 2002). Children do not feel safe, valued, or accepted in a completely permissive relationship (Moustakas, 1959). Limits are a vital and necessary part of all healthy relationships. Individuals are free to grow and develop within the limits of their own potentialities, talents, and structure. Limits are one aspect of an individual's true experience, and identify, characterize, and distinguish the dimensions of a therapeutic relationship. Limits provide the form or structure of an immediate relationship. In a therapeutic relationship, limits provide the boundary or structure necessary for growth to occur. The play therapist's use of consistency and predictability help the child to feel safe within the therapeutic relationship.

Limits (Landreth, 2002) are used in the playroom to: (1) protect the child both physically and emotionally, (2) to protect the therapist and the therapist's acceptance of the child, (3) to facilitate the child's decision-making, self-control, and self-responsibility, (4) to anchor the session to reality and to the here and now, (5) to promote consistency in the playroom environment, (6) to preserve the professional, ethical, and socially acceptable relationship, and (7) to protect the play therapy materials and room. The play therapist words limits in a way that allows the child to achieve self-control. Landreth (2002) outlined the A-C-T method of limit-setting (p. 261):

A – Acknowledge the child's feelings, wishes, and wants.
C – Communicate the limit.
T – Target acceptable alternatives.

All children need to feel understood and accepted. All children experience issues of self-concept maintenance and enhancement, and children will deal with those issues in their own unique way. The child determines the content and direction of the play.

Traumatic Play

Post-traumatic play is a type of play observed in children who have undergone a psychic trauma, such as domestic violence, so intense that their ordinary coping mechanisms and defenses are insufficient to prevent them from being overwhelmed by pain and anxiety. Some of the characteristics of post-traumatic play include compulsive repetition, unconscious link between play and the trauma, literalness of play with simple defenses, and failure to relieve anxiety (Terr, 1983). Findling (2004) outlined five behaviors of traumatic play in the development of Trauma Play Scale. The play of traumatized children, as those who have experienced domestic violence, are often characterized by intensive play, repetitive play, play disruption, avoidant play, and negative affect.

Intense play is defined as play that has a compulsive and driven character. Children engaged in intense play will often appear as though are unaware of the world around them. Repetitive play is defined as play that must be done the same way each time it occurs. Children engaged in repetitive play will repeat the same play theme within session or across sessions. The toys selected may differ (i.e. tigers, snakes, dolls), but the theme or character of the play will remain the same. Play disruption is defined as play that is interrupted by the child as a form of dissociation. Children demonstrating play disruption will abruptly disengage in play that has become overwhelming, and may be intense or repetitive, and switch to another form of play, often play that is comforting. Avoidant play behavior is defined as play in which the child evades the therapist as means of coping with interpersonal relationships. Children engaged in avoidant play may sit with their backs turned to the therapist as they play, remain on the far side of the room, hide behind a puppet theatre, or act in ways that are rejecting to the therapist. Negative affect is defined as play in which the child's affect is either flat or incongruent with the child's play. Children demonstrating negative affect may play out intensively emotional play with a blank expression or smile when playing out themes of anger.

Research has shown that traumatized children engage in post-traumatic play that is secret and ritualistic, with a driven quality to it (Terr, 1981). Through post-traumatic play, children are able to communicate to the therapist how they experienced the trauma (Marvasti, 1994). Awareness of the elements of traumatic play opens a window into the child's inner world and increases the therapist's understanding of the child.

Conclusion

Freud (1999) stated dreams were "the royal road to the unconscious." Play is the royal road to the child's inner world. Through play, children permit the therapist to see their inner worlds, their developmental levels of functioning, and their competency abilities. Children can identify the intricacies of their pain, and express and release their anxieties and concerns through therapeutic play (Hall, 1997). Through play, children can communicate those experiences in their life too difficult or scary for them to face.

Experiencing domestic violence is traumatic to children, often overpowering their defenses and normal coping skills. Play therapy is a developmentally appropriate, curative approach to helping children recover from the experience of domestic violence. The natural elements of play make therapy less threatening for children and can encourage them to be less guarded and more open and spontaneous. Through the empowering process of play therapy, a child can relieve emotional distress (Griffith, 1997) and replenish the feelings of joy and hope (Hall, 1997). Play opens the royal road to healing for a child.

References

Allan, J., & Lawton-Speert, S. (1989). *Play psychotherapy of a profoundly sexually abused boy: A Jungian approach.* Paper presented at the Annual Convention of the American Psychological Association. New Orleans, LA.

Allen, F. (1942). *Psychotherapy with children.* New York: Norton.

Ater, M. K. (2001). Play therapy behaviors of sexually abused children. In G. L. Landreth (Ed.), *Innovations in play therapy: Issues, process, and special populations* (pp. 119-129). Philadelphia: Brunner-Routledge.

Axline, V. M. (1964). Nondirective therapy. In M. Haworth (Ed.), *Child psychotherapy* (pp. 34-39). New York: Basic Books.

Axline, V. (1969). *Play therapy* (Rev. ed.). New York: Ballantine Books. (Original work published 1947.)

Bratton, S. C., Ray, D., Rhine, T., & Jones, L. (2005). The efficacy of play therapy with children: A meta-analytic review of treatment outcomes. *Professional Psychology: Research and Practice, 36*(4), 367-390.

Brooke, S.L. (2007). *The use of the creative therapies with sexual abuse survivors.* Springfield, IL: Charles C Thomas, Publisher, Ltd.

Caplan, F., & Caplan, T. (1974). *The power of play.* New York: Anchor Books.

Carlson, B. (1984). Children's observations of interpersonal violence. In A. R. Roberts (Ed.), *Battered women and their families* (pp. 147-167). New York: Springer.

Cattanach, A. (1992). *Play therapy with abused children.* Philadelphia: Jessica Kingsley Publishers.

Cochran, J. L. (1996). Using play and art therapy to help culturally diverse students overcome barriers to school success. *The School Counselor, 43* (3), 287-297.

Edleson, J. L. (1999). Children's witnessying of adult domestic violence. *Journal of Interpersonal Violence, 14,* 839-870.

Erikson, E. H. (1963). *Childhood and society.* New York: Norton.

Findling, J. H. (2004). *Development of a trauma play scale: An observation-based assessment of the impact of trauma on the play therapy behaviors of young children.* Unpublished dissertation. University of North Texas: Denton, TX.

Freud, A. (1946/1982). *The psychoanalytical treatment of children.* London/New York: Imago/ International Universities Press.

Freud, S. (1999). *Interpretations of dreams* (J. Crick, Trans.). New York: Oxford Press. (Original work published 1900.)

Gallo-Lopez, L. (2000). A creative play therapy approach to the group treatment of young sexually abused children. In H. G. Kaduson & C. E. Schaefer (Eds.), *Short-term play therapy for children* (pp. 269-295). New York: Guilford Press.

Ginott, H. (1959). Theory and practice of therapeutic intervention in child treatment. *Journal of Consulting Psychology, 23*, 160-166.

Griffith, M. (1997). Empowering techniques of play therapy: A method for working with sexually abused children. *Journal of Mental Health Counseling, 19* (2), 130-142.

Hall, P. E. (1997). Play therapy with sexually abused children. In H. G. Kaduson, D. Cangelosi, & C. Schaefer (Eds.), *The playing cure* (pp. 171-194). Northvale, New Jersey: Jason Aronson Inc.

Homeyer, L. (1994). *Play therapy behaviors of sexually abused children.* Unpublished doctoral dissertation, University of North Texas, Denton, TX.

Homeyer, L. E. (1999). Group play therapy with sexually abused children. In D. S. Sweeney & L. E. Homeyer (Eds.), *Group play therapy: How to do it, how it works, whom it's best for* (pp. 299-318). San Francisco: Jossey-Bass, Inc.

Huth-Bocks, A., Schettini, A., & Shebroe, V. (2001). Group play therapy for preschoolers exposed to domestic violence. *Journal of Child and Adolescent Group Therapy, 11*(1), 19-34.

Johnston, S. S. M. (1997). The use of art and play therapy with vicitims of sexual abuse: A review of the literature. *Family Therapy, 24* (2) 101-113.

Klein, M. (1932). *The psychoanalysis of children.* London: Hogarth Press.

Kot, S., Landreth, G., & Giordano, M. (1998). Intensive child-centered play therapy with child witnesses of domestic violence. *International Journal of Play Therapy*, 7(2), 17-36.

Kottman, T. (2001). *Play therapy: Basic and beyond.* Alexandria, VA: American Counseling Association.

Landreth, G. L. (2002). *Play therapy: The art of the relationship* (2nd ed.). New York: Brunner-Routledge.

Landreth, D. S., & Sweeney, G. L. (1997). Child-centered play therapy. In K. J. O'Conner & L. M. Braverman (Eds.), *Play therapy theory and practice: A comparative presentation* (pp. 17-45). New York: John Wiley & Sons, Inc.

Levy, D. (1938). Release therapy in young children. *Psychiatry, 1*, 387-389.

Lloyd, S. A. (1990).Asking the right questions about the future of marital violence research. In D. J. Besharov (Ed.), *Family violence: Research and public issues* (pp. 93-107). Washington, D. C.: AEI Press

Mader, C. (2000). Child-centered play therapy with disruptive school students. In H. G. Kaduson & C. E. Schaefer (Eds.), *Short-term play therapy for children* (pp. 53-68). New York: Guilford Press.

Mann, E., & McDermott, J. F. (1983). Play therapy for victims of child abuse and neglect. In C. E. Schafer & K. J. O'Conner (Eds.), *Handbook of play therapy*, (pp. 283-307). New York: John Wiley & Sons, Inc.

Marvasti, J. (1994). Play diagnosis and play therapy with child victims of incest. In K. O'Connor & C. Schaefer (Eds.), *Handbook of play therapy: Vol. 2 Advances and innovations* (pp. 319-348). New York: John Wiley & Sons, Inc.

Moore, T., Pepler, D., Mae, R., Kates, M. (1989). Effects of family violence on children: New directions for research and interventions. In B. Pressman, G. Cameron, & M. Rothay (Eds.), *Intervening with assaulted women: Current theory, research, and practice.* Hillsdale, NJ: Lawrence Erlbaum Associates.

Moustakas, C. (1959). *Psychotherapy with children: The living relationship.* New York: Harper & Row.

Moustakas, C. E. (1953). *Children in play therapy: A key to understanding normal and disturbed children.* New York: McGraw-Hill.
Mullen, J. A. (2002). How play therapists understand children through stories of abuse and neglect: A qualitative study. *International Journal of Play Therapy, 11*(2), 107-119.
Piaget, J. (1962). *Play, dreams, and imitation in childhood.* New York: Basic Books.
Ray, D., Armstrong, S. A., Warren, E. S., & Balkin, R. S. (2005). Play therapy practices among elementary school counselors. *Professional School Counseling, 8*(4), 360-365.
Straus, M. A., & Gelles, R. J. (1990). *Physical violence in American families: Risk factors and adaptation to violence in 8145 families.* New Brunswick NJ: Transaction.
Sweeney, D. (1997). *Counseling children through the world of play.* Wheaton, IL: Tyndale House Publishers, Inc.
Sweeney, D. S., & Homeyer, L. E. (1999). Group play therapy. In D. S. Sweeney & L. E. Homeyer (Eds.), *Group play therapy: How to do it, how it works, whom it's best for* (pp. 3-14). San Francisco: Jossey-Bass Inc.
Terr, L. C. (1983). Play therapy and psychic trauma: A preliminary report. In C. Schaefer & K. O'Conner (Eds.), *Handbook of play therapy* (pp. 308-319). New York: John Wiley & Sons, Inc.
Terr, L. (1981). Forbidden games: Post-traumatic child's play. *Journal of American Academic Child Psychiatry, 20,* 741-760.
Tyndall-Lind, A., Landreth, G. L., & Giordano, M. A. (2001). Intensive group play therapy with children witnesses of domestic violence. *International Journal of Play Therapy, 10*(1), 53-83.
Webb, N. B. (2002). Play therapy crisis intervention with children: Individual, group, and family treatment (2nd ed.). In N. B. Webb (Ed.), *Play therapy with children in crisis: A casebook for practitioners* (pp. 29-48). New York: Guilford Press.

Biography

Charles Edwin Myers, M.A., LPC, LMHC, NCC, NCSC, RPT-S, is a Licensed Profes- sional Counselor-Supervisor in the State of Texas, a Licensed Mental Health Counselor and Certified School Counselor in the State of Florida, a National Certified Counselor and National Certified School Counselor, and a Registered Play Therapist-Supervisor. Mr. Myers is currently a doctoral candidate at the University of North Texas specializing in play therapy. He works as therapist in private practice at Sharp Focus Centers in Denton, TX and as a Teaching Assistant at the University of North Texas. Mr. Myers has presented at the local, state, and national levels on play and filial therapy, sandtray therapy, diversity, and school counseling. In addition, Mr. Myers has served as a school counselor in rural and inner city schools using play and sandtray therapy, as well as providing play and filial therapy in a homeless shelter in Tampa and crisis counseling in the hurricane shelters in Dallas. Mr. Myers has also served in leadership roles for a number of local, state, and national level professional organizations and currently serves on the Clinical Communications Committee of the Association for Play Therapy.

Chapter 6

THE USE OF PLAY THERAPY WITH CHILDREN IN A DOMESTIC VIOLENCE CONTEXT

JOSHUA A. THOMAS-ACKER AND MARY L. MCGINNIS

Introduction

Play has historically been used in educational and therapeutic environments and has captured quite a bit of interest as to its benefits and insights into children's behavior. Saracho and Spodek (1995) note that pioneers in educational play; Friedrich Froebel (1782-1852), John Dewey (1859-1952) and Maria Montessori (1870-1952) made significant contributions to the use of play in educational contexts and in support of child development. Froebel is known for developing the original concept of kindergarten; Dewey for developing the concept of pre-school education; and Montessori for the Montessori School concepts (Saracho & Spodek, 1995). Freud recognized that play had important therapeutic value for children (Leblanc & Richie, 2001; Sarcho & Spodek, 1995). It was Freud's daughter, Anna Freud, who furthered play in working with children in psychoanalytic theory (Leblanc & Richie, 2001).

The term play therapy can be deceiving. The name, for some, may sound as though there is little therapeutic value in the process. It's important to remember that play therapy is a legitimate approach to a therapeutic intervention that is most frequently applied to working with children. This modality has been carefully constructed, and consideration has been taken for developmental needs of the client or patient (Landreth, 2002). Play therapy has been found to be effective in decreasing anxiety and behavioral problems while increasing self concept and social skills (Ray, 2007; Bratton & Ray, 2000).

Infants, preschool-aged children, school aged children and adolescents show signs of being exposed to domestic violence situations (Stiles, 2002). Children demonstrate the impact of witnessing domestic violence in various ways, depending on their age and development. Infants may show signs of attachment difficulties and cry excessively when exposed to domestic violence (Stiles, 2002). Preschool aged children may show psychosomatic symptoms and display regressive behaviors. School aged children may have a range of ways they demonstrate the impact of domestic violence by such issues as psychosomatic complaints, problems in school, have guilt, and have difficulty with friendships (Stiles, 2002). Adolescents can have interpersonal problems, fatalistic views of the future, risk taking behaviors, and antisocial behaviors (Stiles, 2002). The variations of ways children show the effects of being exposed to domestic violence at various levels of development indicate that there is a need to find appropriate ways to help intervene and provide therapeutic relief that is developmentally suitable for these age categories. Play therapy is one option for finding the most fitting way of intervening at each level of a child's life.

Play therapy offers a viable option for therapists treating children that do not respond well to therapeutic modalities that rely on verbalization (Leblanc & Richie, 2001). It can also be used at some of the most difficult situations, such as when a child is in the process of dying (Glazer & Landreth, 1993). Creative modalities of treatment are also beneficial in allowing children to express their grief over the loss of a loved one (Glazer & Marcum, 2003).

The therapeutic relationship with the child client is very important to the play therapy experience. Central to the therapy is the connection between the therapist and the child (Allan & Brown, 1993; Ray, 2007). In research conducted by Carroll (2002), children were thankful for the items provided by therapists for them to utilize in play therapy. The attention given by the therapist and the opportunity for children to express themselves is quite important.

Theoretical Applications of Play Therapy

There are multiple approaches to play therapy. They are based in therapeutic theoretical perspectives. Child-centered play therapy is one of the most common approaches to play therapy (Gladding, 1996; Peery, 2002). However, other theoretical perspectives have also adapted therapeutic interventions to use with children in a play context. This format prohibits an examination of all theoretical applications of play therapy; however, a few of the more common will be included in this chapter. It is difficult to do justice to the theoretical perspectives in limited space, and it is recommended that readers take advantage of the plethora of articles and books focusing on the theoretical perspectives of interest.

Psychoanalytic theory has been applied to play therapy. As noted earlier in this chapter, Freud is credited with developing some of the early conceptualizations of how play can be therapeutic (Leblanc & Richie, 2001; Saracho & Spodek, 1995). Freud believed that children utilize play as their means of catharsis. Psychoanalysts believe that children can use play as a way to act out situations that have occurred in their lives and learn ways to cope. These theorists believe that when children have been exposed to painful events, they can master their distress by coming to terms with them in play (Saracho & Spodek, 1995, p. 139).

Jungian and post-Jungian therapists believe that children experience a "struggle of opposites" (Allan & Brown, 1993, p. 31). This belief is that the child has an internal world of "drives, desires, and impulses" and an outer world of family, school mates, and other relationships (Allan & Brown, 1993, p.31). A positive therapeutic relationship is central to the Jungian theory and the therapist will simply witness or become involved in play at the request of the child. Throughout the session, the therapist watches and is prepared to articulate the psychological struggles the child demonstrates through play. Interpretations are shared with the child only if the therapist believes the observations will increase the child's understanding.

There are cognitive theories of development. Jean Piaget and Lev S. Vygotsky have contributed to this theoretical area (Saracho & Spodek, 1995). Piaget believed that young children in the earlier stages of development use play to explore objects and learns ways to use them. The next stage of development, age 18 months to about 7 years of age, allows children to pretend or use play in symbolic ways. Older children begin to play games that require learning social conventions and interactions. They use games that require more cognitive development and require rules and usually other people to play (Saracho & Spodek, 1995).

Adlerian play therapy is another common treatment option. Alfred Adler believed that a natural way for child expression was through play, and hypothesis about behavior could be confirmed through observation of the child's play (Yura & Galassi, 1974, p.195). Therapists using this approach monitor or "track" the child's movements and activities and communicate their observations to the child to help the child gain awareness and to aid in communication of feelings (Kottman & Johnson, 1993). The therapist also helps the child recognize the emotion represented by their activities which can help foster deeper understanding by the child of feelings. An important aspect of the Adlerian approach is for the therapist to build relationships through encouragement, and to set limits to help prevent destructive behaviors (Kottman & Johnson, 1993, p.43; Kottman & Warlick, 1989).

Child-centered play therapy is an approach based on Carl Roger's person-centered theory (Ray, 2007; Rogers, 1942). As previously noted, this is one of the most commonly used theoretical perspectives of play therapy, which is supported by a survey of Association of Play Therapy members who identified as child-centered practicing therapists (Ray, 2007; Ryan, Gormory, & Lacasse, 2002). This concept of non-directive therapy, developed by Virginia Axline, a student of Rogers, allows children to express their experiences, relationships, and perceptions while the trained therapist observes and interprets (Axline, 1947; Landreth, 1993; Ray, 2007).

Axline (1947; Brooke, 2006) provided principles essential to the non-directive approach used in child-centered play therapy. The first area Axline (1947) focused on involved the therapeutic environment. She believed children need a safe and friendly environment in which to develop a rapport with their therapist. In addition to an environment conducive to rapport building, she encouraged therapists to have genuine interest and unconditional acceptance of their child client. In order for the therapist to be non-directive, the therapist must trust that the child has the capacity to be responsible and be capable of solving problems. The gradual and non-rushed approach that Axline encouraged meant that limits are set in the therapeutic session only for the purposes of the child developing personal responsibility and for relationships (Axline, 1947, pp. 73-74; Brooke, 2006, p. 66).

Play Therapy Applications in Domestic Violence Context

It is important to recognize that there are multiple ways that domestic violence situations may impact children. Children may face the loss of a parent or caregiver as a result of a domestic violence situation (Huth-Bocks, Schettini, & Shebroe, 2001). This loss may be the result of numerous reasons such as arrest, hospitalization, or through death of a parent or caregiver as a result of domestic violence. Some children may even be witness to the death of a parent at the hands of another parent (Osofsky, Cohen, & Drell, 1995). Lehmann (1997) indicates that Post Traumatic Stress Disorder (PTSD) is a potential outcome for children who witness domestic violence incidents. PTSD basically produces symptoms in three areas such as re-experiencing the event through flashbacks and nightmares; avoidance of situations, people, or locations which remind them of the traumatic experience; and through hyper-arousal, manifested through sleep disturbances and hyper-vigilant behaviors (APA, 2000; Lehmann, 1997, p. 242).

Play therapy has grown as an acceptable way to treat issues related to abuse, mal-adaption, and for developmental issues in children (Kot, 1995; Leblanc & Richie, 2001). Even in such horrific circumstances and environments as concentration camps during the Holocaust, it was observed that play and art were important ways for children to adapt to loss and traumatic circumstances (Glazer, 1999). Play therapy is a particularly good treatment option for children exposed to domestic violence for several reasons. A child participating in this type of therapy can be protected through the safety of toys and a play environment to express situations that were quite scary or dangerous in real life (Griffith, 1997; Landreth, 2002). Children who may be inhibited about speaking about their exposure to a traumatic or stressful situation can feel safety to express themselves in a therapeutic play setting (Cochran, 1996).

Play therapy is also particularly well-suited for working with children exposed to domestic violence because it can be practiced in a variety of settings. Venues such as schools and domestic violence shelters are potential locations where areas can be set-up for therapeutic interactions (Barabash, 2003; Yih-Jiun & Sink, 2002). There are many options for stocking a room designated for play therapy interactions (Guerney, 2001; Landreth, 1993; Kottman, 1995). Generally, it is suggested that the room designated for play therapy be safe for children and be stocked with toys that can represent a variety of people and objects. It is important to recognize that aggression and other emotions may be expressed in the room with the toys, so care should be taken in selecting items for use in this therapeutic setting.

In Kot's (1995) research, she found evidence that self-concept improved, behavior problems were reduced, when intensive play therapy was utilized with children who had witnessed domestic violence situations. Intensive play therapy in this context relates to the number of sessions in a short time period. In Kot's experiment, children were given twelve therapeutic sessions in a two-week time period. Kot found that intensive play therapy was a good match for children who were exposed to inter-parental violence and who had unstable lives due to the short time duration of the treatments (p. 76).

Utilizing parents in therapeutic interactions with children can be effective in assisting with children's issues (Leblanc & Ritchie, 2001). In filial therapy, parents receive training and supervision from professionals in therapeutic interactions with their children (Leblanc & Ritchie, 2001). Bernard and Louise Guerney are credited with advancing the use of filial therapy in the 1960's as a way to train parents in therapeutic play with their children (Bratton, Ray, Rhine, & Jones, 2005). Garry Landreth built upon the work of the Guerneys and developed a structured, supervised protocol for training parents in the role of therapeutic play (Bratton, Ray, Rhine, & Jones, 2005; Landreth, 1993, 2002). Poole (2006) reported that in her study, play therapy was incorporated into a family therapy context where the non-battering parent and children presented Post Traumatic Stress Disorder (PTSD) symptoms at the onset of the study. After treatment utilizing play therapy techniques in the family context, non-battering parents, and children reported reductions in PTSD symptoms.

Filial therapy has been applied following domestic violence situations with custodial grandparents participating in the process (Bratton, Ray, & Moffit, 1998). It stands to reason that after a domestic violence situation, grandparents may have custody of children exposed to the violence. Grandparents, in these cases, would be potential candidates for participating in filial therapy with the children.

Legal and Ethical Issues

As with any therapeutic method, practitioners of play therapy must understand and recognize their legal and ethical obligations (and the distinction between them) to maintain the necessary standards for care and competence, to protect the public, and to avoid becoming the subject of an investigation, complaint, or lawsuit. Discussion of these topics is not meant to dampen the enthusiasm of those who wish to practice creative modalities like play therapy, but more to insure practitioners engaged in this important therapeutic approach remain sensitive to their responsibilities and potential liability.

Mental health professionals, regardless of their specialty, are presumed to realize and comprehend issues related to confidentiality, use and forms of releases, the effect of claiming privilege in an forensic proceeding and who may do so, recordkeeping and documentation (including taping of sessions), record retention requirements, dual relationships, the limitations that may arise when an existing counselor is asked to become an expert witness on behalf of a client, and situations requiring referral to another professional. To maintain the integrity of the profession and specialty, play therapists should have authoritative resources on these subjects available for quick reference and review, particularly references related specifically to this modality (Blau, 1998; Sweeney, 2001).

Additionally, voluntary Play Therapy Practice Guidelines are now promulgated by the Association for Play Therapy (Association for Play Therapy, 2007). These guidelines include references to and have drawn upon the ethical guidelines of many other professional boards and associations. Jackson (1998) has outlined compatibility of the ethical guidelines of the American Psychology Association (APA, 2007) and play therapy practice. However, there appears to be great variation among play therapists about issues such as discussion of fees, theoretical orientation, goals for treatment, confidentiality, and the child's need for treatment (Jackson, Putty, & Lazicki-Puddy, 2001 – Ethical practices reported by play therapists: an outcome study). Guidelines may be enforced by the issuing board or association and adherence required for credentialing or membership, but these are not necessarily statutory obligations unless compliance is mandated by laws and regulations governing the profession. Nevertheless, the wise play therapist will give both ethical and legal obligations substantial weight in daily decision-making and practice.

Becoming "registered" in play therapy may offer the practitioner an added measure of credibility, both to clients served and other professionals who may evaluate the work of the therapist or seek to refer others. APT's Registered Play Therapists and Registered Play Therapists-Supervisors are licensed or certified practitioners who have earned a Master's degree or higher mental health degree, 150 or more hours of specialized play therapy training, substantial clinical and play therapy experience and supervision, and at least 36 hours of continuing education during subsequent three-year renewal cycles (Association for Play Therapy, 2007). The APT website also includes a "Paper on Touch" discussing clinical, professional and ethical issues as further guidance for play therapists (Association for Play Therapy, 2007).

Additionally, the APT contracts with the American Psychological Association (APA) to market, technically edit, publish and distribute its semi-annual, peer-reviewed *International Journal of Play Therapy*. The APA website describes this journal as "dedicated to publishing and disseminating reports of original research, theoretical articles, and substantive reviews of topics germane to play therapy on behalf of psychologists, psychiatrists, social workers, counselors, school counselors, marriage and family therapists, and other mental health professionals" (American Psychological Association, 2007). Those who intend to practice in play therapy are encouraged to review this journal in detail for further skill development and to remain current on issues relevant to this modality.

Play therapy as an intervention for witnesses to or survivors of domestic violence frequently leads to forensic involvement, whether anticipated or not. A basic review of literature published for legal professionals reflects the risk for anyone who attempts to practice play therapy without the appropriate expertise and understanding of the forensic and ethical implications. More than a few attorneys and judges, and even some mental health professionals, may characterize the play therapist's methods as unsubstantiated and lacking credibility (Underwager & Wakefield, 1995; Westfall, 2003). Whether or not this assertion is accurate is less important than the fact that it is a common strategy used by legal professionals attempting to discredit play therapists as fact or expert witnesses.

Therefore, practitioners of play therapy must ensure that methods used, environment, and equipment are proven to be reliable and appropriate for the child and the circumstances. Those who operate without proper understanding of the complexities of play therapy ultimately may risk license suspension or revocation, as one forensic psychologist in New Jersey found after being charged in a state disciplinary complaint of questioning a child in a suggestive, coercive, and/or manipulative manner during a play therapy session (Gallaher, 2007).

Since domestic violence allegations frequently arise in divorce and custody litigation, the play therapy practitioner should anticipate at the outset of treatment the possibility of being called to court, at least, as a fact witness. If the play therapist is qualified for and chooses to accept the more daunting role of "expert witness" in these cases, becoming well-informed of the obligations and expectations of those who will engage you for this purpose is essential (Blau, 1998). Even if the informed consent signed by a parent appears to clarify the practitioner's unwillingness to become involved in litigation, once treatment begins, the mental health professional may be subpoenaed to disclose information gained in play therapy sessions. Helpful resources also are available for practitioners in the United Kingdom (Bond & Sandhu, 2006).

It may be to the practitioner's advantage to establish a relationship, before an emergency need arises, with an attorney experienced in issues relevant to the mental health professional, including subpoena compliance and disclosure limitations and obligations. The attorney should be well-versed in the many laws and administrative regulations governing the therapist's specific profession and how case law has interpreted those laws and regulations. While the practitioner is always responsible for remaining current regarding laws and rules, trying to understand and accurately interpret their meaning in a particular situation may be best left to a competent and experienced attorney.

Competence and Cultural Awareness

Ethical guidelines relevant to mental health practitioners require, at a minimum, sufficient competence to practice generally and in the specialty for which a particular set of guidelines has been developed. Inasmuch as play therapy is practiced with children, it typically falls within the context of family therapy. However, Raimondi and Waters (2004) found low competence levels reported by both program directors and family therapists in the areas of knowledge of individual and family play therapy techniques and in the history of such techniques. Until very recently, few counselor education programs offered specific training or a specialty in counseling with children (Hollis, 1997). Even fewer offer concentrated courses in Play Therapy, leaving the practitioner interested in play therapy to look to outside resources for training necessary required to meet appropriate levels of competence. Child-centered play therapy training increased graduate students' play therapy knowledge and confidence in applying play therapy skills (Kao & Landreth, 1997). Understanding the conceptual framework, creating a welcoming environment, knowing the essentials of play therapy, and providing the minimal requirements for a play therapy session are all important elements of competence (Landreth, Baggerly, & Tyndall-Lind, 1999).

Equally important as an element of competence for play therapists is an understanding of and accommodation for cultural diversity (O'Connor, 2005; Hinman, 2003). According to one literature review, children from ethnically and culturally diverse backgrounds (including Aboriginal groups), those with lesbian, gay, or bisexual parents, and those who come from other minority groups will likely have different issues than children from the dominant culture as related to intimate partner violence (Agar, 2004). With the increasing growth of the Mexican-American population, mental health services, including play therapy, must become more culturally responsive (Flores-Torres, Kranz, Lund, & Ramirez, 2005; Martinez & Valdez, 1992; McCabe, Yeh, Garland, Lau, & Chavez, 2005). In working with Mexican-American children, it is critical for therapists to be sensitive to the cultural nuances that can be part of their play (Garza & Bratton, 2005). Some Asian cultures place a high value on privacy of family matters and may not understand Anglo-American institutions and systems (Preisser, 1999). Baggerly and Parker (2005) describe how child-centered 2-person group play therapy sessions with African American elementary school boys can honor the African worldview and facilitate self-confidence. Play and art therapies have been described as effective with children reluctant to talk due to perceived cultural differences (Cochran, 1996). Play therapists may find helpful O'Connor's (2005) discussion and expansion of Pedersen's (1988) Awareness, Skills and Knowledge model of cultural competence to include general competencies designed to enhance play therapy practice. A play therapist must be sensitive to the ways in which play behavior is understood, valued and shaped in the child's culture (Hinman, 2003; Roopnarine & Johnson, 1994). For example, cultural differences between Korean-American and Anglo-American preschoolers have been observed in the thematic content and communicative strategies used to structure and maintain pretend play (Farver & Shin, 1997). Differences between Finnish and English children have been reported in the use of color in "emotionally characterized drawings," (Burkitt, Tala, & Low, 2007), the type that may well be seen in play therapy used to address domestic violence issues. However, it is important not to over-generalize a child's experience of his or her culture (Gibbs & Huang, 1998).

Conclusion

When considering how best to help children and adolescents exposed to the trauma of domestic violence, specialized approaches may be an important part of assessment and treatment. Play therapy, using developmentally appropriate techniques, may be one option to aid this vulnerable population in telling their stories and expressing their emotional experience. Particularly in cases of domestic violence, the therapist who chooses to use play therapy must be especially sensitive to legal and ethical issues, and to ensure that all practice activities reflect both general and cultural competence. By doing so, the good intentions and substantial efforts of those who practice in this field will also reflect the necessary level of professionalism and integrity

References

Agar, S. (2004, November). *Agar Lit Review 2004.* Retrieved October 27, 2007, from BC Institute Against Family Violence: http://www.bcifv.org/pubs/Agar_Lit_ Review_2004.pdf

Allan, J., & Brown, K. (1993). Jungian play therapy in elementary schools. *Elementary School Guidance and Counseling, 28,* 30-41.

American Psychiatric Association. (2000). *Diagnostic and Statistical Manual of Mental Disorders, DSM-IV-TR.* (4th ed.). American Psychiatric Press: Arlington, VA.

American Psychological Association. (2007). *APA Journals-International Journal of Play Therapy.* Retrieved October 23, 2007, from American Psychological Association: http://www.apa.org/journals/pla/

Association for Play Therapy. (2007). *Paper on Touch.* Retrieved October 24, 2007, from Association for Play Therapy: http://www.a4pt.org/download.cfm?ID= 9971

Association for Play Therapy. (2007). *RPT/S Guide & Application.* Retrieved October 23, 2007, from Association for Play Therapy: http://www.a4pt.org/ps.credentials.cfm?ID=1637

Association for Play Therapy. (2007). *Voluntary Play Therapy Practice Guidelines.* Retrieved October 23, 2007, from Association for Play Therapy: http://www.a4pt.org/download.cfm?ID=21458

Axline, V. M. (1947). *Play therapy.* New York: Ballantine Books.

Baggerly, J., & Parker, M. (2005). Child-centered group play therapy with African American boys at the elementary school level. *Journal of Counseling & Development, 83,* 387-396.

Barabash, K. J. (2003). *Developmental filial therapy: Process-outcome research on strengthening child-parent relationships through play in a setting for victims of domestic violence.* Ph.D. Dissertation, University of Victoria, Canada.

Blau, T. H. (1998). *The psychologist as expert witness.* New York: John Wiley & Sons, Inc.

Bond, T., & Sandhu, A. (2006). *Therapists in Court.* London: Sage Publications and BACP.

Bratton, S. & Ray, D. (2000). What the researchs shows about play therapy. *International Journal of Play Therapy, 9,* 47-88.

Bratton, S., Ray, D., & Moffit, K. (1998). Filial/Family play therapy: An intervention for custodial grandparents and their grandchildren. *Educational Gerontology, 24,* 391-406.

Bratton, S. C., Ray, O., Rhine, T., & Jones, L. (2005). The efficecy of play therapy with children: A meta-analytic review of treatment outcomes. *Professional Psychology: Research and Practice, 36* (4), 376-390.

Brooke, S. L. (Ed.). (2006). *Creative arts therapies manual: A guide to the history, theoretical approaches, assessment, and work with special populations of art, play, dance, music, drama, and poetry therapies.* Springfield, IL: Charles C Thomas, Publisher, Ltd.

Burkitt, E., Tala, K., & Low, J. (2007). Finnish and Engllish children's color use to depict affectively characterized figures. *International Journal of Behavioral Development, 31*(1), 59-64.

Carroll, J. (2002). Play therapy: the children's views. *Child and Family Social Work, 7*, 177-187.

Cochran, J. (1996). Using play and art therapy to help culturally diverse students overcome barriers to school success. *School Counselor, 43*(4), 287-299.

Farver, J. M., & Shin, Y. L. (1997). Social pretend play in Korean and Anglo-American preschoolers. *Child Development, 68*(3), 544-556.

Flores-Torres, L. L., Kranz, P. L., Lund, N. L., & Ramirez, S. Z. (2005). Using Axline's eight principles of play therapy with Mexican-American children. *Journal of Instructional Psychology, 32*(4), 329-337.

Gallaher, M. P. (2007). Stage alleges psychologist coached child on sex abuse in custody case. *New Jersey Law Journal 0028-5803*, NA.

Garza, Y., & Bratton, S. (2005). School-based child-centered play therapy with Hispanic children: Outcomes and cultural considerations. *Journal of Instructional Psychology, 14*(1), 51-79.

Gibbs, J. T., & Huang, L. N. (1998). *Children of color: Psychological interventions with culturally diverse youth.* San Francisco, CA: Jossey-Bass Publishers.

Gladding, S. (1996). *Counseling: A comprehensive profession.* (3rd ed.) Engelwood Cliffs, NJ: Prentice Hall.

Glazer, H. R. (1999). Children and play in the Holocaust: Frieda Dicers-Brandeis - Heroic Child therapist: *Journal of Humanistic Counseling, Education, & Development, 37*, 194-201.

Glazer, H. R. & Landreth, G. L. (1993). When a child is dying. *Educational Digest, 59*, 64-68.

Glazer, H. R. & Marcum, D. (2003). Expressing grief through storytelling. *Journal of Humanistic Counseling, Education & Development, 42*(2), 131-138.

Griffith, M. (1997). Empowering techniques of play therapy: A method for working with sexually abused children. *Journal of Mental Health Counseling, 19*, 130-143.

Guerney, L. (2001). Child-centered play therapy. *International Journal of Play Therapy, 10*, 13-31.

Hinman, C. (2003). Multicultural considerations in the delivery of play therapy services. *International Journal of Play Therapy, 12*(2), 107-122.

Hollis, J. W. (1997). *Counselor preparation: 1996-1998.* Muncie, IN: Accelerated Development.

Huth-Bocks, A., Schettini, A., & Shebroe, V. (2001). Group play therapy for preschoolers exposed to domestic violence. *Journal of Child and Adolescent Group Therapy, 11*(1), 19-34.

Jackson, Y. (1998). Applying APA ethical guidelines to individual play therapy with children. *International Journal of Play Therapy, 7*(2), 1-15.

Jackson, Y., Putty, R. W., & Lazicki-Puddy, T. A. (2001). Ethical practices reported by play therapists: An outcome study. *International Journal of Play Therapy, 10*(1), 31-51.

Kao, S. C., & Landreth, G. L. (1997). Evaluating the impact of child-centered play therapy training. *International Journal of Play Therapy, 6*(2), 1-20.

Kot, S.Y. (1995). *Intensive play therapy with child witnesses of domestic violence.* Ph.D. dissertation, University of North Texas, United States - Texas.

Kottman, T. (1999). Integrating the crucial Cs into Adlerian Play Therapy. *The Journal of Individual Psychology, 55*, 290-297.

Kottman, T., & Johnson, V. (1993). Adlerian Play Therapy: A tool for school counselors. *Elementary School Guidance & Counseling, 28*, 41-52.

Kottman, T., & Warlick, J. (1989). Adlerian play therapy: practical considerations. *Individual Psychology, 45*, 433-446.

Landreth, G. L. (2002). Time limit setting in the Play Therapy Relationship. *Professional Psychology: Research and Practice, 33*, 529-535.

Landreth, G. L. (1993). Child-centered play therapy. *Elementary School Guidance and Counseling, 28*, 17-30.

Landreth, G., Baggerly, J., & Tyndall-Lind, A. (1999). Beyond adapting adult counseling skills for use with chldren: the paradigm shift to child-centered play therapy. *The Journal of Individual Psychology, 55*(3), 272-287.

Lehmann, P. (1997). The development of Post Traumatic Stress Disorder (PTSD) in a sample of child witnesses to mother assault. *Journal of Family Violence, 12*, 241-257.

Leblanc, M., & Richie, M. (2001). A meta-analysis of play therapy outcomes. *Counseling Psychology Quarterly, 14*, 149-163.

Martinez, K. J., & Valdez, D. M. (1992). Cultural considerations in play therapy with Hispanic children. In L. A. Vargas & J. D. Koss-Chioino, *Working with culture* (pp. 85-102). San Francisco, CA: Jossey-Bass Inc.

McCabe, K., Yeh, M., Garland, A., Lau, A., & Chavez, G. (2005). The GANA program: Atailoring approach to adapting parent child interaction therapy for Mexican-Americans. *Education and Treatment of Children, 28*(2), 111-129.

O'Connor, K. (2005). Addressing diversity issues in play therapy. *Professional Psychology: Research and Practice, 36*(5), 566-573.

Osofsky, J., Cohen, G., & Drell, M. (1995). The effects of trauma on young children: A case study of 2-year-old twins. *The International Journal of Psychoanalysis, 76*, 595-607.

Pedersen, P. (1988). *A handbook for developing multicultural awareness.* Alexandria, VA: American Association for Counseling and Development.

Peery, J. (2002). Archetype and object: Primary deintegration and primary love in analytical play therapy with young children. *Journal of Analytical Psychology, 47*, 407-420.

Poole, J. S. (2006). *Reconstructive play-based psychoeducational family therapy: A study of effectiveness. Families exposed to domestic violence.* Ph.D. dissertation, Capella University, United States – Minnesota.

Preisser, A. B. (1999). Domestic violence in South Asian communities in America. *Violence Against Women, 5*(6), 684-699.

Raimondi, N., & Walters, C. (2004). Training family therapists to work with children: Competence, relevance, and interest ratings in the field of family therapy. *The American Journal of Family Therapy, 32*, 225-237.

Ramirez, S. Z., Flores-Tores, L. L., Kranz, P. L., & Lund, N. L. (2005). Using Axline's eight principles of play therapy with Mexican-American children. *Journal of Instructional Psychology, 32*(4), 329-337.

Ray, D. C. (2007). Two counseling interventions to reduce teacher-child relationship stress. *Professional School Counseling, 10*, 428-440.

Rogers, C. (1942). *Counseling and psychotherapy.* Boston: Houghton Mifflin.

Roopnarine, J. L., & Johnson, J. E. (1994). The need to look at play in diverse cultural settings. In J. L. Roopnarine, J. E. Johnson, & F. H. Hooper, *Children's play in diverse cultures* (pp. 1-7). Albany, NY: State University of New York Press

Ryan, S. D., Gomory, T., & Lacasse, J.R. (2002). Who are we? Examining the results of the Association of Play Therapy membership survey. *International Association of Play Therapy, 11*, 11-42.

Saracho, O., & Spodek, B. (1995). Children's play and early childhood education: Insights from history and theory. *Journal of Education, 177*, 129-148.

Schaefer, C. (2003). *Foundations of Play Therapy.* Hoboken, NJ: John Wiley & Sons, Inc.

Stiles, M. M. (2002). Witnessing domestic violence: The effect on children. *American Family Physician, 66*(11), 2052-2066.

Sweeney, D. (2001). Legal and ethical issues in play therapy. In G. Landreth, *Innovations in Play Therapy* (pp. 65-74). New York: Brunner-Routledge.

Underwager, R., & Wakefield, H. (1995). Psychological evaluations you need for trial: What they can and cannot do. *Issues in Child Abuse Accusations, 7*(1), 30-52.

Westfall, G. (2003). *Opinion and Expert Testimony (Texas Rules of Evidence-Title VII)*. Retrieved October 23, 2007, from www.gregwestfall.com: http://www.gregwestfall.com/pdf%20files/opinion%20and%20expert%20testimony.pdf

Yih-Jiun, S. & Sink, C. A. (2002). Helping elementary age children cope with disasters. *Professional School Counseling, 5,* 322-331.

Yura, M. T., & Galassi, M. D. (1974). Adlerian usage of play therapy. *Journal of Individual Psychology, 30,* 194-201.

Biography

Joshua A. Thomas-Acker, MS, LMHC, LPC, NCC, CAP, is a counselor licensed in Florida and Illinois. He has experience in school settings, law enforcement settings, and emergency services settings. His clinical experience is in various environments including: private practice, consultation, training, an inpatient psychiatric setting, and working with children and adults in grief and trauma. Currently, he holds adjunct faculty positions with two institutions, and is living in Tampa, Florida.

Mary L. McGinnis, MA, LMHC, LMFT, NCC, CLA, is a counselor and marriage and family therapist in Florida. She is in private practice, working with children, adolescents, couples and families. She is designated as a Certified Legal Assistant through the National Association of Legal Assistants, with particular experience in the field of marital and family law. She is trained in mediation of family law issues and has been designated as a Parent Coordinator in high-conflict divorce and post-divorce cases. She has held an adjunct faculty position, teaching divorced couples about parenting issues, and lives in Tampa, Florida.

Chapter 7

BEYOND THE BRUISES: THE USE OF PLAY THERAPY WITH CHILDREN EXPOSED TO DOMESTIC VIOLENCE

Brian L. Bethel

Introduction

Tragically, we live in a violent world. Each day individuals are exposed to the media attention of terrorist events, war, and gang related violence. Unfortunately, these images of violence have become common fixtures in our daily routines. In addition to these horrific examples of violence, millions of children are also impacted by the experience of witnessing domestic violence. Although exact figures are unknown, studies have estimated between 3.3 million and 10 million children in the United States are exposed to domestic violence each year (Margolin, 1998).

Despite the numerous efforts to examine the treatment of interpersonal violence, it continues to be a commonly debated issue by mental health professionals. The stigma and complexity associated with domestic violence have only served to reinforce the debate among professionals. According to the American Psychological Association (APA), there is a great diversity regarding counseling strategies for survivors of domestic violence (APA, 2005). Consequently, domestic violence remains an enigma to those in the helping profession.

This chapter will offer an overview regarding the impact of domestic violence in the lives of children. In addition, a rationale for the use of play therapy in working with children exposed to domestic violence will be provided. Several case examples will illustrate the implementation of play therapy techniques in addressing the treatment goals for children exposed to domestic violence.

Domestic Violence

Although several terms have been used in attempting to explain the complexity of domestic violence, most researchers agree that several forms of abuse should be included in the definition (Berry, 2000). For most individuals, the term domestic violence generates thoughts and images of physical violence. However, as Wilson (2006) reported, abuse often encompasses less noticeable signs and frequently involves emotion and/or sexual abuse in combination with the use of physical violence. Similarly, Schecter and Edleson (1999) defined the term domestic violence as "a pattern of assaultive and/or coercive behaviors, including physical, sexual, and emotional abuse as well as economic coercion, that adults use against their intimate partners to gain power and control in that relationship" (p. 135).

Many professionals believe that society has continued to deny the issue of domestic violence and several commonly cited myths have reinforced this denial (Bancroft, 2004). Wilson (2006) reported several misconceptions regarding the issue of domestic violence. It is also believed that society's acceptance of these myths have aided the perpetrators in allowing the abuse to continue thereby taking some accountability away from persons who engage in violent acts against their intimate partners (Dallam & Silberg, 2006).

Regardless of the commonly cited myths, the incidences of domestic violence cannot be ignored. The Center for Disease Control has reported that domestic violence is a serious and preventable health issue that affects at least 32 million Americans annually (Tjaden & Thoennes 2000). Berry (2000) also reported that a woman is battered in the United States every seven seconds. The impact that domestic violence has on female survivors has been well documented for the last few decades (Berry 2000; Wilson, 2006). However, no one is immune from the effects of domestic violence.

As recently as 1999, professionals have cited the limitations in the literature regarding children's exposure to domestic violence (Findlater & Kelly, 1999). Despite the increased awareness over the last decade, it has only been in the last few years that research has begun to focus on the effects children exposed to domestic violence. The traditional response to the issue of domestic violence has focused on adult victims of abuse. Fortunately, over the last several years, more studies have examined the impact of domestic violence on children (Carlson, 2000).

It is important to note that a child's reaction to the exposure of domestic violence is very individualized. Professionals should be cautioned in the assessment process as the adverse effects will vary greatly from one child to the next. Studies have indicated that children may have no negative consequence to their exposure to domestic violence, while other children are not as resilient and exhibit significant signs of maladaptive adjustment (Carlson,

2000; Edleson, 1999). Studies have cited several factors that can increase a child's risk of negative symptoms when exposed to domestic violence. Specifically, children who encounter a greater frequency of exposure typically exhibit more distress (Edleson, 1999) Likewise, children with poor coping strategies also have an increased risk for negative responses. Age related differences have also been reported as a significant factor with younger children displaying higher levels of psychological and emotional difficulties (Wilson, 2006). The presence of additional family stressors such as mental illness and substance abuse have also been documented as factors that contribute to a greater risk of adverse reactions (Margolin, 1998).

The range of symptoms that children can develop as a result of witnessing domestic violence may also vary. Researchers have classified a child's response to domestic violence in several categories. These include behavioral, social and emotional issues, cognitive and academic issues, and long term problems such as trauma related symptoms and adult depression (Berry 2000; Carlson, 2000; Wilson, 2006). Not surprisingly, it has also been reported that a boy's response to domestic violence is more externalized through behaviors such as aggression and acting out. Conversely, female children respond to domestic violence through more internalized behaviors such as withdrawal, isolation, and depression (Carlson, 2000).

Children not only are challenged by the psychological effects of domestic violence but may also experience physical injury. Berry (2000) reported that 50 percent - 70 percent of men who abuse their female partner also abuse children in the home. Although batters and survivors frequently indicate that their children are unaware of the violence, Wilson (2006) stated that 80 percent - 90 percent of children from homes with domestic violence are able to give detailed accounts of the violent episodes. This may precipitate a child's response to protect their parent from the abuser. As Edelson (1999) suggested, these actions may place the child in a position of being directly injured or the child may sustain indirect injuries from the violent incident. The greatest tragedy is that it has been found that domestic violence is the single most precursor to a child's death in the United States (Mills et al., 2000).

Due to the diversity of children's reactions, the treatment interventions for children exposed to domestic violence can be challenging for mental health professionals. As Carlson (2000) indicated, not all children exposed to domestic violence will require therapeutic interventions. Professionals must be cautious in outlining treatment modalities for children who do require therapeutic interventions. As Silvern, Karyl, and Landis (1995) reported, children may require different forms of treatment as children will progress differently through the therapeutic process.

Although treatment must be individualized for the child, several therapeutic goals have been identified in the literature. In her publication, *Too Scared to Cry*, Lenore Terr (1990) indicated that the first goal of therapy after a traumatic event is allowing the child the opportunity for an open discussion of his or her experiences. Groves (1999) supported this hypothesis and stated that allowing children to integrate the traumatic experience into their world is a beneficial component of the therapeutic process. Peled and Edelson (1995) highlighted the importance of using the therapeutic relationship as an avenue for children exposed to domestic violence in expressing their emotions. Utilizing psychoeducational interventions and educating children on the cycle of violence have also been cited as an important therapeutic goal for children affected by domestic violence. Additionally, Groves (1999) emphasized the importance of educating parents on understanding the child's need for consistency in their lives. Finally, Pedel and Edelson (1995) recommended that interventions should encompass conflict resolution skills for children as well as safety planning.

Professionals have explored a variety of treatment modalities in addressing the therapeutic goals for children exposed to domestic violence. Wilson (2006) reported that both individual and group counseling are the most widely used treatment modalities for children affected by domestic violence. However, the most innovative therapeutic approaches for working with children impacted by domestic violence have been in the area of the expressive therapies. Malchiodi (1997) detailed the use of art therapy in working with children exposed to violence in their homes. Likewise, several professionals have documented the effective use of play therapy in treating children adversely affected by domestic violence (Smith & Landreth, 2003; Tyndall-Lind, Landreth, & Giordano, 2001; VanFleet, Lilly, & Kaduson, 1999).

Rationale for Play Therapy

Unlike traditional therapeutic models, play therapy does not require children to cognitively re-visit past traumatic events. Therefore, clinicians can use play therapy as an avenue for children to regain a sense of mastery and control over their environment without necessarily reliving the trauma that they have experienced (Kauson, Cangelosi, & Schaefer, 1997). This is particularly helpful when working with children traumatized by domestic violence. As Smith and Landreth (2003) note, children can be allowed to use play as a means of communicating and gaining control over their traumatic past.

Play therapy offers a unique approach for working with children and adolescents by offering individuals a non-threatening environment in which they can work to regain some sense of stability. With the specialization of play therapists and play therapy techniques, these theories have been popularly implemented over the last fifty years (Kauson et al., 1997). Similarly, Landreth, Homeyer, Glover, and Sweeney (1996) concluded that play therapy is an effective tool for counseling children with a variety of issues. Gil (1994) also stated that most child therapists agree that play therapy is the most effective medium for treating children.

The history of play therapy dates back to as early as 1920 (Gil, 1991). However, Virginia Axline is perhaps the most commonly recognized for the application of child-centered therapy techniques via play in her work with children (Axline, 1947). Child-centered therapy or nondirective therapy grew out of the work of Carl Rogers (1980). This model emphasized the philosophies of unconditional positive regard and being present with the child as foundations of this theory (Rogers, 1980).

Landreth (1991) expanded on Axline's (1947) work and identified the term child-centered play therapy using these same standards. Similar to the work of Rogers (1980), child-centered play therapy focuses on the relationship between the clinician and the child (Landreth, 1991). The use of child-centered play therapy when working with children exposed to domestic violence has also been documented in the play therapy literature (Kot, Landreth, & Giordono, 1998).

Conversely, directive play therapy techniques are typically best implemented to address specific therapeutic goals. Literature has suggested the implementation of directive play therapy techniques to assist children with a variety of issues. Specifically, VanFleet, Lilly, and Kaduson (1999) reported the use of play therapy techniques for individuals traumatized by the effect of domestic violence. The use of directive play therapy techniques may prove beneficial in assisting children in developing safety plans.

Filial play therapy is an additional intervention when working with children and families. Guerney (1964) first developed filial play therapy as a means of involving parents in the treatment of children with emotional and behavioral difficulties. Yet, this practice has been applied in treating a variety of issues. Smith and Landreth (2003) discussed the rationale for the use of filial play therapy with children who have witnessed domestic violence. VanFleet, Lilly, and Kaduson (1999) also documented the implementation of play therapy when working with family survivors of domestic violence.

Case Illustrations

The first case example will show how the use of sand-tray work can assist clinicians in normalizing feeling associated with a child's reactions to violence. Additionally, the case cited will offer an example of how safety plans can be developed from non-directive play therapy. The first case example involves a child who survived the physical and emotional abuse of his father as well as witnessing incidences of domestic violence.

Jason

Jason was an eleven years old when he presented with his mother for services at a community mental health center. During the diagnostic assessment, Jason's mother reported a history of domestic violence with Jason's father being physically and emotionally abusive to both herself and her son. Consequently, Jason and his mother left the home and moved in with relatives where they have remained for the prior six months. Jason's mother addressed a number of concerns during the initial assessment. These included some behavioral problems. Specifically, it was reported that Jason liked to order his mother around. A decline in Jason's academic performance was also reported. However, the most troubling issue for Jason's mother was his on-going ambivalence toward his father. Jason had expressed anger according to his mother but also expressed a sense of loyalty and at times stated he wanted to return home.

The child presented with stoic facial expression and remained silent throughout the initial assessment. He responded via negative body language to his mother's report but failed to respond to any questioning during the first session. The only statement that the child made during his hour and a half visit was;" I don't want to be here." At times the child would move his head from side to side but if questioned about his mother's statement he simply turned away from the clinician.

During our second session, I met with Jason alone and once again his defenses continued. Despite the child's initial opposition, I remained patient and provided him with a tour of the play room. Jason was particularly intrigued by the sand-tray and asked the purpose of using sand in therapy. I explained to Jason that children often times use the sand a miniatures to create their world. Jason asked if he could complete this activity.

Over the next thirty-five minutes, Jason worked on his sand-tray without stating a word. I simply reflected his actions in a non judgmental manner. The child was methodical in the placement of the miniatures in the sand and would re-arrange the miniatures until he was completely satisfied with his finished product. This was a strategic task as the child used a limited number of miniatures. His view of his world became a powerful analogy for therapy. Upon completion of the sand-tray Jason turned and asked; "Do you want me to tell you about my world?" Below is a picture of the sand-tray Jason completed in his second session.

I responded to Jason's question by welcoming him the opportunity to discuss his sand tray as long as he felt comfortable. Jason immediately provided me with a moving and telling account that the impact of domestic violence had in his life. He started by pointing to three miniature horses that he placed in the lower left-hand corner of the sand-tray. The child said; "This is

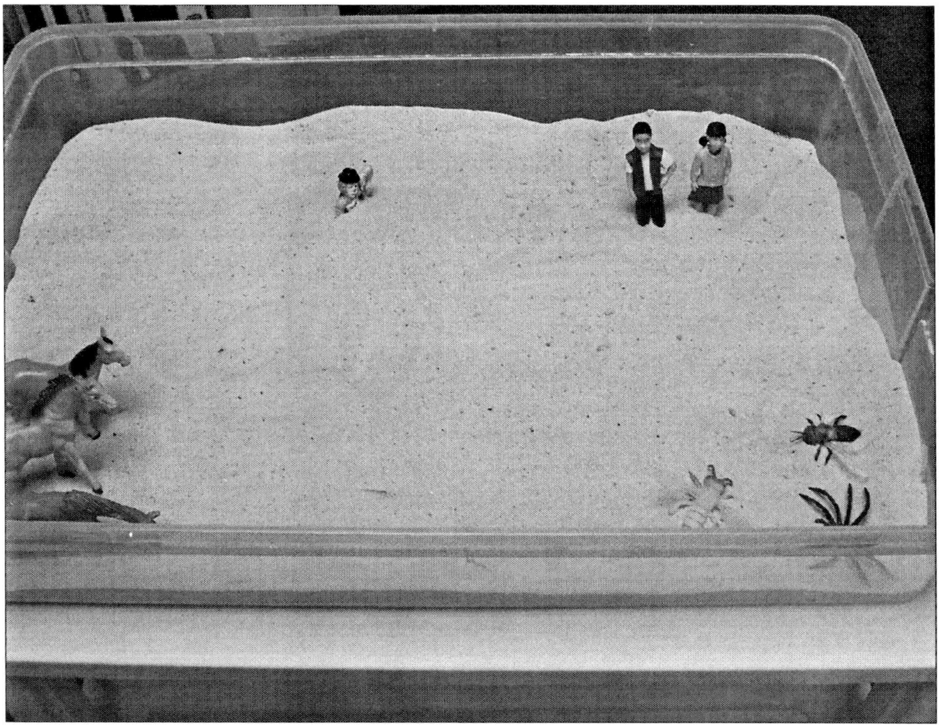

Figure 1. Jason.

me, my mom, and dad when we had happy times." Jason then moved to the lower right hand-corner of the sand-tray where he had placed two flies and a spider. Jason stated; "Sometimes my dad hits mom and me and is dangerous and we have to fly away." Pointing to the human miniatures Jason identified himself as the young boy who was accompanied by is mother. He said; "Mom and I left because my dad hurt us and we're trying to move on, but my dad doesn't realize what he did and he is stuck." The child then pointed to a miniature clown that he had buried in the sand away from the other miniatures.

This sand-tray was photographed and kept in Jason's client record. It became an integral part of therapy for the child as I would frequently refer to the photograph of his world. I used the sand-tray in attempting to normalize Jason's feelings associated with the violence in his home. It was also used as a psycho-educational technique in describing the cycle of violence. Most importantly the analogy of the flies and dangerous spider was used to discuss safety planning. This clinician asked Jason what the flies could do to keep themselves safe from the spider. Through the use of the miniatures this child was more open in discussing issues of violence. Jason's utilization of the miniatures assisted in discussing issues of violence. The use of this technique served to distance Jason from the personal effects of his exposure to domestic violence.

The second case example will offer specific techniques in assessing a child's view of his relationships with family members. The use of a play genogram (Gil, 1994) will be demonstrated. As indicated in the case example this technique can provide a variety of benefits for working with children confronting issues related to domestic violence. The second case example involves a child who also witnessed domestic violence.

Michael

Michael was a seven-year-old child when he was presented with his mother at the community mental health center for treatment. According to Michael's mother, he was physically abused by his father after attempting to intervene during an episode of domestic violence involving his parents. It was reported by Michael's mother that he had been aggressive with her since they moved to the local domestic violence shelter. The child's anger was apparent with his repeated interruption of his mother during the initial assessment.

The child also exhibited a strong need for control during his second appointment and was guarded in the therapy session. I implemented a non-directive play therapy approach based on client's defensive nature. The child used knights and army men creating a battle scene and was aggressive in his play. Michael discussed hitting and hurting the figures in the battle scene. I remained non-judgmental and reflected the child's actions and acknowledged feelings of hurt and anger that he displayed through the figures. I continued to use a non-directive therapy approach until Michael was less defensive.

It was during the fourth session that I implemented the play genogram technique. I assisted Michael in drawing a large genogram on poster board and labeled members of his family. The child was then instructed to choose a miniature that best represented the person listed for each of the diagrams in the genograms. Michael chose a small dog for himself, a baby for his infant sister, a goose for his mother, and an alligator with a snake on top for his father. The picture below will show Michael's play genogram.

Michael reported that his father was "dangerous" and that was the reasoning behind his choosing the alligator and the snake. It was important to note the positioning of the miniatures as the alligator appears to be facing the small dog which was representative of Michael. Similarly, the miniature the child selected for his mother, the goose, was turn away from the dog. The positioning of the miniatures was useful in generating discussion.

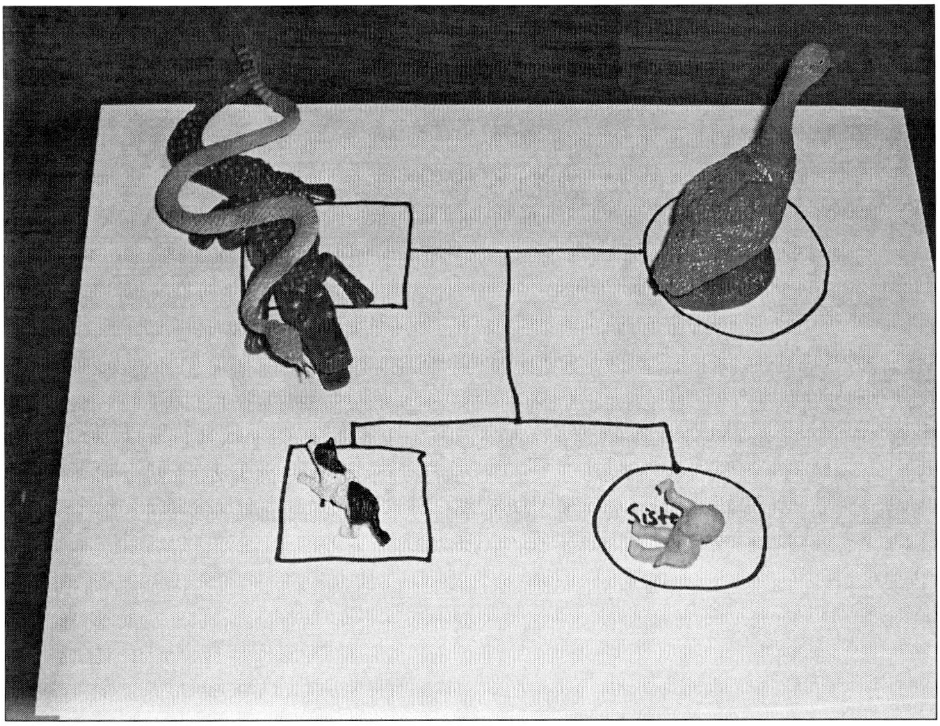

Figure 2. Michael.

Michael was asked what he would like the dog to say to the alligator. The child's response was one of anger and fear. Most telling was the dog's statements to the goose. The child reported that the dog would tell the goose that she had not kept him safe. The use of the play genogram and the child's statement precipitated the hypothesis that Michael was experiencing a great deal of anger direct towards his mother. This was consistent with the initial reports of the child's anger.

The play genogram was also photographed and kept as part of the child's record. The use of the miniatures provided the child an opportunity to gain some mastery over his feelings of anger and fear. Eventually, Michael's mother accompanied him in therapy sessions. The genogram was used to assist Michael and his mother in the development of future safety planning. The parent and child were directed to generate ideas and suggestions for keeping the dog safe. The pair was questioned on how each miniature would respond if faced with violence in the future.

The final example provided addresses the importance of prevention. As Wilson (2006) reported, educational efforts for children serve as the best preventative measure in protecting children and families. The following case examples will show how educational strategies can be implemented through the use of play therapy techniques. The puzzle technique was developed by this clinician for purposes of educating children on the dynamics of healthy and unhealthy relationships.

Two puzzles were created using cardboard and paint. One puzzle represented healthy relationships while the other was used to represent unhealthy relationships. Group members were shown each puzzle as a whole so the picture on each puzzle could be seen. The unhealthy puzzle was broken up into pieces and group members were timed in putting the pieces together. However, members could not take a puzzle piece until they wrote a characteristic of an unhealthy relationship. This same process was repeated using the healthy relationship puzzle. The pictures below are puzzles created for this procedure.

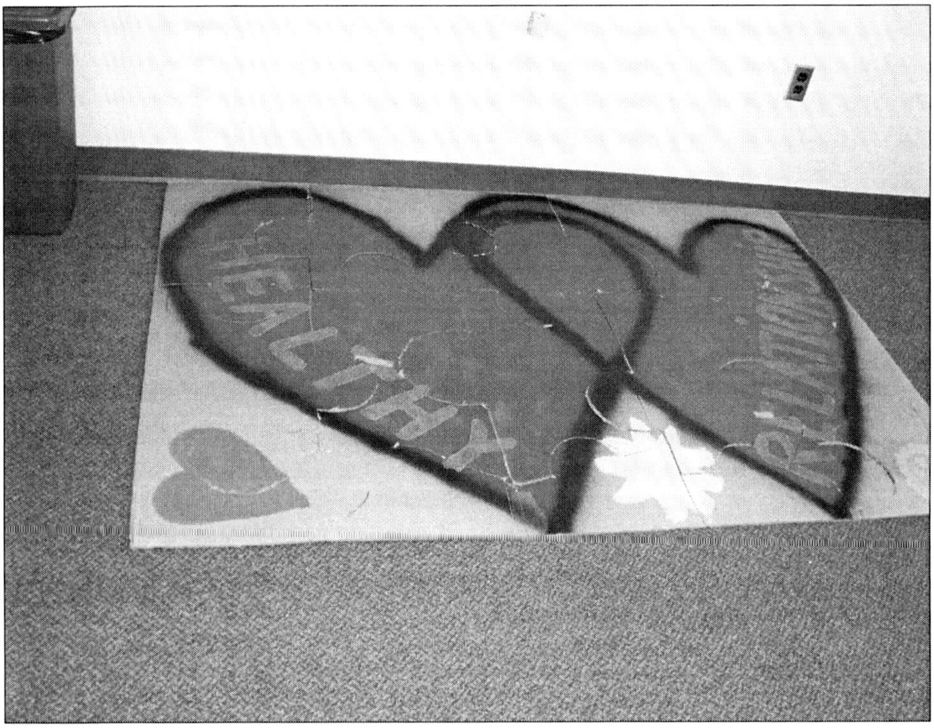

Figure 3. Michael's healthy relationship (see also Plate 9 in color).

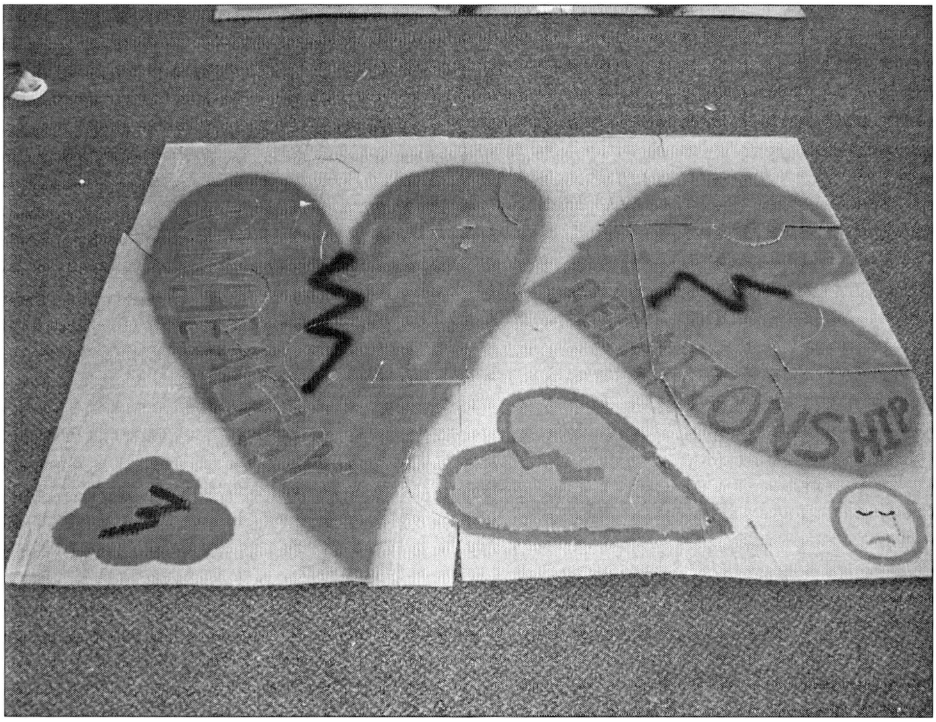

Figure 4. Michael's unhealthy relationship (see also Plate 10 in color).

In summary, counseling children can be extremely challenging. As Gil (1991) stated the work with children can be both very rewarding and yet, challenging. Children who are exposed to domestic violence often share their traumatic experiences and this can present countertransferences issues for clinicians. Therefore, clinicians should be strongly advised to establish appropriate boundaries and utilize appropriate self-care practices.

The treatment of children exposed to domestic violence is a complex and often challenging task. It is important that clinicians explore all available options when counseling this challenging population. Play therapy provides one modality for the treatment of children who have witnessed domestic violence. However, play therapy offers a variety of techniques to assist clinicians in the normalization of the traumatic experience as well as addressing specific symptoms that children may present. The use of play therapy provides children with unique opportunities to gain a sense of control and stability in their often violent and unpredictable worlds.

Domestic violence can have adverse effects on children. The above information offers clinicians examples of play therapy approaches in working with children exposed to domestic violence. Professionals who are dedicated to serving children have the opportunity to utilize play therapy in assisting child survivors of domestic violence in moving beyond the bruises.

Terms

Directive play therapy techniques: Techniques are typically best implemented to address specific therapeutic goals.
Domestic Violence: A pattern of assaultive and/or coercive behaviors, including physical, sexual, and emotional abuse as well as economic coercion, that adults use against their intimate partners to gain power and control in that relationship.
Filial play therapy: A therapeutic intervention that can help children by teaching parents (and other paraprofessionals such as teachers) basic child-centered play therapy principles and methods to use with their children.
Play Therapy: A developmentally sensitive therapeutic modality in which a trained play therapist uses the therapeutic powers of play to help clients prevent or resolve psychosocial difficulties and achieve optimal growth and development

References

APA Online. (2005). *Interesting careers in psychology.* Available at: http://www.apa.org/ science/nonacad_careers.html.

Axline, V. (1947). *Play therapy: The inner dynamics of childhood.* Cambridge, MA: Houghton Mifflin.

Bancroft, L. (2004). *When dad hurts mom. Helping your child heal the wounds of witnessing abuse.* New York: Berkley Books.

Berry, B. B. (2000). *The domestic violence sourcebook.* Los Angeles: Lowell House.

Carlson, B. E. (2000). Children exposed to intimate partner violence: Research findings and implications for intervention. *Trauma, Violence, Abuse, 1*(4), 321-340.

Dallam, S. J., & Silberg, J. L. (2006). Myths that place children at risk during custody disputes. *Sexual Abuse Report, 9*(3), 33-47.

Edelson, J. L. (1999). The overlap between child maltreatment and women battering. *Violence Against Women, 5*(2), 134-154.

Findlater, J., & Kelly, S. (1999). Michigan's domestic violence and child welfare collaboration. In J. L. Edleson & S. Schechter (Eds.), *In the best interests of women and children: Child welfare and domestic violence services working together* (pp. 167-174). Thousand Oaks, CA: Sage.

Gil, E. (1994). *Play in family therapy.* New York: Guilford Press

Gil, E. (1991). *The healing power of play.* New York: Guilford Press.

Groves, B. M. (1999). Mental health services for children who witness domestic violence. *The Future of Children, 9*(3), 122-132.

Guerney, B. (1964). Filial therapy: Description and rationale. *Journal of Consulting Psychology, 20,* 304-310.

Kauson, H. G., Cangelosi, D., & Schaefer, C. E. (1997). *The playing cure.* Northvale, NJ: Jason Aronson, Inc.

Kot, S., Landreth, G. L., & Giordano, M. A. (1998). Intensive Child-Centered Play Therapy with Child Witnesses of Domestic Violence. *International Journal of Play Therapy* 7(2), 17-36.

Landreth, G. L. (1991). *Play therapy: The art of the relationship.* Muncie, IN: Accelerated Development, Inc.

Landreth, G. L., Homeyer, L. E., Glover, G., & Sweeney, D. S. (1996). *Play therapy interventions with children's problems.* Northvale, NJ: Jason Aronson, Inc.

Malchiodi, C. A. (1997). *Breaking the silence: Art therapy with children from violent homes.* (2nd. Ed., rev. & exp.) Bristol, PA.

Margolin, G. (1998). Effects of domestic violence on children. In P. K. Trickett & C. J. Shellenbach (Eds.) *Violent children in the family and in the community,* Washington, D.C.: APA Books.

Mills, L. G., Friend, C., Conroy, K., Fleck-Henderson, A., Krug, S., & Magen, R. H. (2000). Child protection and domestic violence: Training, practice and policy issues. *Children and Youth Services Review, 22*(5), 315-332.

Peled, E., & Davis, D. (1995). *Groupwork with Children of Battered Women: A Practitioner's Manual.* Thousand Oaks, CA: Sage.

Peled, E., Jaffe, P. G., & Edleson, J. L. (Eds.). (1995). *Ending the cycle of violence: Community responses to children of battered women.* Newbury Park, CA: Sage.

Rogers, C. L. (1980). *On becoming a person.* Boston, MA: Houghton Mifflin.

Schechter, S. & Edelson, J. L. (1999). *Effective intervention in domestic violence and child maltreatment case: Guidelines for policy and practice.* National Council of Juvenile and Family Court Judges.

Silvern, L., Karyl, J., & Landis, T. Y. (1995). Individual psychotherapy for the traumatized children of abused women. In E. Peled, P. G. Jaffe, & J. L. Edleson (Eds.), *Ending the cycle of violence: Community responses to children of battered women.* Thousand Oaks, CA: Sage Publications, pp. 43-76.

Smith, N., & Landreth, G. L. (2003). Intensive filial play therapy with child witnesses of domestic violence. *International Journal of Play Therapy, 12*(1), 67-88.

Terr, L. (1990). *Too scared to cry.* New York: Harper and Row.

Tjaden, P., & Thoennes, N. (2000). *Full report of the prevalence, incidence, and consequences of violence against women: Findings from the national violence against women survey.* Washington, DC: U. S. Department of Justice, Office of Justice Programs, 2000. Available from: http://www.ncjrs.org/txtfiles1/nij/183781

Tyndall-Lind, A., Landreth, G. L., & Giordano, M.A. (2001). Intensive group play therapy with child witnesses of domestic violence. *International Journal of Play Therapy, 10*(1), 53-83.

VanFleet, R., Lilly, J. P., & Kaduson, H. (1999). Play therapy for children exposed to violence: Individual, family, and community interventions. *International Journal of Play Therapy, 8*(1), 27-42

Wilson, K. J. (2006). *When violence begins at home: A Comprehensive guide to understanding and ending domestic violence.* Alameda, CA: Hunter House Publishers.

Biography

Brian L. Bethel, M.Ed., PCC-S, LCDC III is the Outpatient Services Director for a community mental health center in south central Ohio. In addition to his supervisory role, Brian specializes in the therapeutic treatment of children, adolescents, and families. He is a Licensed Professional

Counselor with Supervisory Endorsement (PCC-S) and a Licensed Chemical Dependency Counselor (LCDC) with the state of Ohio. Brian earned dual masters degrees in clinical counseling and rehabilitation counseling from Ohio University. Brian also serves as an independent trainer consultant with The Ohio Child Welfare Training Program. He has developed and facilitated professional trainings on a local, state and national level for individuals working with children. As a member of the Association for Play Therapy, Brian has published articles on the use of play therapy for children with a variety of mental, emotional, and behavioral challenges.

Chapter 8

GATHERING VOICES: MUSIC THERAPY FOR ABUSED WOMEN

Sandra L. Curtis

Introduction

While there has been an increasing public awareness of domestic violence, this issue has been relatively neglected within the music therapy profession. This chapter will examine the nature of violence against women in their lives and within their intimate relationships. The politics of naming and explaining the phenomenon will also be explored. In so doing, the connection will be made between this and all other types of male violence against women. The impact of this violence can be profound, both on the personal, and the societal level. The current scope of music therapy practice and its potential in this area will be outlined. There is a critical need for music therapists to have an understanding of the true nature of this violence and to ensure not only that music therapy is available, but also that it is genuinely responsive to the needs of women survivors. The chapter will conclude with a gathering of voices: The voices of music therapists speaking to the emergent trend of feminist music therapy for survivors of violence; and the voices of women empowered through this new approach.

Male Violence Against Women

It is increasingly acknowledged that, whether experienced directly or indirectly, violence forms a part of the very fabric of women's lives (Burstow, 1992; Curtis, 2006, 2000, 1994; Marshall & Vaillancourt, 1993). For those who experience it directly, the violence is serious, extensive, and harmful. For others, it is the threat of violence that impacts their lives. Yet "what about men?" is the frequent response to any work that focuses on violence against women. The answer to this question lies in the very nature of male violence against women and of the patriarchal culture that accepts and condones this violence. Women's experiences of violence differ dramatically from those of men. Women's experiences are more likely to be within their own homes, at the hands of their intimate partners, and with greater risk of sexual abuse (Statistics Canada, 2006). Men are more likely to experience violence in the public sphere at the hands of a stranger (Statistics Canada, 2006). Without a focus on women, dimensions of gender and power are neglected; the sociopolitical underpinning of male violence against women is overlooked. In acknowledging dimensions of gender and power, both a political definition and political solution are possible: "Gender-based violence is perhaps the most wide spread and socially tolerated of human rights violations. It both reflects and reinforces inequities between men and women and compromises the health, dignity, security and autonomy of its victims" (Statistics Canada, 2006, p. 8). In this light, the sociopolitical nature of male violence against women is identified. It is a violence directed at individual women that serves to control all. It is rooted in a culture of inequality that ignores, accepts, condones, and even promotes male violence against women (Curtis, 2007). As such, the solution must include not only zero tolerance of this violence, but also full equality for women (Curtis, 2000; Marshall & Vaillancourt, 1993; Statistics Canada, 2006).

Recognition of the sociopolitical nature of male violence against women also makes it possible to identify the connection between all types of this violence–from child abuse, sexual assault, and stalking, to abuse in intimate relationships. Previously, each type of violence was treated as a unique and unrelated phenomenon. With a sociopolitical understanding, the connection becomes clear. Furthermore, this understanding makes it possible to move from seeking individual solutions for individual problems to seeking political solutions for all (Curtis, 2007; Marshall & Vaillancourt, 1993; Worell & Remer, 2003).

Intimate Male Partner Violence

Having examined the sociopolitical underpinning of and connection between all types of male violence against women, this section will explore the specific experiences of women abused by their intimate male partners. Women's experiences of male violence differ depending on their own particular circumstances. Therefore, an examination of women's experiences of intimate male partner violence can only be done accurately while keeping in mind the diversity of women and of their lives. In looking at this phenomenon, attention must first be directed to the naming of it.

Violence against women within intimate relationships has a long and contentious history around its naming. The issue of naming is a powerful one. Naming reflects, determines, and perpetuates beliefs. Ultimately, it can acknowledge or deny existence. It was not until the 1970s that the term "battered wife" was coined. Until that time, it was a phenomenon with no name (Curtis, 2000; Worell & Remer, 2003; Yllö & Bograd, 1988). This reflects societal views of the time that this was a husband's prerogative, perhaps even duty, rather than abuse. The use of the term battered wife arose out of a struggle to identify this violence as unacceptable, serious, and problematic. This struggle, however, did not end there as a large number of terms subsequently emerged that served to alternately highlight or obscure the dimension of gender and the seriousness of the violence. Currently the term "domestic violence" is widely used. This term truly obscures the dimension of gender, contributing to the myth that men and women are equally violent in their relationships; in reality, 95% of the victims are women (Marshall & Vaillancourt, 1993; Yllö & Bograd, 1988). It also places the violence firmly within the family to the neglect of the sociopolitical underpinnings. The professionalization of the phenomenon with increased involvement of government and social service agencies further de-politicizes domestic violence. Grassroots battered women's shelters with a feminist focus on social change have metamorphosed into professional shelters geared towards achieving personal change (Curtis, 2000 & 1994; Yllö & Bograd, 1988). In the ongoing struggle to highlight the dimensions of gender and power and to include women in a diversity of relationships (e.g., married, divorced, co-habiting, etc.), "intimate male partner violence" is now being used. The term "intimate partner violence" is also being used (Teague, Hahna, & McKinney, 2006); however, this serves once again to mask gender. Subsequently, I adopt the term intimate male partner abuse. It should be noted that this chapter will not address the issue of violence against women within same sex relationships because the dimensions of gender and power in violence of this type differ dramatically in our patriarchal and homophobic culture.

The struggle to name and identify intimate male partner violence has been accompanied by a similar struggle to document its prevalence and severity. Because my music therapy practice has included work in the United States and Canada and because both countries share similarities in the area of violence against women, this chapter will examine the experiences of American and Canadian women. In both countries, there is an increasing awareness of the high incidence of intimate male partner violence. It is a serious and longstanding problem with profound negative impact on personal and societal levels. An examination of the impact has been hindered in the past by the undercounting of violence against women in studies that neglected gender. It continues to be hindered by underreporting of women because of the personal nature of the violence and for reasons of fear, shame, and failure of institutional response (Statistics Canada, 2006; U.S. Department of Justice, 2003). In Canada, one out of every two women reported experiencing male violence at some point in their lives (Marshall & Vaillancourt, 1993), with 52,127 women and 36,840 children admitted to battered women's shelters in 2004 and with the number of shelters increasing from 18 in 1975 to 543 in 2004. Yet, only 36% of women abused in their intimate relationships reported this abuse to the police (Statistics Canada, 2006).Of those women reporting intimate male partner violence, 50% feared for their lives and 40% indicated their children had been present. In the United States, there were 588,490 reports from women of nonfatal intimate male partner violence, with an additional 1,247 women killed by such violence in 2001 (U.S. Department of Justice, 2006). One in four American women reported experiencing intimate male partner violence (National Women's Health Information Center, 2003).The cost for women, children, and the community at large of such violence is incredibly high, with economic costs alone estimated in the billions of dollars (Statistics Canada, 2006; U.S. Department of Justice, 2006).

The high prevalence of intimate male partner violence and its profoundly negative impact raise questions about the underlying cause. This is not a matter of mere curiosity. An understanding of the root cause of this violence determines the solutions sought in eliminating the violence, in working with abused women, and in working with abusive men. Since the original naming of the problem in the 1970s by the women's movement, a slew of explanatory theories have been proposed. This chapter will limit its focus to those that have current strong support in public or in professional circles.

One of the explanatory models with the most long-standing popular appeal is the Medical Model (Curtis, 1994). This model defines intimate male partner violence as a personal problem in which a few individual men with psychological problems are unable to control their anger. Additionally, some supporters of this model identify a further problem of a few aberrant women who like abuse or are attracted to abusive men. With an explanatory model based on personal problems, the resultant solution is personal as well–assistance for abusive men to gain control of their anger and assistance for women in identifying and changing their pattern of selection of and attraction to abusive men. The medical model also informs the widely-held belief of the intergenerational cycle of violence–the belief that violence against women is experienced and then transmitted from generation to generation. Despite widespread support, research does not back up these explanatory models (Burstow, 1992; Curtis, 1994 & 2000; Worell & Remer, 2003). Abusive men are not out of control; they very carefully control and direct their anger at one person–their intimate female partner. Despite their abhorrent behavior, they are not mentally ill, nor are the women they abuse. Identifying the women as being at fault only serves to perpetuate the patriarchal tradition of woman blaming. While there is no doubt that growing up in violent homes has a profound impact on children–an impact that may stay with them throughout their lives–the intergenerational cycle theory does not account for those abused women and those abusive men who have had no previous experience of violence (Burstow, 1992; Curtis, 1994 & 2000; Worell & Remer, 2003).

One explanatory model with support in professional circles is the Battered Woman Syndrome (Curtis, 2000; Walker, 1984). The Battered Woman Syndrome identifies a cycle of violence that leads to the development of learned helplessness. While the Battered Woman Syndrome has been used effectively at times as a defense for women in the legal system, it poses some problems. It continues the tradition of blaming women for the abuse. As well, its description of a cycle of violence ignores the presence of control and non-physical violence throughout all phases of the relationship. Ultimately, abused women do not exhibit helplessness. Rather they seek actively to either leave their abusers or to handle the violence in the best way possible if their circumstances make leaving impossible. There are very real and significant barriers to leaving–social isolation, financial constraints, concern for their children, inadequate response from the legal, health, and social services agencies, and genuine fear–women are at greater risk of being murdered after they leave (Curtis, 2000; Marshall & Vaillancourt, 1993; Yllö & Bograd, 1988).

An explanatory theory gaining acceptance in professional circles and in the community at large is the Feminist Model. This model is reflected increasingly not only in the work of individuals, but also in the very definitions of violence against women by organizations committed to the elimination of such violence (Curtis, 2000 & 2007; Statistics Canada, 2006; United Nations, 1995). The Feminist Model identifies violence against women as rooted in the historical and ongoing inequality of power for women in a patriarchal culture, making it a societal problem rather than a personal one. The solution must consequently be one of social rather than personal change –although personal support for women survivors in recovering from the harm will also be needed. Control and gender are key factors underlying this violence. Intimate male partner violence is not a case of a few men out of control. Abusive men control and carefully direct their anger only toward their female partners. This use of violence is condoned and supported by our sociocultural structures. This violence of some men against women serves to control all (Burstow, 1992; Curtis 2007 & 2000; Worell & Remer, 1993).

This feminist model is reflected in a definition of intimate male partner violence as a "pattern of coercive control over women [by their intimate male partners] that uses diverse methods and leaves women questioning their self-worth and perception of reality" (Yllö & Bograd, 1988, p. 15). The methods or types of violence experienced by women in their intimate relationships and the effects of that violence will be the focus of the section that follows.

Women's Experiences of Intimate Male Partner Violence

In the efforts to document that violence against women exists, is harmful, and should be eliminated, there has sometimes been an over focus on physical violence. It is certainly easier to prove physical violence and to prove the harm of it. Abusers, however, use creative and varied types of violence, each with the purpose of asserting and maintaining control over their intimate partners. Indeed some of these other types are more powerful tools in this coercive control (Curtis, 2000; Burstow, 1992; Worell & Remer, 2003). The types of violence traditionally identified include: physical, verbal, sexual, psychological, and (more recently) systemic violence. Physical, verbal, and sexual violence are fairly self-evident. Psychological violence includes intimidation and threats–threats of violence to the woman, her pets, and her children. Physical violence to cherished possessions and pets (including the killing of pets) are frequent precursors to physical abuse of the woman herself. Systemic violence refers to the violence which results from the failure of the assorted legal, social services, and mental health agencies to meet abused women's needs. Traditionally these systems have depoliticized the issue, making it a family or childcare issue. They have trivialized and even legitimized violence against women. Going beyond failing to help, they have at times made the situation worse. A case in point being abused women who experience increased violence at home after their abusive intimate male partner returns from therapy focused on anger management and self-esteem enhancement (Curtis, 2000; Marshall & Vaillancourt, 1993).

Traditionally these different types of violence have been viewed as hierarchical, with physical and sexual violence being seen as more serious than the other types. The reality of women's experiences would argue differently. Each of these types of violence is harmful and interrelated. Underpinning these is another type of violence frequently overlooked–that is internalized violence. This is the cumulative effect of intimate male partner violence within a culture that devalues women and condones or trivializes their experiences of violence. This is harm to women's core self which causes them to doubt themselves. They come to believe the view of their abuser and society that blames women and excuses men for the violence (Curtis, 2000; Marshall & Vaillancourt, 1993).

In discussing the effects of intimate male partner violence, two important issues must be kept in mind: that these are the result–not the cause–of violence; and that women and their experiences are diverse. Women are not to be pathologized or blamed for the violence. Nor are they to be defined by it. More than strong survivors, they can be empowered women. The impact of violence and the time needed to heal and become empowered varies considerably from woman to woman. This is influenced by the nature of the violence, the availability of resources, personal coping strategies, number and age of children, and the presence of other oppressions (Statistics Canada, 2006; Worell & Remer, 2003). The physical results can include wounds, broken bones, insomnia, and, for some, death. The psychological results can include fear, shame, depression, and addictive coping strategies. Harm to self-esteem can represent one of the most profound and long-lasting effects (Curtis, 2000; Marshall & Vaillancourt, 1993; Statistics Canada, 2006; Worell & Remer, 2003).

Having examined the nature of intimate male partner violence and having seen the profound impact it can have, the next section shall explore the practice of music therapy, current and potential, with women survivors. What can music therapy offer these women and how can it be fashioned to best meet their needs, understand their experiences, and honor their strengths.

Music Therapy with Abused Women

Until recently, the area of violence against women has been relatively neglected by the music therapy profession. This is particularly true of intimate male partner violence. Just emerging now is an interest in the use of music therapy for survivors of violence and an understanding that they represent a growing client population. As a result, the professional literature on the issue is still fairly limited (Curtis, 2006; York, 2006).

The existing music therapy literature specific to intimate male partner violence includes a survey of the practice of music therapy in domestic violence (Cassity & Theobold, 1990). It also includes recent clinical work of music therapy in general (Curtis, 2000; Hernandez-Ruiz, 2003; Whipple & Lindsay, 1999), of Guided Imagery in Music (Rinker, 1991), and of music therapy combined with other creative arts (Teague, Hahna, & McKinney, 2006; York, 2006).

Complementing this literature is research in related areas. This includes a growing body of work in music therapy with children, adolescent, and adult survivors of childhood sexual abuse (Amir, 2004; Brooke, 2007; Clendenon-Wallen, 1991; Curtis, 2007; Curtis & Harrison, 2006; Hammel-Gormley,

1995; Lindberg, 1995; MacIntosh, 2003; Purdon, 2006; Rogers, 1993 & 1995). It also includes music therapy for abused women with specific mental health problems–eating disorders, Post Traumatic Stress Disorder, and depression (Brooke, 2008; Montello, 1999; Rogers, 1994; Ventre, 1994).

Whether addressing intimate male partner violence or some other type of violence against women, the findings of this music therapy literature clearly identify music therapy as a particularly effective intervention strategy (Curtis & Harrison, 2006). Women, who have long been silenced by violence, are able to make use of music's unique capacity to evoke imagery and examine metaphors to find their own true voices (Curtis & Harrison, 2006). Yet, the overwhelming majority of this research is uninformed by a feminist understanding of violence against women. Only four authors incorporate a feminist approach to music therapy based on the feminist understanding of violence against women as sociopolitical phenomenon (Curtis, 2007, 2006, & 2000; Curtis & Harrison, 2006; Purdon, 2006; York, 2006), and only two of those deal specifically with women survivors of intimate male partner violence (Curtis, 2006 & 2000; York, 2006). With the very recent publication of the seminal work, *"Feminist Perspectives in Music Therapy"* (Hadley, 2006), it is exciting to imagine how music therapy might radically transform to truly meet the needs of women survivors of intimate male partner violence.

Feminist Music Therapy with Abused Women

Just as feminism developed in the 1970s as a grassroots movement with no individual leader, so too did feminist therapy. Without any one leader, it was developed by individual therapists after having completed their professional education and training. Finding that their traditional training and approach did not prepare them to adequately meet the needs of their women clients, these individuals began to inform their practice with a feminist understanding of women's lives and experiences (Curtis, 2000; Worell & Remer, 2003). Feminist music therapy is developing similarly, although considerably later, as a grass roots movement (Curtis, 2007 & 2006; Purdon, 2006; York, 2006). Far removed from the traditional music therapy education and training schools, some music therapists are informing their practice with principles of feminism and feminist therapy practice. The recent publication of *Feminist Perspectives in Music Therapy* (Hadley, 2006) points to an emergent trend in music therapy rather than a matter of a few isolated instances. The work of the contributing authors in this book reflects a move beyond a feminist understanding of women to a genuine feminist practice in music therapy. The section which follows will outline the guiding principles, goals, and techniques that make this feminist music therapy unique and that make it uniquely qualified to meet the needs of women survivors of intimate male partner abuse.

In describing the specifics of feminist music therapy, I will turn to a unique approach first developed as part of my doctoral work and then continued as part of my ongoing clinical practice. This feminist music therapy was developed with the purpose of better meeting the needs of women in general; its effectiveness was researched, however, specifically with women survivors of intimate male partner violence (Curtis, 2000). Building on this, York (2006) described a feminist music therapy protocol which also incorporates other creative arts. My work later extended to include feminist music therapy with survivors of childhood sexual abuse (Curtis, 2007). Whether practiced with women survivors of intimate male partner violence, survivors of other violence, or a broader client population, the basic principles, goals, and techniques remain common to all.

Stemming directly out of the tenets of feminism, the guiding principles of feminist music therapy include: the personal is political; egalitarian relationships are desired; and women should be valued (Curtis, 2007 & 2000). More specifically, this means that the major source of women's difficulties is identified as sociopolitical, not personal, resulting from women's experiences of oppression in a culture characterized by institutionalized sexism. These experiences differ as a result of other simultaneous oppressions such as racism, classism, heterosexism, ageism, and ableism. Within feminist music therapy, traditional power relationships and gender roles are rejected. As a result, relationships are to be egalitarian including those of the client, as well as the client-therapist relationship and the personal relationships of the therapist. Women's issues are frequently dealt with in feminist music therapy, and women themselves, their perspectives, their values, and their experiences should be valued both within and outside of therapy.

From these principles of feminist music therapy, derive a number of unique goals (Curtis, 2000). These include: to empower women, increasing their independence and freeing them of gender-role stereotypes; to increase understanding of the sociopolitical context through feminist analysis of power and gender-role socialization; to accomplish necessary social change in light of this understanding; to enable women to value women and to develop relationships characterized by mutuality and equality; and to enable women to recover from the harm of oppression, and ultimately to achieve health and happiness as individually defined.

In feminist music therapy, a number of specific techniques exist to accomplish these goals. A fundamental technique which must be employed before and throughout the therapeutic process is that of demystification. While not unique to feminist music therapy, demystification is critical to its success. It involves an attitude on the part of the therapist as much as it involves action.

Through demystification, the therapist must ensure that the client understands and is an active participant in the therapeutic process–from setting goals and selecting interventions to decisions about outcomes and closure. With demystification in mind, the therapist can then direct attention to use of the other feminist music therapy techniques–feminist analysis of power and gender-role socialization; women's empowerment; and the valuing of women, including facilitation of self-nurturance (Curtis, 2000, 2007).

Feminist analysis of power, gender-role socialization, and the sociopolitical underpinnings of women's experiences is addressed through lyric analysis, songwriting, performance, and creation of music CDs (Curtis, 2000, 2007; York, 2006). Women's music can be a powerful tool in this analysis (Curtis, 2000; York, 2006). It can also provide a marvelous impetus for women survivors in finding their own voices, writing their own songs, and becoming empowered. This is an exciting time in the music industry with an incredible rich diversity of women's music available. Some of it explicitly challenges patriarchal norms; other music by women conforms to these norms but can be used equally well in the hands of a feminist music therapist to subvert the status quo.

Building on feminist analysis, feminist music therapists can work with their clients towards empowerment through a variety of music therapy experiences. One of the most powerful of these involves songwriting and recording by clients. A common experience of women abused by their intimate male partners is the sense of loss of voice. This is underscored by a sociopolitical system which ignores and fails them. Reclaiming their voices–both real and metaphorical–can be powerfully achieved in telling their stories through song, in hearing them in recording, and in sharing them on CD with others. Other music therapy experiences effective in empowering women and building their self-esteem include drumming, singing, performing, and the incorporation of other creative arts (Curtis, 2000, 2006; York, 2006). Ultimately women survivors of intimate partner violence must understand the importance and practice of self-nurturance. Strong societal messages about the necessity of selflessness for women–to stand by their man, and equally to self-sacrifice for their children–can undermine their efforts to leave abusive relationships and can flaw social agencies' attempts to help. In feminist music therapy, abused women can learn that self-nurturance is important for their children's sake (eliminating the harm done in seeing their mother abused) and for their own sake as well. This concept can be addressed through feminist lyric analysis and songwriting, while the practice can be learned through such techniques as music-centered relaxation (Curtis, 2000).

In reviewing intimate male partner violence and the emergent practice of feminist music therapy with women survivors, one thing becomes clear. It takes not only a feminist understanding of male violence, but also a specific practice with goals and techniques rooted in this understanding to most effectively meet the needs of women abused in their intimate relationships. Ultimately, it requires social action on the part of both therapist and client to accomplish change outside of therapy. Research in this emergent feminist music therapy practice documents its effectiveness in transforming women's lives (Curtis, 2000; York, 2006). In closing, this chapter will turn to the voice of one woman and her experience in feminist music therapy.

Molly's Voice

Looking at feminist music therapy through the eyes of one woman can provide rich and contextualized insight. Selecting a single woman, however, is not an easy task because of the diversity of women and their experiences. For this chapter, I turn to Molly–a woman who struggled initially within therapy, but one who ultimately was quite successful. Molly–a 27-year-old African American woman–joined my music therapy group at a local battered women's shelter after fleeing an ex-boyfriend who threatened to kill her.

Molly was involved in feminist music therapy twice weekly for 12 sessions. During that time, she participated in feminist lyric analysis, songwriting, and music-centered relaxation. As well, she joined with the group one evening in a community march against violence. In therapy, Molly had trouble giving voice to her feelings. She was enthusiastic about listening to the women's music and enjoyed the relaxation time. However, in terms of discussion and songwriting she was reminiscent of some of the women in *Women's Ways of Knowing* (Belenky et al., 1986). These silent women, as Belenky named them, had gifts of intelligence but were unable to express themselves, to speak out to protest. Such seemed the case for Molly in many ways. She was successful, with support, in the songwriting, but struggled initially to find her voice, particularly as she saw other group participants writing with ease. Yet ultimately, she found her own completed songs graceful and pleasing. Molly's progress in therapy was considerable. Her self-esteem increased from a pretest level at the 8th percentile to a post-test level at the 50th percentile on the Tennessee Self Concept Scale (Roid & Fitts, 1991). While still struggling with words, Molly's increased self-confidence was evident in her final interview: *"I am very important. . . . Yes, I think I am powerful too."* Her final song, finished only after considerable effort, comprised a single verse, while the other women's songs were of five. Yet, within that one verse, Molly was able to give powerful voice to her resistance (Curtis, 2000).

Molly's Blues
Don't wanna be nobody's victim. Don't wanna be black and blue
Don't wanna be nobody's victim. Don't wanna be black and blue
I'm packing up my bags 'cause baby we're through.

Terms

Battered Woman Syndrome: A concept developed by Lenore Walker (1984) which describes abused women's experiences as a cycle of violence that results in learned helplessness.
Child Abuse: takes many forms, but ultimately involves a "violation of power and control from a position of strength, authority, or trust" (Curtis & Harrison, 2006, p. 195).
Demystification: A technique used by, but not unique to, feminist music therapy. Through this technique, the therapist ensures that the client understands and is an active participant in the entire therapeutic process.
Domestic Violence: used to describe violence in intimate relationships, this term has popular acceptance but either purposefully or unintentionally masks critical dimensions of gender and power.
Feminism: is an ideology of grassroots origins with many definitions, having in common their view of "the relationship between the sexes as one of inequality, subordination, or oppression, that sees this as a problem of political power rather than a fact of nature, and that sees this problem as important for political theory and practice" (Bryson, 1992, p. 1).
Feminist Music Therapy: is a unique approach to music therapy developed to better meet client needs in a patriarchal society. It includes hallmark techniques of feminist analysis of power and gender-role socialization.
Institutionalized Sexism: refers to inequality, subordination, or oppression based on gender that is seen in the structure and functioning of societal institutions.
Intimate Male Partner Violence: a term that more accurately reflects the dimensions of gender and power in women's experiences of violence in their intimate relationships. It involves a "pattern of coercive control over women [by their intimate male partners] that uses diverse methods and leaves women questioning their self-worth and perception of reality" (Yllö & Bograd, 1988, p. 15).
Medical Model of Violence: a model which identifies violence against women as an individual problem on the part of a small number of men with psychological issues and/or on the part of women who are attracted to abusive men.
Physical Abuse: refers to any "hitting, slapping, shoving, grabbing, pinching, biting, hair-pulling, etc. Physical abuse also includes denying a partner medical care or forcing alcohol and/or drug use" (U.S. Department of Justice, 2006).
Psychological Abuse: involves "causing fear by intimidation; threatening physical harm, to self, partner, children, or partner's family or friends; destruction of pets and property; and forcing isolation from family, friends,

or school and/or work" (U.S. Department of Justice, 2006).
Sexual abuse: refers to "coercing or attempting to coerce any sexual contact or behavior without consent. Sexual abuse includes, but is certainly not limited to marital rape, attacks on sexual parts of the body, forcing sex after physical violence has occurred, or treating one in a sexually demeaning manner" (U.S. Department of Justice, 2006).
Stalking: involves "a pattern of repeated and unwanted attention, harassment, contact or any other course of contact directed at a specific person that would cause a reasonable person to feel fear" (U.S. Department of Justice, 2006).
Systemic Abuse: refers to the impact of societal institutions that tolerate, encourage, and even perpetuate abuse of women (Curtis, 2000).
Verbal Abuse: involves "derogatory remarks about a woman's intelligence, abilities, social skills, appearance, education, job, income, childrearing practices, or house maintenance abilities" (Canadian Panel on Violence Against Women, 1993, p. 7).

References

Amir, D. (2004). Giving trauma a voice: The role of improvisational music therapy in exposing, dealing with and healing a traumatic experience of sexual abuse. *Music Therapy Perspectives, 22*, 96-103.

Belenky, M. F., Clinchy, B. M., Goldberger, N. R., & Tarule, J. M. (1986). *Women's ways of knowing: The development of self, voice, and mind.* New York: Basic Books.

Brooke, S. L. (2008). *The creative therapies and eating disorders.* Springfield, IL: Charles C Thomas, Publisher, Ltd.

Brooke, S. L. (2007). *The creative therapies with sexual abuse survivors.* Springfield, IL: Charles C Thomas, Publisher, Ltd.

Bryson, V. (1992). *Feminist political theory: An introduction.* London: Macmillan.

Burstow, B. (1992). *Radical feminist therapy: Working in the context of violence.* Newbury Park, CA: Sage Publications.

Canadian Panel on Violence Against Women. (1993). *Without fear: A facilitator's guide.* Ottawa, Canada: Author.

Cassity, M., & Theobold, K. (1990). Domestic violence: Assessments and treatments employed by music therapists. *Journal of Music Therapy, 27*, 179-194.

Clendenon-Wallen, J. (1991). Use of music therapy to influence the self-confidence and self-esteem of adolescents who are sexually abused. *Music Therapy Perspectives, 9*, 73-81.

Curtis, S. L. (2007). Claiming voice: music therapy for childhood sexual abuse survivors. In S. Brooke (Ed.), *The use of creative therapies with sexual abuse survivors* (pp. 196-206). Springfield, IL: Charles C Thomas, Publisher, Ltd.

Curtis, S. L. (2006). Feminist music therapy: Transforming theory, transforming lives. In S. Hadley (Ed.), *Feminist perspectives in music therapy: Empowering women's voices* (pp. 227-244). Philadelphia: Barcelona Publishers.

Curtis, S. L. (2000). *Singing subversion, singing soul: Women's voices in feminist music therapy.* (Doctoral dissertation, Concordia University, 1997). *Dissertation Abstracts International, 60*(12-A), 4240.

Curtis, S. L. (1994). Killing us softly: Male inner violence against women. In S. G. French (Ed.), *Interpersonal violence, health, and gender politics* (2nd ed., pp. 287-306). Dubuque, IA: W. C. Brown.

Curtis, S. L., & Harrison, G. C. T. (2006). Empowering women survivors of childhood sexual abuse: A collaborative music therapy-social work approach. In S. Brooke (Ed.), *Creative modalities for therapy with children and adults* (pp. 193-202). Springfield, IL: Charles C Thomas, Publisher, Ltd.

Hadley, S. (2006). *Feminist perspectives in music therapy.* Gilsum, NH: Barcelona Publishers.

Hammel-Gormley, A. (1995). *Singing the songs: A qualitative study of music therapy with individuals having psychiatric illnesses as well as histories of childhood sexual abuse.* (Doctoral dissertation, New York University, 1995). Dissertation Abstracts International, 56(10B), 5768.

Hernandez-Ruiz, E. (2005). Effect of music therapy on the anxiety levels and sleep patterns of abused women in shelters. *Journal of Music Therapy, 42*(2), 140-158.

Lindberg, K. A. (1995). Songs of healing: Songwriting with an abused adolescent. *Music Therapy, 13*(1), 93-108.

MacIntosh, H. B. (2003). Sounds of healing: Music in group work with survivors of sexual abuse. *Arts in Psychotherapy, 30*(1), 17-23.

Marshall, P. F., & Vaillancourt, M. A. (1993). *Changing the landscape: Ending violence - achieving equality. Final report of the Canadian Panel on Violence Against Women.* Ottawa, Canada: Minister of Supply & Services Canada.

Montello, L. (1999). A psychoanalytic music therapy approach to treating adults traumatized as children. *Music Therapy Perspectives, 2,* 74-81.

Purdon, C. (2006). Feminist music therapy with abused teen girls. In S. Hadley (Ed.), *Feminist perspectives in music therapy: Empowering women's voices* (pp. 205-226). Philadelphia: Barcelona Publishers.

Rinker, R. L. (1991). Guided imagery and music (GIM): Healing the wounded healer. In K. Bruscia (Ed.), *Case studies in music therapy.* Gilsum, NH: Barcelona Publishers.

Rogers, P. J. (1995). Childhood sexual abuse: Dilemmas in therapeutic practice. *Music Therapy Perspectives. Special Issue. International Music Therapy, 13*(1), 24-30.

Rogers, P. J. (1994). Sexual abuse and eating disorders: A possible connection indicated through music therapy? In D. Dokter (Ed.), *Arts therapies and clients with eating disorders: Fragile board* (pp. 262-278). Philadelphia: Jessica Kingsley Publishers Publishers.

Rogers, P. J. (1993). Research in music therapy with sexually abused clients. In H. Payne (Ed.), *Handbook of inquiry in the arts therapies: One river, many currents* (pp. 197-217). Philadelphia: Jessica Kingsley Publishers Publishers.

Roid, G. H., & Fitts, W. H. (1991). *Tennessee self-concept scale (TSCS): Revised manual.* Los Angeles: Western Psychological Services.

Statistics Canada. (2006). *Measuring violence against women: Statistical trends 2006.* Commissioned by the federal/provincial/ territorial ministries responsible for the status of women. Ottawa, Canada: Statistics Canada.

Teague, A. K., Hahna, N. D., & McKinney, C. (2006). Group music therapy with women who have experienced intimate partner violence. *Music Therapy Perspectives, 24*(2), 80-86.

U. S. Department of Justice. Office of Justice Programs. (2003). *Intimate partner violence, 1993-2001.* Retrieved January 3, 2007 from U. S. Department of Justice, Office of Justice Programs, Bureau of Justice Statistics website: http://www.ojp.usdoj.gov/bjs/pub/pdf/ipv01.pdf

U. S. Department of Justice. Office on Violence Against Women (2006). *About domestic violence.* Retrieved January 7, 2007 from U.S. Department of Justice, Office of Violence Against Women website: www.usdoj.gov/ovw/domviolence.htm.

United Nations. (1995). *Platform for Action and Beijing Declaration.* Retrieved January 7, 2007 from United Nations Division for the Advancement of Women website: http://www.un.org/womenwatch/daw/beijing/beijingdeclaration.html

Ventre, M. (1994). Healing the wounds of childhood abuse: A guided imagery and music case study. *Music Therapy Perspectives. Special Issue. Psychiatric music therapy, 12*(2), 48-53.

Walker, L. E. (1984). *The battered woman syndrome.* New York: Springer.

Whipple, J., & Lindsey, R. S. (1999). Music for the soul: A music therapy program for battered women. *Music Therapy Perspectives, 17*(2), 61-68.

Worell, J., & Remer, P. (2003). *Feminist perspectives in therapy: Empowering diverse women.* New York: Wiley.

Yllö, K., & Bograd, M. (Eds.). (1988). *Feminist perspectives on wife abuse.* Newbury Park, CA: Sage

York, E. (2006). Finding voice. In S. Hadley (Ed.), *Feminist perspectives in music therapy: Empowering women's voices* (pp. 245-265). Philadelphia: Barcelona Publishers.

Biography

Sandra L. Curtis, Ph. D., MT-BC, MTA, is Director of the School of Music and Coordinator of Music Therapy at the University of Windsor in Canada. She received a bachelor's degree in music from McGill University, Canada, a master's in music therapy from Florida State University, USA, and an interdisciplinary Ph.D. in music therapy and feminist therapy from Concordia University, Canada. Her published articles, chapters, and reviews appear in the *Journal of Music Therapy, Music Therapy Perspectives, Voices: A World Forum for Music Therapy,* the *Journal of Palliative Care, Feminist Perspectives in Music Therapy* (Barcelona Publishers, 2006), *Creative Modalities in Therapy for Children and Adults* (Charles C. Thomas, 2006), *Interpersonal Violence, Health, and Gender* (W.C. Brown, 1994), and *Research in Music Therapy: A Tradition of Excellence* (AMTA, 1994). Dr. Curtis also serves on the editorial board of the *Journal of Music Therapy.* She has been actively engaged in social justice work in Canada and the United States for more than 15 years.

Chapter 9

MUSIC THERAPY WITH CHILDREN WHO HAVE WITNESSED DOMESTIC VIOLENCE

Amy Clarkson

Introduction

For women and children who have lived within the fearful and controlling environment of a home scarred by domestic violence, music can be a powerful and effective medium for healing (Cassity & Theobold, 1990; Hernandez-Ruiz, 2005; Sutton, 2002; Whipple & Lindsey, 1999). Music offers a sense of safety and support through predictable structures, freedom, and opportunity for authentic expression of thoughts and emotions, and a new means for connecting with and relating to others. Drawing on existing theory and research and clinical case examples, this chapter will explore different ways in which music therapy can help children to move forward in their healing process following the trauma of domestic violence. In order to protect the anonymity of the children mentioned in this chapter, names, and other identifying information have been changed. Some case examples reflect a composite of more than one child.

Child Survivors of Domestic Violence

The problem of child exposure to domestic violence is both deep and broad. Rossman, Hughes, and Rosenberg (1999) estimate that at least 15 percent of children in the United States are exposed to some form of aggression between their parents. From her work in the Child Witness to Violence Project, Groves (2002) states that domestic violence is the "most toxic form of violence for children" (p. 50). With one parent as aggressor and the other as frightened victim, the child is left with no one to provide the sense of stability and safety needed for healthy development. Documented effects of children's exposure to domestic violence include impairment in emotional development, social functioning, ability to learn and focus in school, capacity for intimate relationships in later life, and increased risk for antisocial behavior, substance abuse, mental illness, and direct physical injury (Groves, 2002). From their review of relevant research, Rossman, Hughes, and Rosenberg (1999) conclude that children exposed to domestic violence show significant emotional and behavioral differences with regard to both internalizing and externalizing behaviors. Internalizing behaviors, such as withdrawal, depression, and anxiety are common in children who have witnessed domestic abuse, as are symptoms associated with Post Traumatic Stress Disorder. Externalizing behaviors take the form of aggression toward others and hyperactivity.

Jeffrey and Frisone (2003) cite the cognitive adaptations often employed by children in order to endure living in a home environment of on-going violence. These adaptations include denying the reality that the violence has occurred, feeling responsible for the violence, and having an altered sense of time, place, and person. They state: "Exposure to domestic violence may harm children's abilities to engage in the cognitive activity and exploration necessary for the construction of reality and selfhood, the de-centering that is fundamental to moral cognition, and the curiosity and hopefulness that is central to productive thinking" (p. 7).

Jeffrey, Frisone, and Owens (1999) have documented statistically significant improvement in the behavioral profile of children exposed to domestic violence following participation in a program that included intensive therapy and case management services. Through art and drama therapy, children in the program were given a safe space in which to experience and express emotion, to make choices, to experience being valued, and to review and reenact past events in ways in which the child retained a sense of control. Drawing on Gruber's (1980) evolving systems theory, Jeffrey and Frisone (2003) suggest that the child recovering from the trauma of domestic violence needs to go through his or her own unique process of constructive repetition, review, and reinterpretation of the traumatic events. They stress the importance of engaging the child's thinking, creativity, and imagination within a safe and supportive therapeutic environment in order to help the child arrive at a new understanding of him or herself and the traumatic events.

The emotional availability of the non-offending parent has been shown to have an important impact on children's recovery from the trauma of domestic violence (Groves, 2002). Parenting practices and the quality of attachment between parent and child are also factors that impact the child's level of emotional security, self-esteem, and social competence (Cummings & Davies, 1994). Having the parent survivor of domestic abuse involved in the recovery process of her child as well as her own recovery process, seems to be of critical importance.

Clinical Context

The context in which I provide services to child survivors of domestic violence is similar to that described by Jeffrey, Frisone, and Owens (1999). Supported by a state-funded grant, PALS (Peace, A Learned Solution) offers comprehensive services to children who have been exposed to domestic violence. Services provided through the program include creative arts therapies, family therapy, case management services, and a parenting support and education group for the non-offending parent, based on a program titled *Compassionate Parenting* (Stosny, 2001). Many of the non-offending parents are involved in their own individual or group counseling in addition to the parenting support group. While not exclusively, the vast majority of the non-offending parents are the children's mothers. The children, ages four to twelve years old, participate in the program for six months and occasionally, up to one year, receiving both individual and group therapy in two different creative arts modalities. Parent-child dyad sessions are offered as clinically indicated.

A *Compassion Workshop* (Stosny, 1995) is a separate group that is available for abusers who are pursuing their own process of change and recovery. The abusers are only involved in family therapy in the rare cases in which they complete the *Compassion Workshop* and are assessed by the facilitator as being safe and committed to their own process of change and recovery. Communication among those working with the different members of the family is viewed as essential to effective intervention. This comprehensive approach is seen as having the greatest potential for the recovery of the children, with the long-term goal of breaking the cycle of violence.

From Stosny's (2001) work, a key concept that is present in the healing process is that of core hurts and core value. Core hurts are seen as being the root cause of anger, anxiety, and obsessions, with all harmful behaviors being caused by the motivation to avoid or numb core hurts. These core hurts include feeling disregarded, unimportant, accused, guilty, devalued, rejected, powerless, and inadequate or unlovable. The core hurts mask the experience of core value, an instinctual sense of self-worth present at birth. The foundation of personal security, well being, and self-esteem, core value is an emotional awareness that no problem, event, or behavior can reduce one's value as a person. It is my role and the role of the other treatment team members, then to create a safe and supportive therapeutic environment and therapeutic relationships in which children have the repeated experience of feeling regarded, important, free of judgment, innocent, valued, included, empowered, adequate, and lovable.

Bannister (1997) describes a child-centered approach to work with traumatized children, which draws on both psychodrama theory and object relations theory. Her emphasis on following the agenda of the child, while providing empathic understanding and clear boundaries resonates with my own approach. She states, "When trauma enters our lives we merely exist and we cannot live as fully as we would wish. Our creativity is stifled at traumatic times but, with encouragement, it can grow and be used to heal the hurt" (p. 71). The development of spontaneity and creativity are central to psychodrama theory, with spontaneity being, "an adequate response to a new situation, or the novel [and adequate] response to an old situation" (Moreno, 1993, p. 336). Children recovering from domestic violence need a safe place within which to discover their core value and to develop their innate spontaneity and creativity so that they can gradually move from a place of pain, anxiety, and confusion to a place of healing and peace.

Music Therapy with Child Survivors of Domestic Violence

Within the context of a therapeutic environment, there are many different types of musical experiences that hold potential for healing and growth for child survivors of domestic violence. These experiences include musical improvisation, listening to songs, singing or playing songs, composing, music supported story telling, and music supported relaxation. Through a therapeutic relationship within a musical context, children can move toward a state of increased spontaneity and creativity, reduced anxiety, an improved ability to regulate and express emotions, healthier patterns of thinking, and an ability to develop new, healthier relationships with others and within oneself.

Assessment

Through a process of assessment, one can begin to understand the particular ways a child has been affected by exposure to domestic violence, to discover how the child relates within musical experiences, and to learn about musical preferences, significant songs, and prior musical involvement. Lowey's (2000) *Music Psychotherapy Assessment* has been a useful means for gathering relevant information about the child through engagement in musical experiences. Lowey (2000) outlined 13 areas of inquiry to be explored through both structured and unstructured musical experiences: awareness of self, others and the moment, thematic expression, listening, performing, collaboration/relationship, concentration, range of affect, investment/motivation, use of structure, integration, self-esteem, risk taking, and independence. Information is gathered in a descriptive manner related to each of the 13 areas of inquiry.

> Assessment information is shared among members of the treatment team. The child and the child's parent are asked to give input during the goal setting process as a means of encouraging parent and child to take ownership of their recovery process. We have developed a bank of goals based on the needs that the children in the program have presented over a period of several years. The goals fall within six overarching categories that reflect the main areas of focus for treatment: safety, emotional regulation and expression, communication, conflict resolution, relationships, self-esteem, and coping with change and loss. (p. 49)

Decisions regarding types of musical experiences and interventions to use with a child also grow out of the assessment process and are based on several factors. As delineated by Bruscia (1991), factors that influence the selection of musical experiences include the ways in which the experience relates to the goals, the client's preferences and the client's musical abilities. For the purposes of this chapter, different types of musical experiences will be discussed separately in order to demonstrate the unique potential of each one. Within the therapy itself, a variety of musical experiences are interwoven throughout the process, based on the leading of the child.

Music Improvisation

In music improvisation, music is newly created in the moment. Sutton (2002) has found that the way in which music can be experienced in the body as emotion and through time holds particular relevance for the child recovering from trauma. She notes that because music is experienced at a pre-symbolic level, it has the potential to express and reflect the chaos and fragmentation of the traumatic experience. It is the role of the music therapist, then to provide a safe, containing musical space to support the child in gradually creating form and structure out of the chaos and confusion. By improvising music with a child that is grounding and containing, which holds the child's music without being controlling, the music therapist lets the child know that neither the adult nor the child will be consumed by the expression. Improvising provides a means for children to learn that they have the ability to regulate their own expression. This learning opens up new possibilities for a child who is used to an all or nothing, overwhelming or shut down experience of emotion common to those recovering from trauma (Austin, 2002).

Often children who come from homes affected by domestic violence have not developed healthy patterns of communication because such communication has not been modeled within the home. It may be very difficult, for example, for the child to listen to what someone else is saying without interrupting. Improvisations between two children or between a child and therapist can focus on and help develop an improved ability to listen and to respond, to enter a pattern of call and response, to maintain the boundaries necessary for effective communication.

Ruud (1998) discusses the concept of *void* in relation to music improvisation. Of relevance here is the suggestion that the improvisational experience provides a blank slate, an opportunity to clear old meanings and create something new. The environment of domestic abuse is one in which the cycle of violence often makes it difficult for either parent to see or hear the child clearly, it is an environment in which the child's ideas and emotions may be neither validated nor safe to express. Children often learn to cope in this environment by holding their own thoughts and emotions in. The act of improvisation helps a child, at her own pace, to learn to express herself and relate in ways that were not possible within the controlled and intolerant environment within which she had been living.

For children who have learned to disconnect from their feelings in order to cope with the trauma they have experienced, improvisation can provide a safe means to touch and stay with emotions that have previously felt too overwhelming to be near. Metaphor and imagery can help such a child to improvise in ways that access emotion. For example, I will sometimes suggest that a child or a group improvise a piece that has three parts: "The Calm Before the Storm," "The Storm," "After the Storm." Children have given titles to their improvisations such as "The Giant," "The Jungle," "The Monster," "The Butterfly." These images may be suggested by the child before, during or after an improvisation. The imagery can move a child forward in his or her process in a way that is powerful, and often times more accessible than dealing more overtly with his or her feelings in relation to the abuse witnessed.

The following case examples provide a sense of the ways in which music improvisation can be approached to address a range of different challenges and goals within the unfolding treatment process.

Jared and Evan

Jared (7) and Evan (6) were both having difficulties at school in controlling and regulating aggressive impulses. Challenges with attention and focusing were evident for both boys, and neither boy had a very positive sense of self. Jared had recently moved from a different region of the country with his sister and mother, who were fleeing from the violence of his father. Evan saw his father weekly for visitation. He often found himself caught in the middle of parental issues and disagreements.

When they began attending music therapy, Jared and Evan showed difficulties with impulse control in relation to the playing of the musical instruments. Each liked to play the instruments in a loud and chaotic manner, showing little awareness of the music being made by the other child or therapist. Allowed to express the internal chaos each was feeling, the boys seemed to greatly enjoy the experience of banging loudly on the large gathering drum. The auditory and vibrational feedback was satisfying to them. Jared had the idea of adding cymbals, hanging the cymbals on either end of the keyboard stand. This physical arrangement meant that the boys shared the large drum, and each boy had his own cymbal to crash. The boys were also in close proximity to me, face to face. By experiencing both a sense of closeness and connection and by maintaining their own space on the cymbals, the boys found the needed balance of autonomy and support.

Out of the chaotic rhythms that were typical of the pair, Jared developed a repeated rhythmic motif consisting of two eighth notes and a quarter note on the large drum followed by a half note on the cymbal. As he repeated this motif over and over, Evan joined him, synchronizing with Jared's rhythm. I had begun the improvisation by maintaining a steady pulse on the keyboard to offer support and grounding for the experience. I then moved to synchronizing with the rhythmic pattern which was now shared by Jared and Evan, providing supportive mirroring in order to further affirm the musical idea and emphasize the experience of musical connection.

Through the improvisation, the boys discovered their ability to regulate and control their music making and to relate their responses to the music made by one another and by me. There was a quality of power and strength to the music, along with a quality of listening and connection. This experience of 'positive power' was significant for these boys who had witnessed power as being something used to control, to hurt, to keep for oneself. The boys returned to this rhythmic pattern repeatedly in future sessions and it became a means through which focus and connection was possible. Over time, the boys also grew in their ability to play and listen to soothing sounds. While there continued to be challenges with emotional regulation at school and home, the boys had a successful experience with regulation, positive power, and self-control within the music. The need for proximity, consistency, and containment was shared with the boys' mothers as they sought positive parenting strategies to use with their sons. The parental role was viewed as key to generalizing the improved ability to relate and regulate that had begun to emerge in the music therapy sessions.

Peter

Peter was eleven years old when he began coming for music and art therapy. Peter's father had been emotionally abusive to his mother throughout

Peter's life and his parents had recently separated. Peter was seen in a dyad session with another boy. An adult male musician, experienced in using music therapeutically was also present in the sessions. Peter played the saxophone at school, so he had some knowledge of note reading. It was very difficult for him to improvise music. He spent considerable time writing, crossing out, and rewriting notes to play or he relied on small fragments of songs that he could play from memory on the piano. The idea of musical expression without notation seemed to be anxiety provoking for him. He did not want to make mistakes or create music that did not sound "good." It seemed that he was responding to his lack of control over his family's situation by attempting to be perfect.

In relation to his father, Peter's attempts to seek his father's love and approval were frequently met with criticism. I experienced in him a desire to please and to be approved. His life was full of many activities from which he seemed to derive some satisfaction, but which left him little time to relax and to reflect on the recent changes in his family. There was a great deal of structured activity within the family, which seemed to be a way to cope with the pain.

The music therapy sessions became a place within which Peter, over time, learned to let go to a greater degree, to experiment, to relax, and to be comfortable without a prescribed task or precise direction. The first breakthrough came when he switched from playing the keyboard to playing a large drum together with his peer. Within the drumming experience, Peter was able to let go of his anxiety over "getting it right" and played with freedom, energy and a sense of mutual enjoyment with his peer. Following this positive experience with the drum, Peter became more willing to experiment musically through improvisation. He developed an interest in the guitar and began to experiment both within and outside of the sessions on the guitar. He continued to grow in his ability to be more free and expressive in his music.

What seemed to be most significant for Peter about the improvisational experience, was that he came to anticipate each week, a time that had no particular demands or expectations, a free space, a blank slate, in which his spontaneity and creativity was given an opportunity to be expressed freely. Within this free musical space, he experienced unconditional positive regard from both a male and female adult as well as a strong, positive bond with his peer. He experienced a different means of relating between a male and female adult than he had become accustomed to within his own family. My co-facilitator and I were intentional in modeling flexibility of roles within the music. We communicated with one another in a respectful and open manner within the group. A balanced sense of power and interdependency, rather than dominance or dependency, was modeled.

Within this environment of freedom, positive regard, and honest, respectful communication, Peter was able to develop new insights into the dynamics of his family. He found a means to express his confusion, anger, and hurt in an environment that was affirming of his internal experience. He grew in his acceptance of the losses that he had sustained, and at the end of his time in the program, he expressed gratitude, reported feeling a greater sense of peace within himself. He came to recognize and to begin to accept the limitations of his father and the permanency of his parents' divorce.

Rebecca

When a child is approaching a readiness to directly express emotion in relation to a person in his or her family or in response to the abuse s/he has witnessed, the child is in both a courageous and vulnerable place. I have found the psychodrama technique of doubling useful in such cases. Doubling means that the therapist joins with the client, expressing through "I" statements, inner thoughts, and feelings that are difficult for the child to express on his or her own (Hoey, 1997). Musical doubling through improvisation was the technique I used with Rebecca during the session described below.

Rebecca had been witness to her father's rage and physical aggression. She talked about a time when she was young and in the care of her father, traveling with him while he was working and not really being noticed or attended to. She made a statement, with little emotion in her voice, that she had felt like she had been "drug in the dirt." I began to improvise at the piano and sing "feels like I'm being drug in the dirt" in Phrygian mode, a pattern of tones which has greater dissonance and tension than a major or natural minor scale. By repeating the rhythmic pattern of the words, "drug in the dirt," using the tones of the Phrygian mode, I was able to reflect the heaviness, the anger, the hurt that I sensed were present under the surface of Rebecca's words. Rebecca played rhythmic patterns that matched the rhythm of the words I sang, and when I left space in the music, she accented the end of some phrases with a large cymbal crash. Her focused, deliberate energy in the music and the way in which her playing was so connected with mine let me know that my musical doubling was accurate for her. The repetition of her statement, the musical tension, and the physical act of beating the drum and cymbal all helped Rebecca to be in touch with a core hurt in an emotionally connected way.

The session with Rebecca continued, moving through a number of different statements toward her father. The last improvisation of the session was based on her statement, "I am here! I am not invisible! I am here!" These were significant statements for Rebecca of her own right to be, to be who she is and not pretend to be who she thinks others want her to be or not be. I sang these statements out in a strong and repeated manner, accompanied by open octaves on the piano, with occasional contrast of a slow, pensive mood, in which I quietly sang, "sometimes I feel invisible when you don't pay attention to me." Rebecca again, with cymbals and strong percussion, joined in with the rhythmic pattern of the words "I am here!" and through her music, expressed her inner strength and right to be. Each of the improvisations was recorded so that Rebecca could listen over again as often as she would like to her internal process that she had courageously expressed. Rebecca clearly felt good about herself and the risk she had taken. She asked to play the tape for a few peers in the program with whom she had been in group and she received an affirming response from her peers. In this way, the expression of a core hurt, being disregarded, was met with an experience of being regarded and valued.

Use of Songs

Music therapists have found that listening to songs helps survivors of domestic violence to access and express emotion (Cassity & Theobold, 1990; Whipple & Lindsey, 1999). Children are naturally drawn to songs that reflect emotional content that resonates with their own internal experience. Because the song is sung by another, there is a distance that makes the experience tolerable and safe enough for the child. By discovering and listening to songs that hold meaning for them, children may feel less alone, and may experience validation of their emotions. As described by Kaser (1993), internal conflicts that are unconscious, subconscious, or too scary to share directly may be revealed through song choices made by the child.

Often a child will bring in a song, saying, "I like the beat," or "I just like the way it sounds," unaware or not ready to directly talk about how the song is related to his or her own life and internal struggle. For the child who has coped with the domestic violence by disconnecting from his or her emotions, listening to songs can be a first step toward accessing his or her inner emotional life.

Tricia

Tricia was a 10-year-old who almost always had a smile on her face. She had become very skilled at masking her own pain. Songs became one way to begin to permeate the mask, to glimpse beneath the surface, and to be honest and real about the pain beneath. Tricia brought in the song *Losing Grip* by Avril Lavigne (2002). Through her identification with this song, Tricia found a tolerable way to touch her own pain. Lavigne sings, "I was left to cry there, waiting outside there, grinning with a lost stare. That's when I decided why should I care? Cause you weren't there when I was scared, I was so alone." While Tricia did not yet feel safe enough to directly seek emotional support from me or from the other group members, she had found a source of support through the song. The music of the song conveyed an emotional intensity that resonated with the reality of Tricia's internal life. By sharing the song with the group, Tricia took a beginning step toward connection and toward sharing her secret inner world. The song then became a link between Tricia and her peers, who also liked and were able to relate to the song.

Anna

Songs serve at times to catalyze and at other times reflect the child's forward movement in his or her healing process. At the start of her music therapy group, eight-year-old Anna and her peers were asked to share a song with the group that was important to them. Anna chose the song *Yesterday* by Lennon and McCartney (1965). The song suggested a number of ideas that gave insight into Anna and her struggles. The first idea that was striking about the song was that it sounded "old." One would typically expect an eight-year-old child to be looking toward tomorrow rather than longing for yesterday. It was my hunch that she was holding on to a fantasy about returning to an earlier time which she imagined must have been happier than the way she was feeling now. A dichotomy of old and young was evident in Anna and, yet, she did not seem to be happy or comfortable with being an eight-year-old girl. A line in the song seemed particularly significant, "Why she had to go, I don't know. She wouldn't say. I said something wrong now I long for yesterday." I sensed that Anna was feeling guilty and responsible for the violence between her parents and for the fact that her father had left. It is also interesting that the song is sung by a solo male singer, with fairly sparse musical accompaniment. Her focus and identification seemed to be with that which was lost and perhaps taking on the guilt and responsibility that belonged to her father.

Being part of a group, Anna had the benefit of listening to and growing into songs brought in by the other group members. One song that became significant for Anna and the group was *Breakaway* by Gerrard, Benante and Lavigne (2004). In contrast to *Yesterday*, which has a sense of resignation about it, *Breakaway* is full of messages that are encouraging of change. The song suggests that one has the capacity to live differently: "I'll take a risk, take a chance, make a change, and break away." The song is sung by a young female singer, Kelly Clarkson, with the chorus being supported by a cluster of female voices. The group of female voices was reflective of the all-female group of which she was a part.

In order to help Anna and her peers more fully take in the messages expressed in this song, I created a simple, orchestrated arrangement of the song, including parts for different instruments requested by the girls. Anna initially strummed an open chord on the guitar for the song. Over time, she began to sing some of the words. She then tried out different roles that had been modeled by her peers, such as drumming the rhythmic pattern of the opening phrases of the song or playing long sustained notes on the keyboard during the chorus, and singing. As she moved toward musical roles which required increasing levels of involvement, focus, practice, and skill, Anna took on new challenges, took new risks, and by doing so, was living out a piece of the song's message.

The growth Anna had been making was clearly evident when she next brought in a song of her own choosing to share with the group. From the soundtrack of *Shrek 2*, the song *Changes*, sung by Bowie and Boucher (1971) is musically varied and complex. While *Breakaway* has a steady, 6/8 rhythm, providing a feeling of predictability and safety which Anna had needed to begin her growth process, the time signature, timbre, texture, and feel of *Changes* shifts throughout the song, creating a feeling of unrest, and movement. The repeated line in the chorus, "turn and face the stranger," suggests that Anna was now feeling more ready to get to know her true self, herself as an eight-year-old girl. The line, "Where's your shame, you've left us up to our necks in it," seems to be directed toward parental figures. In the sessions following the one in which Anna brought in this song, she was able to move into direct discussion and musical expression around the ways in which her father had frightened her and emotionally scarred her. Her musical expressions continued to involve increased risk taking and a greater sense of confidence in herself.

Singing

Austin (2002) discusses the healing potential of singing for trauma survivors, including a sense of relaxation which results from diaphragmatic breathing and a release of emotion and energy blockages through the internal vibrations which occur when one sings. Through the discovery of his or her own singing voice, the child survivor is able to access his or her own instrument of self, and to experience a freedom of expression which may not have felt possible in the controlling environment of the abusive home. While many of the children with whom I work are initially reluctant or not willing to sing, it is an experience that I encourage and draw out when possible. One of the most effective means to encourage a child to find and develop her own voice is having another peer within a group setting who does sing. I also model vocal freedom and expressiveness. Frequently, a child will sing timidly beside me at first. As the child grows in vocal confidence, I will continue to maintain a vocal presence as long as the child needs, but I will quiet my voice gradually as the child's voice grows in confidence and strength. Singing may take the form of vocal improvisation, vocal warm ups on sustained vowel sounds, singing pre-composed songs, or singing original songs. Following a discussion of the songwriting or composition process, a case example will illustrate a child's growth through both songwriting and vocal development.

Songwriting

Often children who have witnessed domestic violence have felt silenced and powerless. Songwriting is one means by which child survivors can express their own truth. Ruud (2005) states that "Songwriting provides an aesthetic context inviting clients to explore, within a new play-frame, their own life, their possibilities, their losses and their aspirations" (p. 10). It generally takes time for children to feel ready to write down and perform or sing their own songs. The process of writing a song involves significant risk and self-exposure. Through songwriting, a child is able to tell his own story in his own way. A child is also able, through songwriting, to consolidate ideas and healthier patterns of thinking that have begun to evolve.

Again, a group experience can provide the needed catalyst and support to help make the risk of songwriting more possible. In a group setting, the children's ideas can build upon one another. The challenge of working together on a joint task can help children learn to negotiate with one another, to clarify their own thoughts, and to support and encourage one another. Humor sometimes plays a valuable role in the process of eliciting increased expression through songwriting. Through songwriting, one group of three girls, ages six to nine, found their voices in a new way. A strength and unity of expression emerged out of a humorous phrase brought in by one group member.

Eva, Sarah, and Jillian

Eva told the group a story about a conversation she had had with a friend. Eva said, "My friend had something she wanted to say, but she was having trouble saying it, so I told her to spit out the hairball!" The other girls in the group thought that statement was hilarious. Sensing the positive focus of energy through the metaphor of spitting out a hairball, I asked each girl to share about a time in her life when she felt like she had a hairball sitting in her throat, blocking what she wanted to say. The ideas began to build as each girl shared about a time when it was hard to say what she really wanted to say. I was very mindful throughout the process of how each of the girls had felt silenced by the fear associated with the domestic violence that had occurred in her home.

Sarah contributed the line, "When you tell a lie, you get nervous, and keep it in all the time." Eva said "When you want to say something to someone older, but you're nervous to say it." The energy of the song grew through the repeated line of the chorus, "Spit out the hairball, BLAH, BLAH BLAH!" The melodic movement of the chorus was minimal, so that it was almost a chant. Its simplicity and the humor found by the girls in shouting out "BLAH, BLAH" led to a greater strength and confidence in singing than I had seen in them before. In fact, Sarah had never sung before in group. The act of creating and singing the song, then, paralleled its life message of empowerment, of speaking out in moments when it felt risky to do so, thereby growing in one's own sense of personal strength. The song affirmed for the girls, both their right and ability to speak up for themselves rather than swallow their own thoughts and feelings as they had been accustomed to doing.

The group recorded the song and they were each given copies to take home. They also sang the song for their mothers. The song led into an important moment of communication, when Sarah's mother shared, tears in her eyes, about how difficult it had been for her to tell Sarah and her brothers the truth when she and their father had decided to separate. In this way, Sarah was affirmed in her risk taking by her mother taking a risk in honest, emotional communication, something that was hard for her to do.

"Spit out the Hairball" was followed by another original song. In this song, Sarah took even greater vocal risks, singing several lines solo, alternating back and forth with her peer who was more vocally confident. In this song, written near the end of the program cycle, Sarah and Jillian (Eva was out that day) wrote about falling off and holding on. The song was inspired by a moment in which Sarah fell off of her chair in the session. Both girls were facing realities within their family situations that would continue to be stressful. Communication between the parents around visitation and other parental issues is often tense and the children continue to find themselves at times, caught in the middle of challenging parental interactions. The act of falling off the chair led me to think about the fact that there would be times in these girls' futures when they would feel like they were falling, when life would feel difficult and painful, and when the support of the PALS program would feel far away. I asked them to think about what they could hold onto when they felt like they were falling. They came up with a variety of wonderful metaphors. Again the song was recorded for them to have at home. The song included the lines, "Hold on to your friends and the people you love, never let them go. Let go of the stress, hold on to the warmth. Hold on to the things you know."

Music-Supported Dramatic Play

Play is the natural means through which young children communicate and make sense out of their world (Bannister, 1997). As described by Bannister (1997) and Hoey (1997), through dramatic play, children can recreate, often through metaphor and imagery, aspects of the traumatic experience, while retaining a sense of control over the play. By improvising music to support the dramatic play, the therapist is able to reflect, support, aid and at times exaggerate the emotional content of the play.

Kyle, Connor, Haley and Victoria

Kyle, Connor, Haley, and Victoria were a group of four and five-year-olds who were drawn to the experience of dramatic play and who used the dramatic play as a means to play out their internal conflicts and emotions in a way that was safe, supportive, and often, fun. Having been trained in psychodrama as well as music therapy, I was eager to engage the group through both music and drama. The group had the benefit of a co-facilitator, Sara, a senior music therapy student who was doing her practicum work with me. Each week, following an opening time of connection through song, the group would move into an experience they came to know as "story time."

As the story was getting started, I invited each child to choose an animal that they would like to be in the story and I suggested that all stories have a problem that the characters face. The idea evolved among the group members that there would be a bridge, which was built with a row of small chairs. Connor knocked two of the chairs over and stated that the bridge was broken. The broken bridge became the opening problem faced by the group. While the group set about trying to fix the bridge in a number of ways, I improvised song lyrics to reflect the actions of the group and provided a steady, driving musical accompaniment to support the notion of working hard on a difficult problem. After a significant period of time had elapsed, Haley (the kitten) said, "The bridge is broken and it cannot be fixed." I musically echoed and repeated her statement several times, slowly, deliberately, with a feeling of heaviness. I was aware that the children had just acted out their central concern and that Haley had stated a profound truth, that the brokenness which had occurred in each of their families was beyond their own power to fix.

The story continued to evolve each week. Though it was never stated or prescribed that we were continuing the same story, each week the children seemed to naturally want to pick up where we had left off the week before. It was as if there was a magical window in the room that we walked through together each week, a free space, a safe place, where their imaginations were given permission to reconstruct, through their own images, the fears and conflicts that they carried within. I was eventually cast as a monster who was thrown in jail by the children for "stealing the sun." There was a sense in which the brightness of the children's lives had been dimmed by the lurking fear of violence. From behind the jail bars, I sang out a lament, an apology for the wrongdoing I had done, sensing that "I'm sorry" was something the children needed to hear and may not in real life. Sara, the music therapy student, supported my singing on the keyboard. She also played dissonant chord clusters on the keyboard, musically supporting and validating the children as they expressed their anger toward the monster.

As the group drew to a close, I asked the children how they would like to end the story. They decided that they would like to release the monster from jail, provided that the monster returned the sun to the sky. I again viewed this idea as a means for the children to have a corrective experience that may or may not be possible in real life. In the surplus reality of the drama, I was the repentant monster. I was aware that the children were drawing closer to me, that they no longer seemed afraid of me. I took the opportunity to share a "special secret" with the children from the role of the monster:

> 'Sometimes each of us has feelings that hurt deep inside and that can feel as mean and big and wild as a monster. I didn't know how to take care of those feelings, so I did a terrible thing. But, there are ways that you can care for even the most monstrous feelings so that nobody gets hurt and so that you feel better.'
>
> 'Like cry when you feel sad?' asked kitten.
>
> 'Yes,' said the monster.
>
> 'How about punch a pillow when you feel angry?' asked the polar bear.
>
> 'That can sometimes help too,' said the monster. 'Let someone you trust know how you are feeling. Once you let a feeling out in a safe place and don't keep it squashed up inside, it loses its monstrous power.'

For the final session, I wrote the story in a form that consolidated the tale that had been told over the previous six months. I thought it important for the children to have an opportunity to look back on it, to have their mothers read the story to them, to recall the process they had been through.

Music-Supported Relaxation

The level of stress and anxiety experienced by both children and their mothers who have recently moved from domestic violence situations is generally very high. Mothers often feel overwhelmed in the face of aggressive behaviors in their children. Strategies that mothers can help their children to practice and use in moments of high stress or aggressive impulses can reduce the sense of overwhelm and lead to more adaptive means of coping. Hernandez-Ruiz (2005) found that preferred music paired with progressive muscle relaxation resulted in significant decreases in anxiety and improved sleep patterns for abused women living in a shelter. She notes that some of the women in the study played the relaxation CD for their children and observed improvements in the children's stress levels.

Helping a child to choose preferred music and relaxation techniques empowers the child with alternative choices to violent or withdrawn behavior when stressed. Based on the need, interest, and level of readiness, I introduce a variety of relaxation strategies with the children. Diaphragmatic breathing, progressive muscle relaxation, imagery, yoga stretches, and simply getting cozy and still in a beanbag chair with dimmed lighting are some of the relaxation strategies that I have used. I play different types of relaxation music and help the children to identify which music feels relaxing to them. For children who identify preferred relaxation music, I burn CDs for them to use at home in moments of stress. We talk very practically and specifically at times about strong feelings, about the desire to hurt oneself or another, and about alternative behaviors and mediating thoughts that can be of help in those moments. Sometimes I will loan out instruments for children to use at home as a means to redirect aggressive impulses or strong feelings. Mothers are encouraged or helped to purchase an instrument if it seems particularly soothing for her child. One mother shared her excitement and joy over the fact that her son, who had taken to hitting her when he felt angry or upset, was now in those moments, going to the piano and playing loud, strong note clusters or other improvisational playing.

Parent Involvement in the Music

Groves (2002) stresses the importance of emotional availability on the part of the non-offending parent toward her child. Musical experiences that emphasize relaxation and shared enjoyment can help facilitate positive communication and interaction between parent and child. Channels of communication can be opened and the mother can be supported in responding to her child in an open and emotionally available way. Oftentimes the mothers, who are going through their own process of recovery and healing from the scars of abuse, need support and practice in responding to the emotional struggles of their children in validating ways. Helping mothers to respond to the core hurts that lie beneath aggressive or anxious behaviors is a key component of the parenting support group. Sometimes, music or art experiences are introduced into the parenting support group to help the parents to gain an increased understanding of how art, music, and drama are being used to support the children's healing. Sometimes a personal experience of creative arts therapy can help parents feel more comfortable in carrying over the use of creative modalities in the home as a means to build positive, open communication. A fellow music therapist in the program engaged the mothers in writing a song to communicate those things to their children that they felt were important for their children to know. Rewriting the lyrics to Jewel's song, *Hands* by Kilcher and Leonard (1998), the mothers communicated messages of love and support for their children and sang out their own feelings of strength:

> If I could tell my children just one thing, it would be you are specialand unique. I cherish you, I really love you, and always believe inyourself. I won't be made fun of or despised. I won't be idle withsadness or fear. I'll gather myself around family and faith, for lightdoes the darkness most fear.

When the children see their mothers as strong and able to cope, it frees them from the need that many of them feel to take care of their mothers. Helping mothers to be strong in their parenting role, setting needed boundaries, and providing emotional support and proximity needed by their children is vital to the children's recovery process. Often still dealing with the abusive behaviors of the children's fathers in relation to parenting issues, it takes a great deal of courage and determination on the part of the mothers to parent effectively. The group songwriting experience was one means of affirming their own courage and determination to give their children the stability, support and love they need.

Bridget and Andrea

A mother may sometimes request or be invited to join her child in a music therapy session or sessions. The goal again is to foster positive communication between child and parent and to help the parent become more comfortable in supporting the emotional expression of her child. Bridget was a 4-year-old girl who was having a great deal of trouble getting to sleep at night. She developed many different behaviors that delayed going to sleep, so that the getting to bed ritual was experienced as long and stressful for Bridget's mother, Andrea. Andrea relied on the hours when Bridget was asleep to do work related to her home-based business and she was becoming frustrated in that Bridget was not responding to the limits she was setting around getting up for drinks, getting out of bed, and so forth. It was my sense that Bridget was experiencing fears and anxieties that she did not know how to express to her mother and that Andrea needed help to create an environment in which Bridget felt safe enough to express her fears. Emotional expression was an area of challenge for Andrea.

Through instrumental improvisation, Bridget was encouraged to play out the sounds of a thunderstorm that had felt scary to her. Bridget was told that she could invite her mother to play with her if she wanted to. Bridget was eager to involve her mother in the music making, and she seemed to relish having her mother's full attention. Following the music, this therapist modeled questions and responses to Bridget that allowed her to say more about her fears. Given modeling, instruction and the freedom to respond differently to her daughter, Andrea became more playful and emotionally available.

Together, we planned a bedtime ritual, which included listening to songs that we recorded together prior to bedtime. Weeks later, Andrea reported that bedtime had been going much more smoothly, that the behaviors had lessened significantly, and that Bridget was getting to sleep much more quickly than before. She also mentioned that Bridget had verbalized her fear that her mother would die and that she would then be alone. Once voiced, the fear was less paralyzing for Bridget, and Andrea had a greater sense of empathy in relation to her daughter's fears. Despite her own uncertainties regarding her safety due to the unpredictable nature of her abuser, Andrea let Bridget know in a variety of ways that she was a strong and capable mother and that she had taken measures to help both of them to be safe in their home.

Conclusion

It is hoped that the stories shared within this chapter provide a window into the courage and resilience with which so many children and parents approach the recovery process following exposure to domestic violence. While more research specific to music therapy intervention with child survivors of domestic violence is needed, current music therapy literature and clinical experience point to music as a viable and effective treatment medium for these children. Relating within musical experience provides many possibilities for affirming the uniqueness of each child, for helping the child move, in his or her own way, along the road of healing and recovery from the trauma of domestic violence.

Terms

Core hurts: Psychological and emotional wounds, such as being disregarded, devalued, rejected, made to feel guilty, powerless or inadequate. These wounds can cause feelings of anger and anxiety. The motivation to avoid or numb core hurts leads to all harmful behavior (Stosny, 2001, p. 17).

Core value: An instinctual awareness of one's own self-worth which is present at birth and which leads to the expectation that one's emotional needs will be met by primary caregivers (Stosny, 2001, p. 17).

Doubling: A psychodramatic technique in which the therapist joins with the client, tuning in to and voicing the client's inner thoughts and feelings (Hoey,1997, p. 17). In musical doubling, the therapist creates music which reflects the inner emotional state of the client in order to encourage the client's own emotional expression through music, movement and/or voice.

Improvisation: Within the context of music therapy, improvising refers to the spontaneous process through which a music therapist and/or client simultaneously create and play music or sound forms (Bruscia, 1987, pp. 5-6).

Music therapy: "An interpersonal process in which the therapist uses music and all of its facets–physical, emotional, mental, social, aesthetic, and spiritual–to help clients to improve, restore or maintain health" (Bruscia, 1991, p. 5).

Object relations theory: A theoretical framework which focuses on how the child perceives or internalizes, consciously or unconsciously, the relationship between him/herself and significant others or love objects, particularly the primary care giver (Sharf, 2004, p. 37).

Phrygian mode: A scalar pattern of notes in which the second note of the scale is lowered by a half step from the diatonic scale on which most Western music is based. This shift in the scalar pattern creates greater dissonance and tension in the music.

Post-Traumatic Stress Disorder: "Extreme reactions to a highly stressful or traumatic event. . . . Resulting behaviors may include being easily startled, recurrent dreams or nightmares, or feeling estranged from or afraid of others" (Sharf, 2004, p. 629).

Psychodrama: "A form of psychotherapy in which participants enact life situations and problems in order to gain new insight, release emotion, and change previously ineffective behaviors. A variety of techniques are used to help participants explore and examine their roles from multiple points of view" (Sharf, 2004, p. 549).

Spontaneity: "An adequate response to a new situation, or the novel [and adequate] response to an old situation" (Moreno, 1993, p. 336).

Supportive mirroring: "Supportively reflecting the client's music in a way which highlights a particular aspect" (Bruscia, 1987, p. 344).

Void: "A space without categories . . . to empty old meaning in order to create a new space, which in turn is filled with new meanings" (Ruud, 1998, p. 123).

References

Austin, D. (2002). The voice of trauma: A wounded healer's perspective. In J. P. Sutton (Ed.), *Music, music therapy and trauma* (pp. 231259). Philadelphia: Jessica Kingsley Publishers Publishers.

Bannister, A. (1997). *The healing drama.* New York: Free Association Books.

Bowie, D. (1971). Changes [Recorded by Boucher, B. & Bowie, D]. On Shrek 2 [CD]. USA: EMI Music Publishing, Ltd., Tintoretto Music and Moth Music.

Bruscia, K. (1987). *Improvisational models of music therapy.* Springfield, IL Charles C Thomas, Publisher, Ltd.

Bruscia, K. (Ed.). (1991). *Case studies in music therapy.* Phoenixville, PA: Barcelona Publishers.

Cassity, M. D., & Theobold, K. A. (1990). Domestic violence: Assessments and treatments employed by music therapists. *Journal of Music Therapy, 27*(4), 179-194.

Cummings, E. M., & Davies, P. (1994). *Children and marital conflict: The impact of family dispute and resolution.* New York: Guilford Press.

Gerrard, M., Benante, B., & Lavigne, A. (2004). Breakaway [Recorded by J. Rothschild, K. Clarkson & J. Shanks]. *On Breakaway* [CD]. New York: RCA Records.

Groves, B. M. (2002). *Children who see too much.* Boston: Beacon Press.

Gruber, H. (1980). The evolving systems approach to creative scientific work: Charles Darwin's early thought. In T. Nickles (Ed.), *Scientific discovery: Case studies* (pp. 113-130). Dordrecht, Holland: D. Reidel Publishing Company.

Hernandez-Ruiz, E. (2005). Effect of music therapy on the anxiety levels and sleep patterns of abused women in shelters. *Journal of Music Therapy, 42*(2), 140-158.

Hoey, B. (1997). *Who calls the tune? A psychodramatic approach to child therapy.* New York: Routledge.

Jeffrey, L. R., & Frisone, J. D. (2003). *The PALS project: Evaluation of an intensive intervention program for children exposed to domestic violence.* Manuscript submitted for publication.

Jeffrey, L. R., Frisone, J. D., & Owens, K. A. (1999). *Evaluation of a program of comprehensive treatment services for child witnesses to domestic violence: Peace: A learned solution (PALS) project.* Summary of report given at the Fifth International Conference on Children Exposed to Family Violence, Vancouver, British Columbia.

Kaser, V. A. (1993). Musical expressions of subconscious feelings: A clinical perspective. *Music Therapy Perspectives, 11*, 16-23.

Kilcher, J., & Leonard, P. (1998). Hands. On *Spirit* [CD]. USA: Atlantic Recording Corporation.

Lavigne, A. (2002). Losing grip. On *Let Go* [CD]. New York: Artista Records.

Lennon, J., & McCartney, P. (1965). Yesterday. On *Help!* [CD]. Hollywood, CA: Capitol Records.

Lowey, J. (2000). Music psychotherapy assessment. *Music Therapy Perspectives, 18*(1), 47-58.

Moreno, J. L. (1993). *Who shall survive? Foundations of sociometry, group psychotherapy and sociodrama.* McLean, VA: American Society of Group Psychotherapy and Psychodrama.

Rossman, B. B., Hughes, H. M., & Rosenberg, M. S. (2000). *Children and interparental violence.* Philadelphia: Brunner/Mazel.

Ruud, E. (1998). Soundtracks of our life. In F. Baker & T. Wigram (Eds.), *Songwriting: Methods, techniques and clinical applications for music therapy clinicians, educators and students* (pp. 9-10). Philadelphia: Jessica Kingsley Publishers.

Sharf, R. S. (2004). *Theories of psychotherapy and counseling: Concepts and cases* (4th ed.) Belmont, CA: Thomson Brooks/Cole.

Stosny, S. (2001). *Compassionate parenting.* Germantown, MD: CompassionPower.

Stosny, S. (1995). *Compassion workshop.* Gaithersburg, MD: CompassionPower.

Sutton, J. P. (2002). *Music, music therapy and trauma.* Philadelphia: Jessica Kingsley.

Whipple, J., & Lindsey, R. S. (1999). Music for the soul: A music therapy program for battered women. *Music Therapy Perspectives, 17,* 61-68.

Biography

Amy Clarkson, MMT, MT-BC, CP, LCAT earned a Bachelor of Arts in Music Therapy from Montclair State University and a Master of Music Therapy degree from Temple University. She is a board certified music therapist and a certified practitioner of psychodrama, sociometry, and group psychotherapy. She works with child survivors of domestic violence through SAFE in Hunterdon, formerly Women's Crisis Services of Hunterdon County, New Jersey, where she helped to launch their PALS: Peace, A Learned Solution Project. Amy teaches music therapy courses and provides fieldwork supervision for the music therapy department of Montclair State University. She also serves young children who are on the autistic spectrum in an inclusive preschool setting on the campus of Montclair State. She has presented her work with child survivors of domestic violence at local, regional, and national conferences. Previous publications appear in *Music Therapy Perspectives* (2000), and in *The Journal for Psychodrama, Sociometry and Group Psychotherapy* (1993).

Chapter 10

DANCE/MOVEMENT THERAPY INTERVENTIONS IN DOMESTIC VIOLENCE: STILL A PARADIGM OF ACTION

MEG CHANG AND FERN LEVENTHAL

When the following chapter was published in the *American Journal of Dance Therapy* in 1991, it was the sole dance therapy publication about spousal/partner violence, as well as the first description in the United States of treating *Post-Traumatic Stress Disorder (PTSD)* with dance/movement therapy (Leventhal & Chang, 1991). Since then, theoretical advances and diverse treatment domains have necessitated an updating of the original article. The basic premise remains sound: dance/movement therapy is an efficacious and integrative therapy that provides a necessary body-mind intervention for those who have been subjected to physical and emotional abuse from an intimate partner. In fact, research in the psychophysiology of trauma indicates that recovery and healing is compromised unless treatment includes the body-mind component (van der Kolk, McFarlane, & Weisaeth, 1996).

This chapter provides a theoretical framework for dance/movement therapists who work with victims of intimate partner and domestic violence. Dance/movement therapy (DMT) offers a paradigm of action to address the physical and behavioral patterns of immobilization commonly found in victims of intimate partner violence, which includes same-sex partners as well as battered women. Domestic violence takes place across all races, ethnicities, ages, and social classes, as well as within genders.

The field of *intimate partner violence*–also termed *domestic violence*–now recognizes that physical or psychological abuse occurs in 25 percent to 33 percent of all same-sex intimate relationships. For gay males, intimate partner violence is acknowledged as the third largest health threat to gay men after substance abuse and HIV/AIDS (Cruz & Firestone, 1998; Island & Letellier, 1991; Peterman & Dixon, 2003). Men or women involved in violent relationships are subject to similar interpersonal dynamics of fear and dominance, shame, and isolation seen in abusive heterosexual relationships (Peterman & Dixon, 2003).

Nonetheless, women remain statistically the most likely to be affected by intimate partner violence at a rate of 1 in 6 women (Gelles, 1997, Lawson, 2003). Treatment resources such as domestic violence shelters and support groups are directed toward female clients, whether heterosexual or lesbian (Peterman & Dixon, 2003). Therefore, in this article female pronouns will primarily be used, although the information about consequences of abuse and treatment can apply to victims of any gender.

Within the gay and lesbian community, reluctance to address violence within relationships has been attributed to *homophobia* and avoidance of the issue in wider society (Peterman & Dixon, 2003; Renzetti, 1992). Such a discriminatory bias has several negative consequences for the individual seeking help. On one hand, there is denial that same-sex relationships exist in the majority culture, therefore intimate abuse is not considered or discussed. Conversely, in the gay and lesbian communities, partner abuse shatters the myth that same-sex relationships are inherently more harmonious than heterosexual ones; consequently abuse is ignored or minimized, particularly when violence takes place between female partners.

Feelings of *internalized homophobia* can occur for gay men, women, bi-sexual, or transgendered individuals, which is the "direction of societal negative attitudes toward the self" (Meyer, 1995, p. 40). In such cases, the abused believes that being mistreated confirms the worst suspicions of the dominant culture. Another factor that interferes with treatment is the absence of shelters for gay men seeking refuge from violent relationships, although some programs provide hotel vouchers. When one member of a lesbian couple seeks refuge and can be accommodated in domestic violence shelters, they are discriminated against just because the word lesbian produces fear in others. Depending on the degree of homophobia present within an agency, abuse shelters may be discriminatory toward gay men, lesbians, bi-sexual, or transgendered individuals (Peterman & Dixon, 2003).

Victims of abuse often respond to a threatening situation by entering "a state of suspended animation in which no element of the situation can change" (Martin, 1976, p. 82). The psychological concept of "learned helplessness" (Walker, 2000) aptly describes how abused persons' submissive behaviors and passive attitudes are determined by their perceptions of reality. Such perceptions affect not only a man or woman's decision to alter an abusive situation, but also the capacity to take the steps necessary to reorganize his or her life.

"Battering is a pattern of coercive control that one person exercises over another" (Schechter, 1987, p. 4). More specifically, a "battered woman is a woman who is repeatedly subjected to any forceful physical or psychological behavior by a man in order to coerce her to do something he wants her to do without any concern for her rights" (Walker, 1979, p. xv). The phenomenon of battering includes physical violence, emotional abuse, financial deprivation, or sexual coercion as means of enforcing domination. Whether heterosexual or homosexual relationships, control of the victim is established and maintained through fear and intimidation.

Physical abuse is the most obvious form of battering. It is evidenced by black eyes, bruises, and broken bones. Less obvious manifestations of physical intimidation include pushing, kicking, slapping, choking, shoving, punching, biting, and destruction of property.

Emotional abuse denotes verbal threats to kill, maim, or disable the victim. In more subtle forms of intimidation and humiliation, emotional abuse serves to undermine the self-confidence and independence of the abused. Threats against children, pets, and other family members are also common. The primary intention of the verbal interaction is to induce fear and compliance.

Sexual abuse may take the form of coercive and violent sex that force the abused partner to take part in sexual acts against his or her will. Sexual abuse is also perpetuated through verbally accusing the partner of having affairs or by the abuser having affairs, through enacting excessively jealous scenes, and by treating the partner as a sexual object (Walker, 2000). In gay and lesbian relationships, sexual abuse may also take the form of the abuser threatening to "out" the partner's sexual identity, which has multiple consequences for the victim, least of which is fear of the consequences of mainstream homophobia.

Financial abuse occurs at all socio-economic levels and all genders of intimate partnerships. Enforced by the threat of violence, economic deprivation effectively reinforces dependence on the abuser and limits residential options the victim can take on their own behalf. Economic abuse can take several forms. An economically persecuted partner may be forced to be the main financial support for the family or couple; or conversely, may be prevented from earning income, holding personal bank accounts, or having any financial responsibility.

These different types of abuse may occur separately or in combination, and a woman who is battered is likely to encounter at least three incidents a year (Gelles, 1997). Although physical abuse is the most reported type due to its obvious manifestations, it does not serve as the sole criteria of battering. "Battered women themselves are the best judges of whether or not they are being battered . . . if a woman has reason to suspect she is being battered, she probably is. If she errs in judgment at all, it is in denying or minimizing the battering relationship" (Walker, 1979, p. xiv).

Historical Perspective

Although some early human societies were female dominated, in patriarchic societies throughout recorded time, women have been regarded as men's property. Chastity belts and bound feet are historical examples of culturally approved means of controlling women's bodies. Until very recently, physical punishment for infractions of a husband's orders and desires has been legally sanctioned. The "rule of thumb"–derived from an 1824 Mississippi statute–states that a husband may "chastise his wife with a whip or rattan no bigger than my thumb, in order to enforce the salutary restraints of domestic discipline" (Calvert, 1974, p. 88). Legally, a husband's property included his wife and children. Prevailing judiciary structures legitimized an abusive man's attempts to control and penalized a battered woman's efforts to leave. For example, the act of rape has been specifically condoned within the confines of marriage since seventeenth century England. In 1993, although rape in marriage was designated as a criminal offense in all 50 states, husbands were given a special exemption from rape prosecution in 33 states; cohabitors are exempt in four states (Bergen, 1999). The legal protection relegates rape in marriage to a lesser crime, ignores the repeated nature of the offense, and minimizes the severe psychological trauma to the victim (Bergen, 1999; Harden, 1987).

Traditionally, members of the medical profession, legal system, organized religion, law enforcement, and even psychotherapy and counseling believed that "it is better to draw the curtain, shut out the public gaze, and leave the parties to forget and forgive" (Calvert, 1974, p. 88). These attitudes have been so universally accepted that it was not until the 1970s that the issue of conjugal violence became a legitimate social concern. In a similar pattern of denial, it was not until the 1990s that two accessible self-help books for gay men–*Men Who Beat the Men Who Love Them*–(Island & Letellier, 1991) and lesbian victims of intimate partner violence–*Violent Betrayal: Partner Abuse in Lesbian Relationships*–(Renzetti, 1992) brought the problem of same-sex partner violence into the open. Legal procedures for gay men and lesbians, such as attaining an Order of Protection against a violent partner, are further complicated by ignorance, homophobic reactions, and restrictions of family law (Peterman & Dixon, 2003).

The women's movement led the way in highlighting personal and social inequities in relationships between men and women. In March 1976, the National Organization for Women established a task force to address wife abuse. In 1979, psychologist Lenore Walker published *The Battered Woman*, which helped the medical and psychological community as well as the public to acknowledge the seriousness of domestic violence. Gradually, both law enforcement agencies and the judicial system began to intervene actively to protect women from domestic violence. A promising study in Minneapolis suggested that arrest and brief imprisonment was the most effective deterrence to repeated battering (Berk & Sherman, 1984). Recent research confirms anecdotal evidence from clinicians and victims of intimate partner violence that victims of intimate violence themselves are the most accurate predictors of repeated violence (Heckert & Gondolf, 2000).

Psychological Perspective

To understand the battered man or woman it is crucial to look at both intrapsychic characteristics and interpersonal behaviors. Walker's (1979, 2000) now classic conceptualization of the *Cycle Theory of Violence*, described the interactive component within the couple's violent interplay. A period of escalating interpersonal tension culminates in a violent episode. The abusive outburst is followed by a "honeymoon period" when reconciliation, calmness, or loving behaviors predominate. Once this pattern has been repeated twice, the battering cycle is established (Walker, 1979, 2000).

Unable to alter the abuser's behavior and burdened by the effects of constant aggression the victim perceives few alternatives for change or escape. Repeatedly subjected to situations in which one's actions do not reliably predict or control the violence, the abused person becomes increasingly passive and compliant. As a result a negative cognitive set is adopted regarding ones' ability to manage or alter the violence. The role of the victim is internalized and the inevitability of the abusive behavior is established. Psychological paralysis results from the process of victimization according to Walker (1979, 2000).

Efforts to place the *battered woman's syndrome* within traditional psychiatric classifications generated extensive controversy until the diagnostic category of Post Traumatic Stress Disorder (PTSD) was adopted for victims of intimate partner violence (Walker, 1989). Post Traumatic Stress Disorder emphasizes psychosocial stresses rather than individual psychopathology (Galliano & Nichols, 1988; Walker, 1991). The essential feature of PTSD for victims of intimate partner violence is the occurrence of an extreme and life-threatening event in which danger to one's physical integrity or sense of human coherence is directly experienced. This event is commonly re-experienced by distressing recollections or dreams and dissociative states in which the abusive event is relived. Symbolic aspects of the event may trigger intense psychological distress. Responsiveness to the external world is usually marked by feelings of detachment, restricted affect, an overall sense of foreboding, and/or an avoidance of stimuli associated with the trauma, which may lead to impairment in social, work, or family functioning. Lastly, this disorder can be characterized by persistent symptoms such as insomnia, hyper-vigilance, irritability, difficulty concentrating, or "psychic numbing" (APA, 2000, pp. 463–464).

Being both somatic and psychic, *dissociation* allows the victim to encapsulate the persistent fear and hopelessness and reinforces the tendency toward denial, inaction, and magical thinking. During repeated incidents of abuse, physical sensation becomes blunted and restricted, consistent with PTSD symptomatology (Walker, 1979; van der Kolk et al., 1996). Victims of repetitive trauma develop an ability to cut off the physical sensations of pain during an attack and perceive themselves as objects at the mercy of the abuser. Unable to control the violence or defend against it, psychophysical detachment becomes routine. Feelings of love and affection for the abuser are split off from other intensely negative emotions (Paley, 1988). Unwanted emotions, such as anger, rage, sadness, and loss, are disowned and projected onto the abuser (Gillman, 1980). By assigning anger and aggression to the abuser, expression of such feelings by the victim are ignored, minimized, and projected.

The victim begins to fear and accept the abuser as strong, powerful, and all-knowing, compared to whom the victim feels incompetent, weak, and ineffective. The loss of an integrated, autonomous self, in the context of unpredictable violence, leads to feelings of *helplessness.* According to Maccoby and Jacklin (1974), "the possibility exists that females show immobilization and other 'passive' behavior primarily when they are afraid" (quotations in original) (Maccoby & Jacklin, p. 167). "In contrast to their dreams, in which they actively attempted to protect themselves, the waking lives of these women were characterized by overwhelming passivity and inability to act" (Hilberman, 1980, p. 1341).

Ambivalence, another factor in the psyche of battered women and men, is experienced as indecision about whether to stay or to leave the battering relationship (Rounsaville, Lifton, & Bieber, 1979). The victim of domestic violence is often isolated by the abuse and begins to accept the abuser's depiction of being worthless, stupid, ugly, or undesirable. A distorted, negative self-image develops and as self-esteem is undermined, the ability to make autonomous decisions declines. The dearth of socio-economic resources that are available to women on their own is a practical consideration which underscores the difficulty of leaving (NiCarthy, 1982).

In addition, when one or both of the partners is a *person of color* or an immigrant, ambivalence takes on a sociocultural valence. Feelings of solidarity and need to stand together against the forces of racial and ethnic discrimination within African-American, Asian-American, Native-American, and Spanish-speaking communities often make it difficult for victims of domestic violence to speak out against their abuser. A prevailing attitude is that people of color have been victimized and brutalized by institutional racism, which is often perpetuated by law enforcement or social service agencies (Artichoker & Gullickson, 2003; Sen, 1999). For immigrants, the decision to invoke the law is further conflicted by realist fears of deportation or other legal sanctions against either the victim or the abuser simply by calling attention to their presence (Sen, 1999).

Isolation may also be induced by the abuser's pathological jealousy, which serves to quarantine the woman from even casual contacts (Walker, 1979). In addition, the battered woman's traditional network of support disintegrates as the abusive situation intensifies. Traditional family values may lead family members to urge the woman to "stay and work it out." Scared of involvement, frightened of the physical violence, or in the case of immigrant communities a reluctance to endanger citizenship status, friends and family withdraw their vital sources of nourishment and confirmation.

The picture that emerges is one of an isolated, fearful, immobilized, and ambivalent victim. Lacking confidence in the ability to change the dangerous situation in any substantive manner, victims of interpersonal violence feel helpless and powerless. Social seclusion further tips the balance of power in the relationship. This permits the abuser's violent threats or behaviors to continue without interference. The perpetuation of the cycle of violence increases the victim's belief that they have little control over life events. Such dependence and loss of control may be reinforced by the social institutions-law enforcement authorities, the legal system, or welfare agencies, all of which may be ineffective, unresponsive, or disbelieving–especially in the case of same-sex violence–to the victim's needs (Peterman & Dixon, 2003; Renzetti, 1992; Schecter, 1987).

Intervention

Dance, as a short-term or in-depth psychotherapy intervention, mobilizes physical, cognitive, and emotional aspects of the individual. Creative movement supports simultaneous exploration on both concrete and symbolic levels that are needed for this population's dual practical and psychological needs. Because dance/movement therapy can be applied within a wide range of theoretical approaches it provides an approach that can operate conjunctively and cooperatively with other paradigms present in clinical settings.

The correlation between physical movement and psychological dynamics is a basic tenet of dance/movement therapy. An assumption underlying both assessment and treatment is "that body movements reflect such personality characteristics as ego strength, maturity, capacity and range of affect, flexibility and ability to relate to others" (White & Schmais, 1974, p. 25). An explicit goal of dance/movement therapists is to:

> integrate the body and the mind through the use of action techniques and projective psychological methods. One concept . . . is the belief that involving the body and musculature in the therapeutic process evokes unconscious psychological material and deeply held emotions. (Levy, 1988, p. 12)

In dance/movement therapy, the creative experience of dancing has as much significance as the resulting dance form. "Because the materials of art are derived from reality, the integration of thought, feeling and action which is present in a dance has a direct relationship with life itself and the life of the creator" (H'Doubler, 1940, p. 166). As the unconscious material is brought to conscious engagement via dance, movement, or body awareness, it can be structured so as to "bring about deeper psychophysical awareness, catharsis, and possibly insight" (Levy, 1988, p. 12). Dance/movement therapy evokes symbolic representation of unconscious images as well as illustrates cognitive beliefs. Once thoughts and feelings are "structurally represented, an idea or emotion can be apprehended, contemplated, analyzed or connected to other symbolic material. The symbol can shed light on old issues, articulate current concerns and anticipate the future" (Schmais, 1985, p. 34).

To make personal and life changes of the magnitude required of victims of domestic violence, an alteration of one's external actions needs to take place concomitantly with modifications of internal perceptions. As described by Edward T. Hall, "when behavior changes, perception changes, and when perception changes, then insight results" (Davis, 1978, p. 38); elucidates the process of an action-oriented intervention.

Dance/movement therapy methods of *externalization* and *physicalization* (Evan, 1991; Mettler, 1990) are *creative dance* mechanisms through which behavior, perception, and insight interface. *Externalization* is a dance or movement process that makes internal feelings or sensations tangible. *Physicalization* is specifically putting an idea into action at the body level, which brings complex internal states into awareness. Such somatic awareness lays a psychophysical foundation for insight. The ability to embody independent actions and take ownership of the conscious choice to move is a matter of vital importance to victims of abuse who have previously been immobilized and cut-off from bodily sensations.

Whereas, therapeutic change can be assessed by alterations in: mobility, perceptions, patterns of behavior and interaction, the effectiveness of intervention is ultimately measured by observable changes in a victim's life. When the battered man or woman's self-deprecation is replaced by self-esteem, positive steps such as returning to school or seeking more rewarding employment may result. The survivor of violence may be able to leave the abusive situation or remain in the relationship with assurance of increased safety and the means to mitigate the abuse. Research has confirmed (Heckert

& Gondolf, 2000) that only the person in the relationship can judge the best and safest action to take.

Beginning Treatment

Intrapsychic change is desirable; yet, not always feasible with a population that is by necessity seeking immediate solutions. A short-term, psychosocial plan of dance/movement therapy intervention addresses primary concerns of immobilization and isolation. Battered women can receive dance/movement therapy in shelters where the immediate survival needs of the client predominate. In on-going groups or individual treatment, personal issues evoked by the battering experience can be addressed through a more long-term, insight-oriented approach that addresses the victim's coping style. Intrapsychic considerations of autonomy and individuation, self-esteem, and distortions of reality can be explored through targeted dance directives, some of which will be described later in the chapter. A psychodynamically oriented dance/movement treatment plan augments the initial, short-term crisis intervention, and leads to substantive alteration in patterns of victimization.

Breaking the self-imposed or social isolation is an initial consideration. It is crucial that a victim's first contact reinforce the fact that she is not alone in her distress. Thus, group treatment, because it promotes social interaction and interpersonal learning (Yalom, 1975), has traditionally been the method of choice. Often disconnected from friends and family by the abuser, a woman benefits from hearing the experiences of others. Indeed, "the realization that their situation is not uncommon reduces their shame and feelings of personal inadequacy, and the group setting reduces the social isolation which compounds the depression and feelings of helplessness characteristic of these women" (Lewis, 1983, p. 56).

Introducing Elements of Dance/Movement

Direct involvement of physical movement with others, clarified by the dance therapist's interventions, challenges psychophysical distortions, and provides immediate feedback to the client. Pragmatic solutions to life problems are explored through guided exercises and movement metaphors. With skills that are distinctive to dance/movement therapists, a client can be guided to embody his or her specific physical characteristics, become aligned with actual body image, and physicalize life options, sources of emotional support, or vocational resources. DMT with victims of trauma can be used to lessen magical thinking, establish boundaries, and make reality confrontations where necessary.

For example, "reaching for what you want" not only defines the actual physical boundary of a person's arms, but also stimulates thinking about improved life options. Using this phrase as a directive led one battered woman to fantasize escaping from her financially and physically abusive boyfriend. She had often spoken to the group about her desire to end the relationship; yet, was unable to do so. As she reached toward the open window, the movement spontaneously developed into her "wanting wings to fly away." It became obvious to both her and the dance/movement therapist that this was not physically possible, as the client's arms tired quickly and she remained fixed to the floor. After discussing more effective options, the client decided to alter her work schedule so that she would be less available to the abuser. Creative movement behavior sensitized her to perceive her physical limitations from which insight developed into realistic planning of how she could establish safer boundaries.

Dance/movement therapy process expands the victim of trauma's *range of motion*, leading to increased physical activity, which can be generalized to increased interaction. Living in an abusive and constrained relationship leads to a limited coping style characterized by a person's restricted use of space, minimal movements, and over-controlled body action (Bartky, 1980; Gray, 2001). Expanding a client's movement repertoire is directly linked to changes in self-concept and interpersonal dynamics (North, 1972). For example, in a dyadic movement or dance exercise, a battered woman is often surprised by her own strength when she is encouraged to push against a partner. Experiencing her muscular strength in a safe and controlled situation, she experiences concordance with the therapist's observation that she is not such a "pushover" as she thought. This enables her to interact more assertively with the important figures in her world. Bartky (1980, p. 135) confirms that "without the active use of weight, there is little hope that these women will ever be able to stand up for themselves."

Exploring the *use of space* is another way of altering self-perception. One emotionally abused woman, an academic administrator, discovered her own link between action and insight as she used the space around her in an expansive movement. She experienced this improvisational movement as "freeing" when she changed her habitually restricted posture. As she raised her arms over her head in full extension, she stated, "I'm stretching towards a new life." This is an example of the DMT theory that "changes often occur in movement before they occur in other areas"(Schmais, 1974, p. 11). After moving, the client talked about interests that had been dormant during her marriage and made plans to contact former colleagues. This woman's small; yet, realistic change should not be minimized. It is through manageable, progressive steps that a victim of intimate partner violence can raise self-esteem and reduce feelings of helplessness.

Encouraging feelings of cohesion and safety while maintaining self-identity and sense of agency can be easily demonstrated in DMT, which occurred in a staff group at a battered women's shelter, where many of the staff were former battered women. Each woman was asked to develop a full-body movement phrase that felt relevant and comfortable. They were then directed to one-by-one form a whole, with the option to make physical contact, until they were all moving together in a cohesive *kinetic group machine.* Asked to retain the central core of their own movements, group members were reminded to pay attention to how they adapted their own original phrases in order to accommodate the larger group whole. Within this structured framework, the members experienced unity with others while simultaneously preserving their individuality.

Psychodynamic Development

Battered women come to treatment with hopes for immediate change. However, crisis intervention alone does not assure permanent change. Women, particularly those who have other mental health problems in addition to Post Traumatic Stress Disorder, may require a long-term approach (Lawson, 2003; Walker, 1991). Clients, who have been traumatized by long standing histories of physical abuse, sexual abuse, or neglect by their family of origin, are especially at risk (Herman & Schatzow, 1984; Rosenthal, 1988, Snyder & Fruchtman, 1981). As with all victims of trauma, a basic level of trust in oneself, intimate relationships, and the environment has been lost. No longer in immediately dangerous situations, survivors of trauma may still be absorbed with prior injury, a negative self-image, and the need to guard against further harm. For this group of clients, there is a need to help them internalize a positive body image and subsequently change their self-concept. A safely mediated experiential approach, with emphasis on body awareness and personalized movement, is a natural medium to promote in-depth psychological change.

Abused clients move through stages of growth, demonstrating varied needs and treatment strategies as the therapy progresses (Gray, 2001; Huston, 1984). Although an initially supportive therapeutic stance is recommended, the importance of the domestic violence victim's increased independence and autonomous functioning must be recognized and validated within the therapeutic relationship. The dance/movement therapy technique of *mirroring* can be used to establish initial trust, to promote a therapeutic alliance, and to support clients with weak ego functioning (Levy, 1988). Analogous psychotherapy theories are person-centered and Gestalt therapy, in which the therapist encourages the client to direct the session (Peterman

& Dixon, 2003). Care must be taken not to reinforce dependency on the leader and undermine the client's autonomous initiation; rather, independent dance/movement interventions are advised. "Victims of violence need to be encouraged to take control of their lives, and learning to share control of their therapy is a beginning step toward that goal" (Walker, 1989, p. 701). Though the therapist has a responsibility to provide the tools and information needed to change the client's situation, insistence on a particular course of action reinforces passivity (Bowen, 1982). A victim of partner violence needs to generate options, assess alternatives, and seek personalized solutions. All of these can be creatively embodied.

A creative movement process that unites victims of violence around a common action theme can reduce self-blame and decrease alienation. For example, in a co-led group with a dance/movement therapist and a playwright, the residents of a domestic violence enacted the Harriet Tubman story, which was well-known to the African-American clients. Ms. Tubman escaped slavery as well as an abusive husband and became one of the legendary "conductors" on the Underground Railroad during slavery. The battered women incorporated elements of her legend into their own personal stories. They danced and discussed their own long and arduous journeys from abuse to safety.

The inventiveness and activity inherent in dance/movement therapy can replace ingrained habits of immobilization. Cognitive patterns of self-denigrating rumination and rigid thinking dominate the victim's thought processes. For these clients "taking a step forward" is much more than a figure of speech. Accustomed to passivity and immobilization, taking a step in any direction can be frustratingly difficult and even unimaginable. As a victim of intimate violence is helped to experiment with a variation of "steps," they begin to see themselves as capable of action. One woman in a short-term group described how she responded when arguing with her female lover. "Something happens to me when she starts yelling at me. I know I should just get up and leave, but my feet are frozen." This *movement metaphor* was a symbolic representation of her immobility. The client was encouraged to *externalize* through a movement directive based on non-verbal observation of her tension level. Once the physical sensation of frozenness was experienced through the client's movement, her breath became deeper and her muscle tone relaxed.

Even when the immediate danger has been reduced, the dissociation, and *depersonalization* that are commonly reported responses to life-threatening abuse may continue. This depersonalization is a protective defense that remains in the muscles and the psyche. An abused person can be helped to re-inhabit his or her body through gradually building tolerance to the physical and emotional sensations that were previously disowned. For example, sensitization to the breathing process can help a client monitor how his or her breath rate is altered by both thoughts and external situations (Saltonstall, 1988). If the client has disowned or minimized their instinctive reactions to fear or anger, this type of exercise can help them more accurately distinguish between present danger and old fears. Learning to trust one's own instincts and perceptions is supported by learning specific techniques. Focusing on the breath is a way to bring the client back to the present while exploring the fears of the past.

However, in the following example, a leader's suggestion to try a simple breathing and relaxation exercise had an unexpected outcome of triggering images and memories of powerlessness. A support group of battered women, not currently in life-threatening situations, were complaining of anxiety and insomnia. The leader asked them to close their eyes and begin to breathe deeply. Within minutes, one woman stated that she felt panicked. Another woman described her inability to ride the subway; a third revealed that on many days she felt unable to leave her apartment. Sensing the group's mounting anxieties, the leader suggested that group members focus on their surroundings, notice the presence of others, feel the temperature of the air against their skin, and sense the chair under them. In the discussion that ensued, the women openly shared strategies for managing their perceived "weaknesses." A higher level of functioning was supported by verbally processing the non-verbal experience and emphasizing a *here and now* orientation.

It is important to help the client experience a continuum of physical and emotional sensation without becoming overwhelmed by feelings and defending. The dance therapist needs to be aware that relaxation exercises or cathartic movement designed to put an individual in touch with repressed emotions may reactivate overwhelming feelings of rage or powerlessness. The trauma victim's unexpressed feelings of explosiveness may be associated with the abuser's acts of violence. Likewise, the intensity of indulgent sensations may evoke negative connotations of engulfment, loss of autonomy, helplessness, and shame. "When the work is deep, each experiential phase may uncover another layer of experience or aspect of self, often for the first time in a recognizable form. Time should be allowed between phases for quiet and natural integration of what has gone on before" (Mackay, 1989, p. 300). It is therefore imperative that the client determines the pacing and intensity of the non-verbal experience. By gradual expression of feelings the victim reconnects to somatic sensation and so gains control of his or her internal processes and sense of latent strength.

Female clients who have become conditioned to rigid modes of relating may react to the dance/movement therapist's movement directives with either compliance or rebellion.

> The one area over which the battered woman does have total control is that of her body . . . it is important for her to begin to build self-esteem and sense of power through body exercise. It is also important to help the battered woman recognize and control her anger. She should be encouraged to experience anger each time it occurs . . . she needs to be taught to feel her anger, control it, and utilize it. (Walker, 1979, pp. 238–239)

When expressing anger, the dance therapist needs to be mindful of how movement directives are worded, as illustrated in the following vignette from a dance/movement therapy session in a domestic violence shelter. At first, the dance therapist reflected the group movement and said "let's just kick him away." Obediently the group made a few explosive movements that quickly diminished into unfocused, peripheral gestures. However when told to "just make noise with your feet and legs and use all the space in the room," exuberant movement and spontaneous group rhythm emerged. The second set of movement directives allowed each woman to express her own version of strength without feeling subtly coerced by the leader's expectations.

Incorporating a DMT approach that encourages self-directed action not only defuses the charged issues surrounding control but also taps sources of individual choice and creativity that reinforce autonomy. While improvising in dance, a survivor of violence creates personal metaphors and makes meaningful connections between dance and life. However, as seen in the example above, premature interpretation of symbolic and non-verbal communication are ". . . liable to foreclose individual process" (Mackay, 1989, p. 300). Open-ended dance directives–i.e., exploring movement polarities such as near and far, quickly and slowly, etc.–stimulate individuality even within the support of the group setting. As the client responds, without superimposed movement from the therapist or group, individual resources are contacted, which in turn generates a personal "route to change" (Blanche Evan, personal communication DMT training class, October, 1982).

Relationship in Treatment

When treating trauma survivors in either short-term or long-term settings, the therapist needs to recognize the influence of his or her preconceptions, associations, and fantasies. Countertransference is a "trap" (Chu, 1988) that diminishes the effectiveness of the treatment and fuels therapist burnout. Identification with the victim can lead to a merging and blurring of the boundaries between client and therapist. Therapists with rescue fantasies may direct clients toward premature or inappropriate decisions. Involvement in power struggles may reenact the abusive relationship, stimulating hostility or dependency. Avoidance of trauma victims' anger and rage can immobilize both therapist and clients. The following vignette demonstrates several countertransferential elements.

Jane, a lawyer, bitterly recanted her history of abuse during a battered woman's support group. Her hostile demeanor and angry diatribe was accompanied by a lack of visible breathing, muscular rigidity, and strong, intense jabs with her hands. "How can I get rid of my anger at my ex-husband? He ruined my life, running up thousands of dollars of debt. . . . I had cancer when I was pregnant. . . . I feel like my life is a deck of cards that could fall apart if any one part is touched." Jane's story was an especially dramatic one. The therapist's impulse was to rescue the client and to resolve her problems quickly. In an attempt to pacify the client by gratifying her desire to "get rid of my anger," the therapist suggested a walking warm-up that "might begin with a little kick." Jane grew uncomfortable, increasingly tense, and even found walking difficult. Unable to mobilize at the therapist's suggestion, Jane demanded, "How do I bend my knees?"

The therapist, intimidated by the client's hostile tone and defensive posture, was surprised to find herself immobilized. Like the client, the therapist was unable to move her legs or bend her knees. Shifting her attention to movement cues from another more responsive group member, the therapist suggested a dancer strategy, "use your whole foot when you walk." Jane responded by retracting her toes, locking her jaw, and eventually sat silently for the remainder of the session. She did not return for future treatment. Feeling attacked, the therapist felt helpless, blocked, and was not able to assist the client with effective movement interventions. The therapist's inability to successfully monitor her countertransference prevented her from connecting to the client's affect, and both lost confidence in the dance/movement process.

With repeated validation, the victims of interpersonal violence can perceive themselves to be capable of action, achievement, and love. "[they] may be able to accept superficially that they are people of worth, but it takes positive experiences over time for them to internalize this concept" (Ibrahim & Herr, 1987). Dance/movement therapy uses a physical, action-oriented approach to address the trauma victim's practical needs while concurrently attending to psychological concerns. Thus, dance/movement therapy promotes psychodynamic growth while supplying a needed dynamic–the ability to move.

Conclusion

This chapter highlights the contributions that dance/movement therapy can make to the treatment of battered women. Dance/movement interventions help a victim of trauma internalize a positive self-concept as well as gain physical and emotional control. Interacting through dance can resurface feelings of openness and child-like powerfulness that are frequently repressed by those burdened by intimate partner violence. With the support of the therapist and other group members, victims of intimate violence can invent, enact, and incorporate desired change. By motivating victims of domestic violence to act, dance/movement therapy addresses patterns of helplessness, ambivalence, and inactivity.

References

American Psychiatric Association. (2000). *Diagnostic and statistical manual of mental disorders-IV-TR* (4th ed.). Washington, D.C.: Author.

Artichoker, K., & Gullickson, V. (2003). *Raising public awareness of domestic violence in Indian country.* (Available from the National Resource Center on Domestic Violence, 6400 Flank Drive, Suite 1300, Harrisburg, PA 17112-2791.)

Bartky, C. (1980). *A comparison of the movement profiles of battered, ex-battered, and non-battered women: A pilot study.* Unpublished master's thesis, Drexel University Hahnemann Medical College, Philadelphia.

Bergen, R. (1999, March). Marital rape. *VAWnet: National Resource Center on Domestic Violence.* Retrieved March 15, 2007, from http://www.vawnet.org/DomesticViolence/Research/VAWnetDocs/AR_mrape.pdf

Berk, R, & Sherman, L. (1984). *The Minneapolis domestic violence experiment.* Washington, D.C.: The Police Foundation.

Bowen, N. (1982). Guidelines for career counseling with abused women. *The Vocation Guidance Quarterly, December,* 123-127.

Calvert, R. (1974). Criminal and civil liability in husband-wife assaults. In S. K. Steinmetz & M. A. Straus (Eds.), *Violence in the family.* New York: Harper and Row.

Chu, J. (1988; December). Ten traps for therapists in the treatment of trauma survivors. *Dissociation, 1*(4), 24-32. Retrieved February 1, 2007 from http://hdl.handle.net/1794/1393

Cruz, M. J., & Firestone, J. M. (1998). Exploring violence and abuse in gay male relationships. *Violence and Victims, 13*(2), 159-173.

Davis, M. (1978). An interview with Edward T. Hall. *Kinesis, 1*(1), 6-15.

Evan, B. (1991). *Collected works by and about Blanche Evan.* San Francisco: Anne Krantz, Blanche Evan Dance Foundation.

Gelles, R. J. (1997). *Intimate violence in families* (3rd ed.). Thousand Oaks, CA: Sage.

Galliano, G., & Nichols, M. (1988). Mental health professional as expert witness. *Journal of Interpersonal Violence, 3*(1), 29-41.

Gillman, I. (1980). An object-relations approach to the phenomenon and treatment of battered women. *Psychiatry, 43,* 346-358.

Gray, A. E. (2001). The body remembers: Dance/movement therapy with an adult survivor of torture. *American Journal of Dance Therapy, 23*(1), 29-43.

Harden, J. C. (1987). Marital rape: Drive for tougher laws is pressed. *New York Times,* May 13, p. A16.

H'Doubler, M. N. (1940). *Dance: A creative art experience.* Madison: University of Wisconsin.

Heckert, D. A., & Gondolf, E. (2004). Battered women's perceptions of risk versus risk factors and instruments in predicting repeat reassault. *Journal of Interpersonal Violence, 19,* 778-800.

Herman, J., & Schatzow, E. (1984). Time-limited group therapy for women with a history of incest. *International Journal of Group Psychotherapy, 34*(4), 605-616.

Hilberman, E. (1980). Overview: The "wife-beater's wife" reconsidered. *American Journal of Psychiatry, 137*(11), 1336-1347.

Huston, K. (1984). Ethical decisions in treating battered woman. *Professional Psychology: Research and Practice, 16*(6), 822-832.

Ibrahim, F. A., & Herr, E. L. (1987). Battered women: A developmental life-career counseling perspective. *Journal of Counseling & Development, 65*, 244-248.

Island, D., & Letellier, P. (1991). *Men who beat the men who love the: Battered gay men and domestic violence.* Binghamton, NY: Haworth.

Lawson, D. M. (2003). Incidence, explanations, and treatment of partner violence. *Journal of Counseling & Development, 81*(1), 19-33.

Leventhal, F., & Chang, M. H. (1991). Dance/movement therapy with battered women: A paradigm of action. *American Journal of Dance Therapy, 13*(2), 131-145.

Lewis, E. (1983). The group treatment of battered women. *Women and Therapy, 2*(1), 51-58.

Levy, F. (1988). *Dance/movement therapy: A healing art.* Reston, VA: The American Alliance for Health, Physical Education, and Dance.

Maccoby, E. E., & Jacklin, C. N. (1974). *The psychology of sex differences.* Palo Alto, CA: Stanford.

Mackay, B. (1989). Drama therapy with female victims of assault. *The Arts in Psychotherapy, 16*, 293-300.

Martin, D. (1976). *Battered wives.* New York: Pocket Books.

Mettler, B. (1990). Creative dance--art or therapy. *American Journal of Dance Therapy, 12*(2), 95-100.

Meyer, I. (1995). Minority stress and mental health in gay men. *Journal of Health and Social Behavior, 36*(1), 38-56.

NiCarthy, G. (1982). *Getting free: A handbook for women in abusive relationships.* Seattle: The Seal Press.

North, M. (1972). *Personality assessment through movement.* Boston: Plays, Inc.

Paley, A. N. (1988). Growing up in chaos: The dissociative response. *American Journal of Psychoanalysis, 48*(1), 72-83.

Peterman, L., & Dixon, C. (2003). Domestic violence between same-sex partners: Implications for counseling. *Journal of Counseling & Development. 81*(1), 40-48.

Renzetti, C. M. (1992). *Violent betrayal: Partner abuse in lesbian relationships.* Newbury Park, CA: Sage.

Rosenthal, K. (1988). The inanimate self in adult victims of child abuse and neglect. *Social Casework: The Journal of Contemporary Social Work*, Oct., 505-510.

Rounsaville, B., Lifton, N., & Bieber, M. (1979). The natural history of a psychotherapy group for battered women. *Psychiatry, 42*, 63-78.

Saltonstall, E. (1988). *Kinetic awareness: Discovering your bodymind.* New York: Publishing Center for Cultural Resources.

Schechter, S. (1987). *Guidelines for mental health practitioners in domestic violence cases.* Washington, D.C.: National Coalition Against Domestic Violence.

Schmais, C. (1974). Dance therapy in perspective. In K. Mason (Ed.), *Focus on dance VII: Dance therapy.* Reston, VA: AAHPERD.

Schmais, C. (1985). Healing processes in group dance therapy. *American Journal of Dance Therapy, 8*, 17-36.

Sen, R. (1999, Spring). Between a rock and a hard place: Domestic violence in communities of color. *Colorlines, 2*:1. Retrieved March 10, 2007, from http://www.colorlines.com

Snyder, D. K., & Fruchtman, L. A. (1981). Differential patterns of wife abuse: A data-based typology. *Journal of Consulting and Clinical Psychology, 49*(6), 878-885.

van der Kolk, B. A., McFarlane, A. C., & Weisaeth, L. (Eds.). (1996). *Traumatic stress: The effects of overwhelming experience on mind, body, and society.* New York: Guilford Press.

Walker, L. (1979). *The battered woman.* New York: Harper and Row.
Walker, L. (1989). Psychology and violence against women. *American Psychologist, 44*(4), 695-702.
Walker, L. E. (1991). Post Traumatic Stress Disorder in women: Diagnosis and treatment of battered woman syndrome. *Psychotherapy, 28*(1), 21-29.
Walker, L. (2000). *The battered woman syndrome.* (2nd ed.) New York: Springer.
White, E., & Schmais, C. (1974). Training for dance therapists: An experimental masters program at Hunter College. *Monographs of the American Dance Therapy Association*, 23-36.
Yalom, I. D. (1975). *The theory and practice of group psychotherapy.* New York: Basic Books.

Biography

Meg Chang, Ed.D., LCAT, NCC, ADTR has worked as a dance-movement therapist in psychiatric facilities, medical and wellness settings, Domestic Violence support groups, and private practice. Publications include, Mobilizing Battered Women: A Creative Step Forward, in Fran Levy (1995) *Dance and Other Expressive Art Therapies*, and How do dance/movement therapists bring awareness of race, ethnicity, and cultural diversity into their practice? in S. Koch & I. Bräuninger (2006) *Advances in Dance/Movement Therapy. Theoretical perspectives and empirical findings.* On faculty of graduate dance therapy programs including the Creative Arts Therapy Certificate Program at the New School University, New York City and the School of Education, Northern State University, South Dakota. Presented numerous DMT workshops and Mindfulness-Based Stress Reduction classes in Europe and East Asia. Formerly on staff at the Stress Reduction Clinic, University of Massachusetts Medical Center, now a Mindfulness-Based Stress Reduction consultant to hospitals and organizations. A life-long dancer, current focus is intercultural praxis of dance as healing.

Fern Leventhal, Ph.D. is a clinical neuropsychologist at New York State Psychiatric Institute as well as an assistant clinical professor of medical psychology at Columbia University. Her responsibilities include the neuropsychological assessment of adults and adolescents as well as the training of psychology interns, medical students, and psychiatric residents. In addition, Doctor Leventhal maintains a private practice in Westchester County, specializing in pediatric assessment. Her educational history includes a BA from Washington University in St. Louis, Missouri, a MA in Dance Therapy from New York University, and a PhD in Psychology from Teacher's College, Columbia University. As a dance therapist, Doctor Leventhal co-edited a book on clinical issues in the creative arts therapies and co-authored an article with Doctor Chang. She has more recently worked with other professionals to write a chapter on autistic spectrum disorders, author a book on ADHD, and publish several articles in areas of neuropsychology.

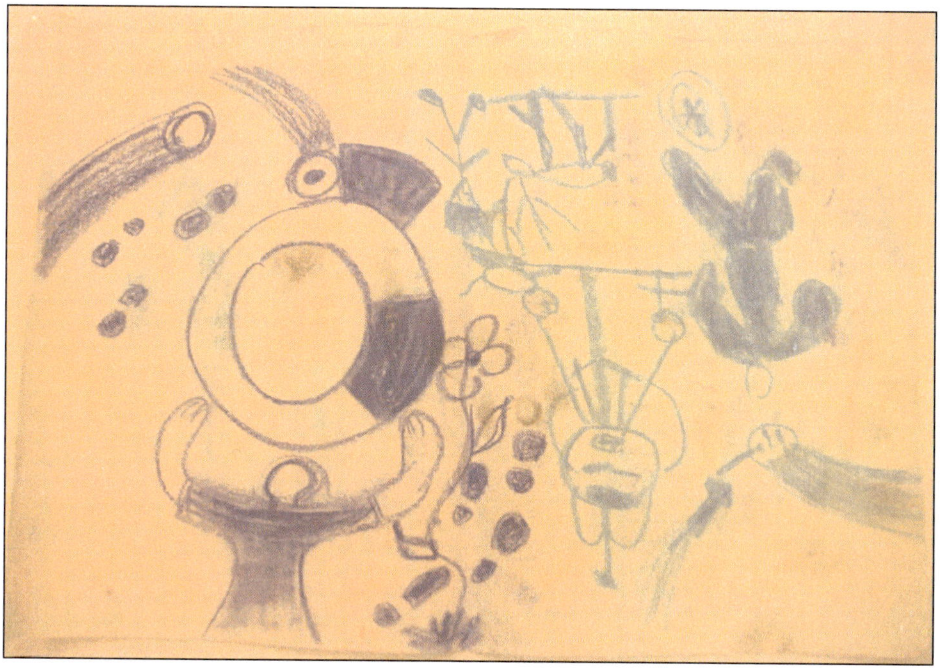

Plate 1. Dual Drawing.

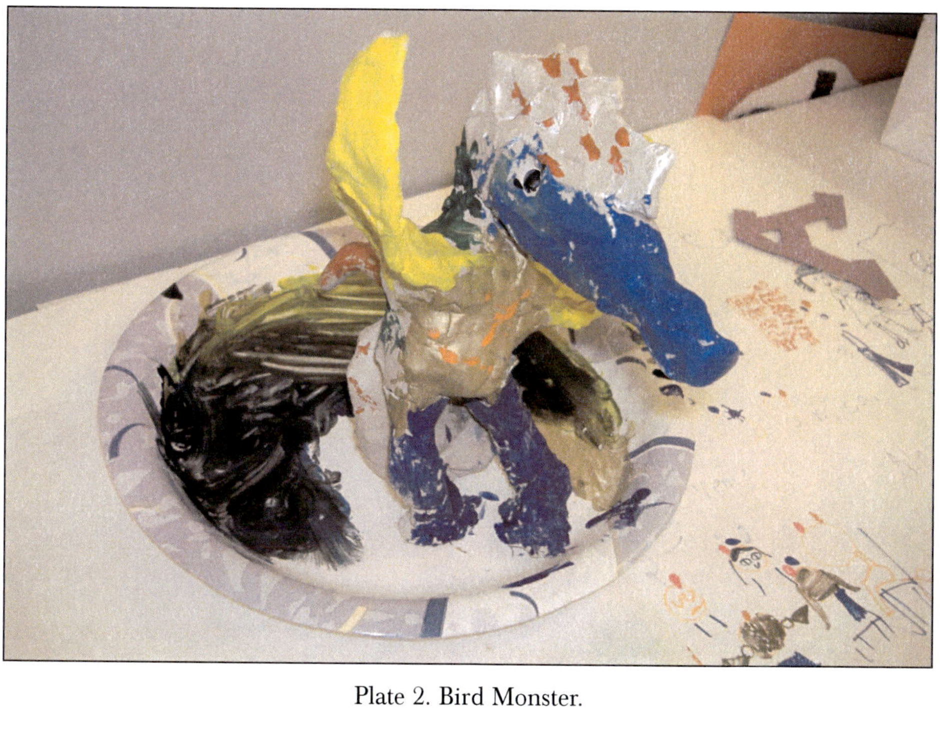

Plate 2. Bird Monster.

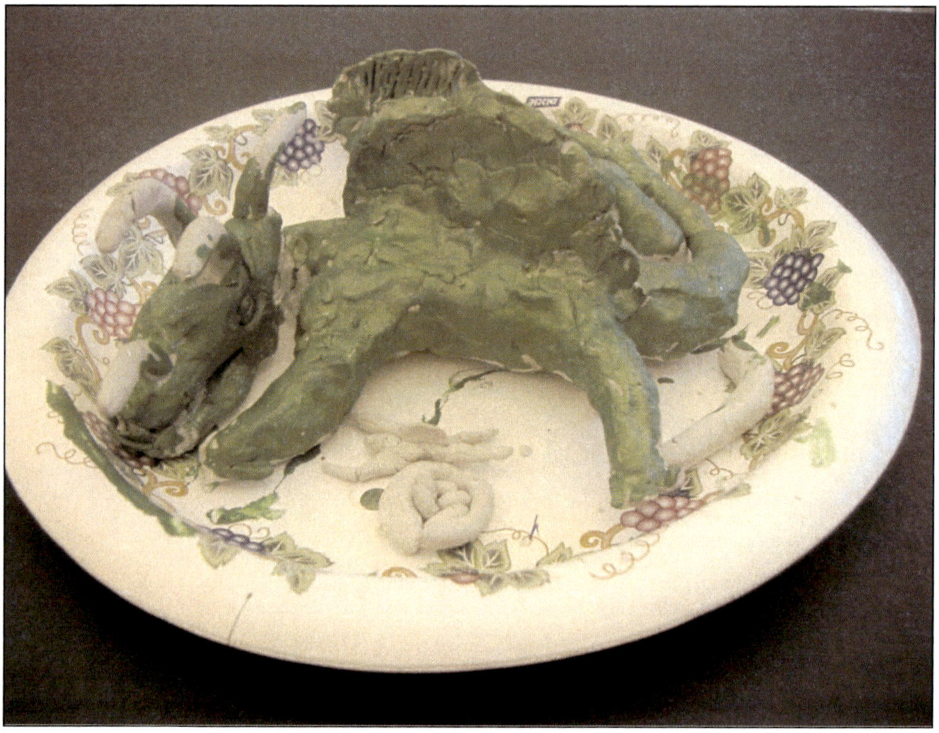

Plate 3. Horn Lizard.

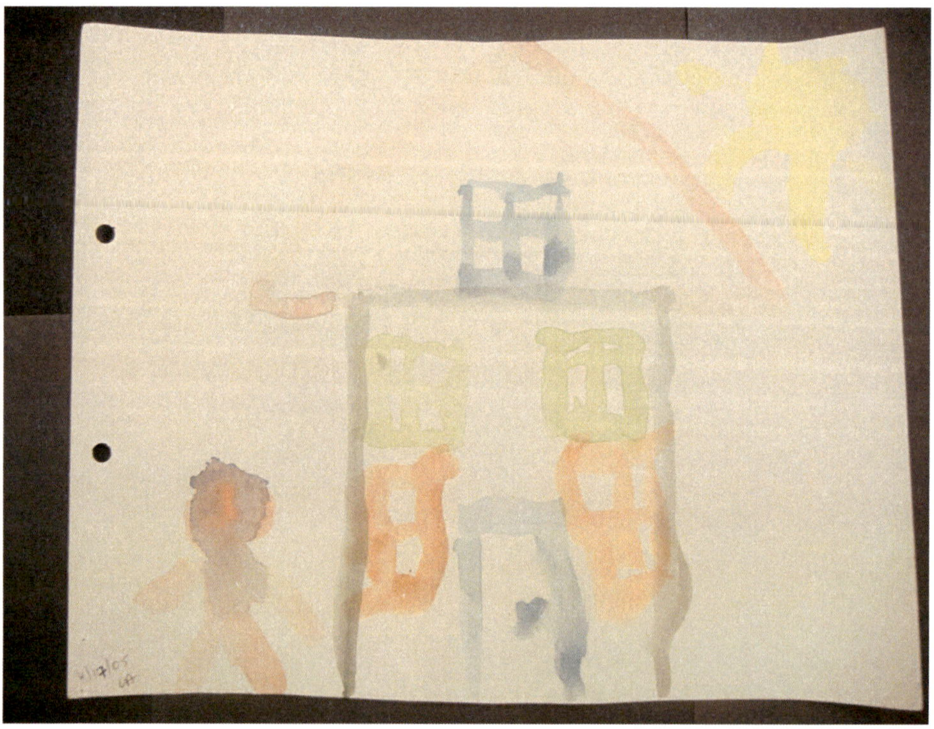

Plate 4. Watercolor House.

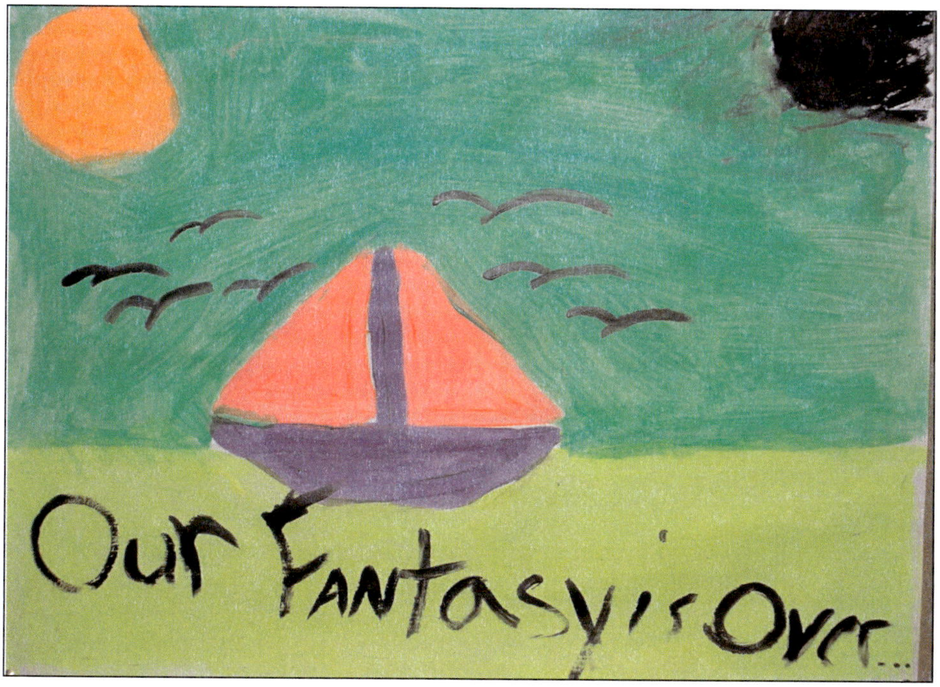

Plate 5. Painting created by 11-year-old boy in PALS program.

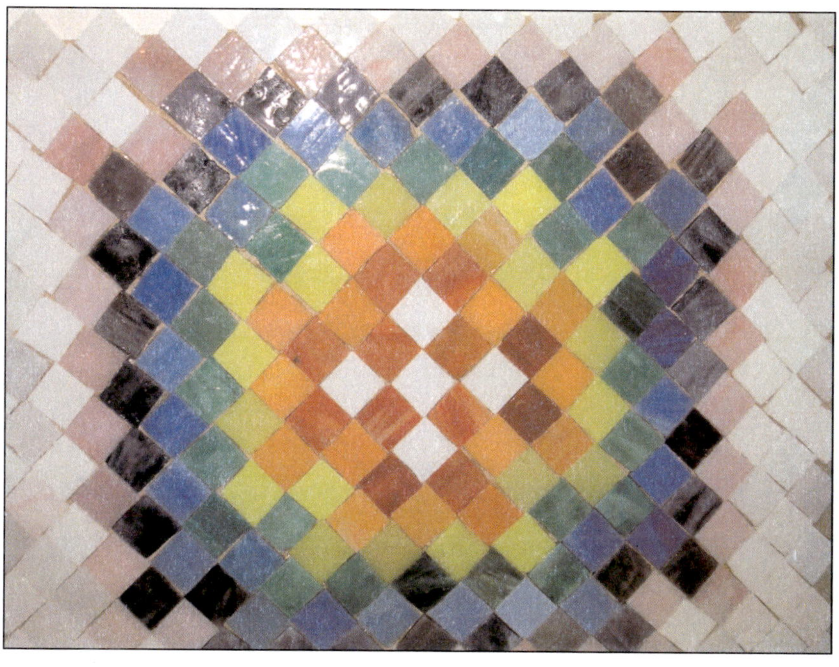

Plate 6. Mosaic created by 11-year-old boy in PALS program.

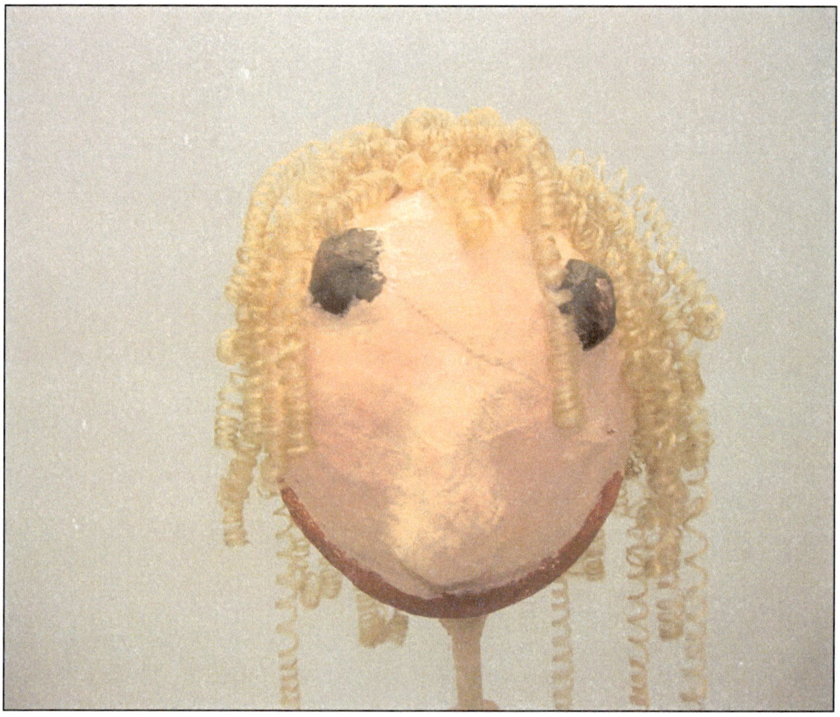

Plate 7. Puppet created by 7-year-old girl in PALS program.

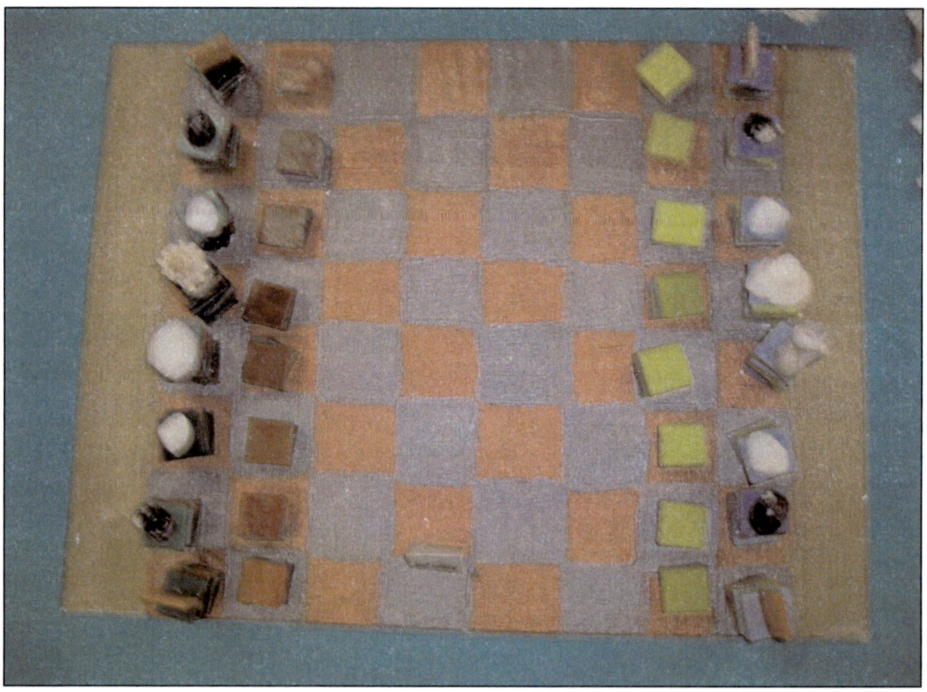

Plate 8. Chess set created by 10-year-old boy in PALS program.

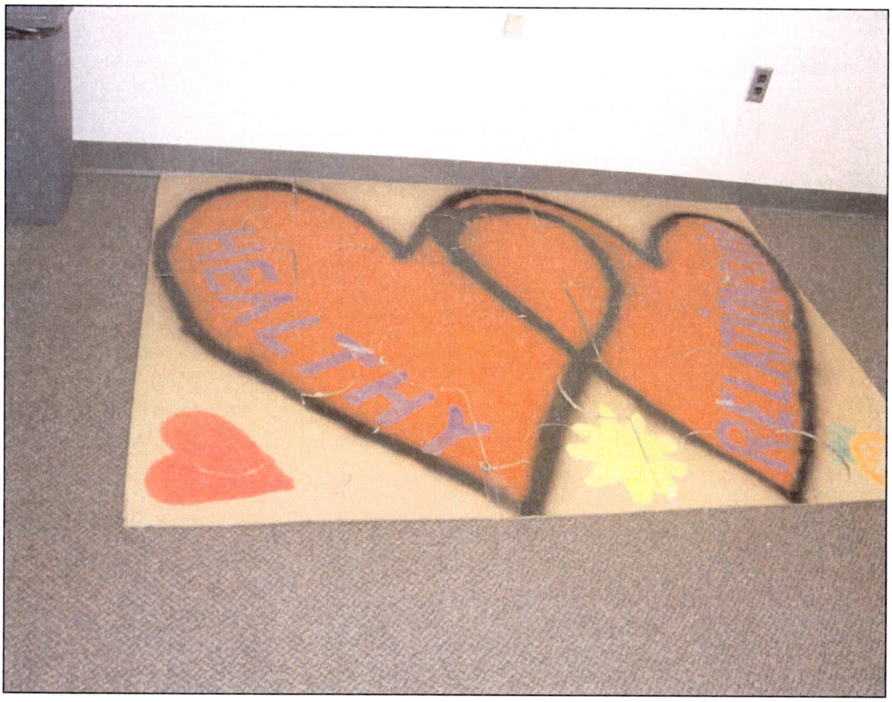

Plate 9. Michael's healthy relationship.

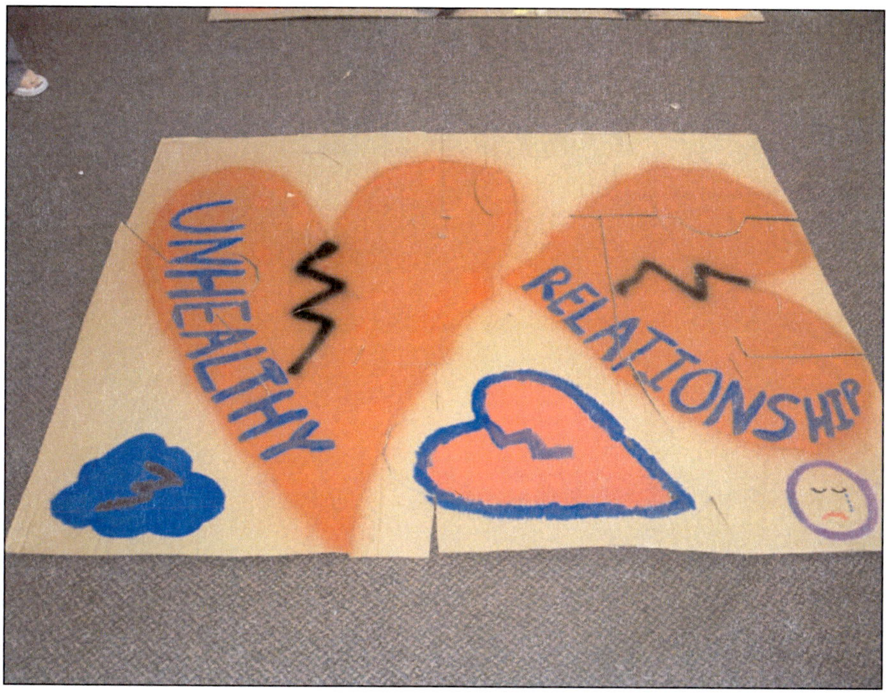

Plate 10. Michael's unhealthy relationship.

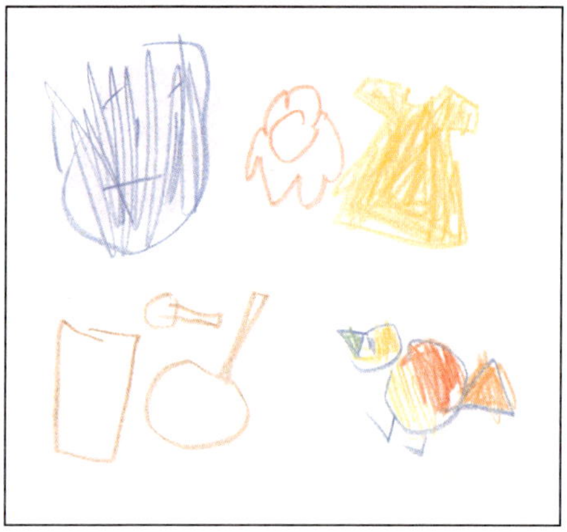

Plate 11. Multicolored Bird.

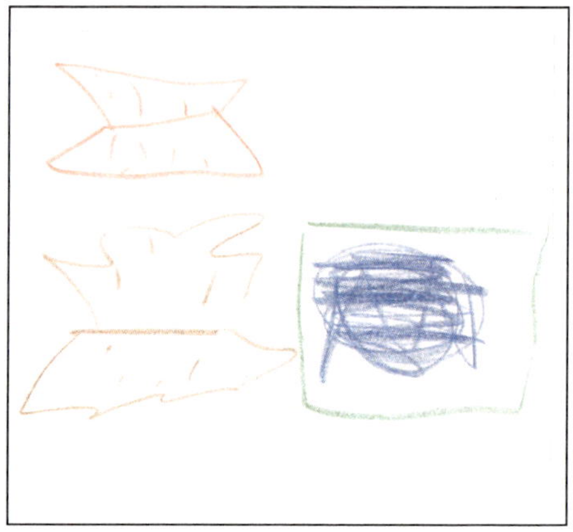

Plate 12. Torn Book.

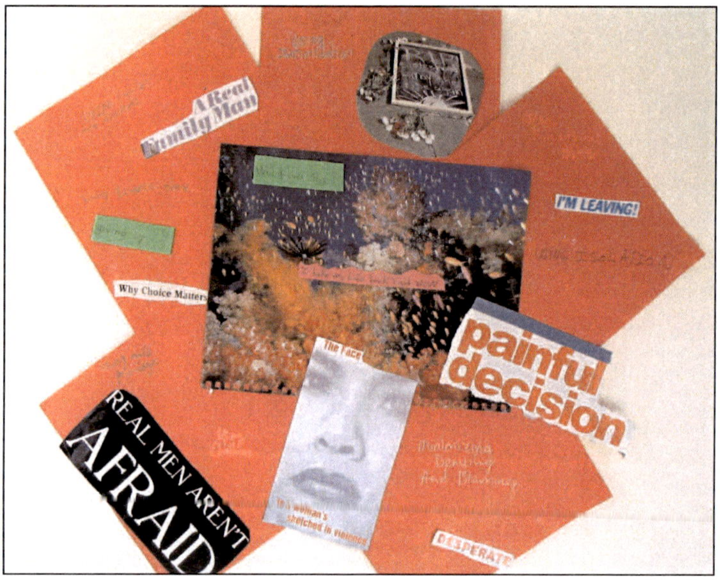

Plate 13. Sample Collage from Power and Control Wheel.

Chapter 11

DEVELOPMENTAL PLAY THERAPY WITH CHILDREN WHO HAVE WITNESSED DOMESTIC VIOLENCE

SONALI SENROY

I am not the battered caterpillar any more,
I am the beautiful butterfly and I am free
(member, domestic violence therapy group)

Introduction

The chapter is an attempt to illustrate the research the author did on using the process of a developmental play therapy modality with children who have witnessed domestic violence in a shelter home in Kolkata, India. The chapter begins with a very brief outline of the impact of domestic violence on the children in India and describes some of the legislation in place for the protection of the children at risk. It then gives information about the shelter home, where this research takes place. The chapter continues by explaining the Embodiment-Projection-Role Play Therapy Approach that formed the basis of the therapeutic work. The group session vignettes attempt to explain the process and shares the outcomes of this work the children and the therapist undertook together. The aim of the research was to use the non-threatening approach of Embodiment-Projection-Role Play therapy technique to provide a therapeutic environment to fragile emotional state of the children to explore their feelings around domestic violence and feeling unsafe. The goal was also to regain and redevelop healthy, trusting relationships with the adults and see them as positive role models and caregivers in a safe environment. The chapter finishes with a conclusion, glossary, followed by bibliography. Due to the nature of the client group, information about the setup and the art made by the group have been changed and modified to respect their confidentiality as well as to adhere to the Data Protection Act.

The Setting

All Bengal Women's Unio is one such non-governmental organization in Kolkata, which tries to ensure the survival, protection and development of exploited children, specifically the girl child. The organization runs three shelter homes housing 160 children between the ages of 6-14. During their stay, the children are sent to the integrated schools and trained in various vocational skills.

The Juvenile Justice (Child Care and Protection) Act of India consolidates and amends the law relating to juveniles in conflict with law and children in need of care and protection. Providing for proper care, protection, and treatment by catering to their development needs is stressed under this law. Adopting a child-friendly approach in the adjudication and disposition of matters in the best interest of children and for their ultimate rehabilitation through various institutions established under this Act (Social welfare department, Government of India 2000).

Subsection (1) and (2) of section 39 of the Juvenile Justice Act states that restoration of and protection to a child shall be the prime objective of any children's home. The children's home or a shelter home, as the case may be, shall take such steps as are considered necessary for the restoration of and protection to a child deprived of his family environment temporarily or permanently (Social Welfare Department, Government of India, 2000).

At the time of this research, according to informal statistics in this centre, 29 girls in the age group of 4–8 years who had witnessed domestic violence were being housed in the shelter home. According to UNICEF, an estimated number of children exposed to domestic violence range about 27.1 to 69 million (UNICEF, 2006). Children in homes where there is domestic violence are also abused or neglected. Although the woman is usually the primary target, domestic violence is sometimes directed toward children (Indian Child, 2007).

Domestic Violence is not just hitting, or fighting, or an occasional argument. It is an abuse of power. The abuser tortures and controls the victim by calculated threats, intimidation, and physical violence. Although both men and women can be abused, in most cases, the victims are women (Indian Child, 2007). According to the National Crime Records Bureau of India (2005), one crime against women is committed every three minutes, one rape every 29 minutes, one dowry death case every 77 minutes, and one case of cruelty by husband and relatives every nine minutes.

For the purpose of this research, four girls in the age range of 5–7 years were chosen to participate in a twelve, weekly play therapy program. The intake questionnaires revealed that the forms of abuse ranged from physical to emotional to sexual abuse. The perpetrators identified by the girls were most often their fathers, brothers, stepmothers, uncles, etc.

The 12-week program was used to provide space for these girls to explore topics around domestic violence and work on the theme of self-esteem related activities. Upon the initial intake, the psychologists found that all these girls were very quiet, introverted, and had a very low self-esteem. They found it challenging to say anything positive or good about themselves. They were able to express themselves through drawings. Tears, hangers, belts, bruised faces, and bloodied lips were some of the images they drew to show the violence they had experienced themselves. They also spoke briefly of seeing their mothers and siblings being hurt and then being taken away and separated from the family.

Some of the challenges that were faced while facilitating this project were about disclosure. These girls were not able to say how recent or old the incidents of abuse were. When new disclosures were shared, it was difficult to report it to the proper authorities because the girls did not know their perpetrators' last names or their addresses. They were rescued by the police from different parts of India and since they spoke the language of the region and were able to identify some geographical landmarks they were transferred to this facility. Neither of them had any schooling so they were not able to read or write and the post traumatic stress disorder was high enough for them to recollect any important and vital information about their family. The only information available was that all of them had run away from home due to domestic violence.

The Approach

A way to start to empower a group to work through the medium of play following the developmental processes in the way children learn to play. Development in playing processes can often be accompanied by changes in cognitive, emotional and interpersonal developments. Hence, the client, for example, can develop emotionally or cognitively through crossing of developmental drama stages in drama therapy (Jones, 1996). This process evolves through three stages: Embodiment play, projective play, and role-play (Cattanach, 1996).

The project is based on the concept of Embodiment, Projection, Role or E-P-R developed by Doctor Sue Jennings (2007), a pioneer in drama therapy from England. It is a developmental paradigm, which uniquely charts the progression of dramatic play from birth to seven years. After initial psychological assessment of these children and a careful evaluation of the embodiment-projection-role-play modality, it was concluded that this would be the appropriate model for intervention.

By engaging in this type of play therapy, children are instructed in areas of problem solving and conflict resolution, giving a child the experience and skills to be part of the social world. E-P-R can be used are the markers of life changes which are ritualized through playing and drama from one stage to the next (Jennings, 2007). Through this process, the child discovers symbols and metaphors, which are embodied, projected, and enacted through the world of developmental play (Cattanach, 1993).

The Structure of Sessions

Each session was structured through a warm-up, main event, and grounding. The children learned how to recognize different kinds of abuse, express emotions, create a safety plan, and make good decisions. The sessions were planned to address feelings related to the violence in families, conflict resolution, enhancing self-esteem, exploring personal space, etc. The sessions created a safe place for these children to share ideas about the best ways to solve problems, think together about feelings that kids have, cope better with their experience and share positive ideas about families. The aim of the session was to provide the children with ways to cope with their experiences and with opportunities to learn new skills to express their feelings using the Embodiment-Projection and Role Play modality.

The Session Vignettes

Embodiment Stage

The first four sessions focused on working with the Embodiment stage. Embodiment in dramatic play therapy involves the way the self is realized through and by the body. For instance, the body often is used as a communication tool to express on an unconscious as well as conscious, level (Jones, 1996). This is through gesture, expression, and voice (Ellam, in Jones, 1996). During the Embodiment stage, one can see how the child's early experiences are made physical and are mainly expressed through bodily movement and the senses. A child's embodiment development can be distorted being violated through physical or sexual abuse; the child's bodily boundaries are invaded with resultant trauma and confusion; there is often fear and anxiety and avoidance of either physical contact or inappropriate physical rage or touch violating body boundary (Jennings, 2007). Exploring personal space was the theme of this stage.

Some Embodiment techniques include working with gross and fine body movements incorporating rhythms games and simple dance improvisations. Various "props" such as hoops, string, or silk scarves are often used to establish contact that is not too personal yet is distanced (Jennings, 2007).

Session 1

In session one, the first step was to get the group going through icebreaker games. The girls all sat quietly in different parts of the room. They sat huddled up and did not have any kind of eye contact. Their body language communicated as if they were nervous and anxious. The session started with inviting the girls to come and sit in a circle. The author explained the session structure, the confidentiality aspect of this session, and mentioned that all participation was voluntary but they were encouraged to explore the activities, as this was a safe space for any kind of expression, keeping in mind mutual respect for each other. A name game was done to help warm up and relax the girls and the same time start to build up group dynamics. Initially, the girls did not have any eye contact and were barely audible. The author had to repeat the game, encouraging the girls with directions and modeling. As the game progressed, they were beginning to use their voices a bit louder. Their body movement and postures were very small their personal space very close to their body but attempting to take the risk of connecting with another group member. The final step of the game was a discussion on their names. The group talked about who gave their names, did they have any nicknames, did they know the meanings of their names, did they like their names, etc. By this time they felt little relaxed and were willing to work on this in the next session. The session finished after a quick feedback about how much did they like the games or what are the areas that they were not comfortable. The issue of confidentiality was repeated and the girls were encouraged to talk to their assigned counselor in-between sessions if needed.

Session 2

Session number two started with a breathing exercise. This helped the girls to start focusing on the here and now and warm up. As they stretched and exhaled, they were invited to vocalize sounds, expressions, and feelings. The group had their eyes closed and faced way from each other thus giving each individual personal space so that they would not feel threatened. The exercises led to an activity where they had to move in different ways and explore the room to explore not only the surrounding physical space but also each other's spaces. They were encouraged to move as animals, as objects, as things in the nature, etc. They were also given opportunities where they had make eye contact, begin to make connections with a partner and as a whole group. The activity was taken to another level where they had to use their bodies to express feelings, like being happy, being sad, being nervous, or being angry. The response was mixed. Two of them had hardly any idea about the body parts can be used as tools of expression. The girls were unconsciously using their bodies to express their feeling but now they were beginning to understand how to recognize and be aware of their own body language. They were beginning to understand that even if they did not speak, their bodies spoke. Their bodies showed if they felt comfortable or not, in a situation. One girl lay down on the floor in a fetal position, other one said that she needed a blanket to cover for feeling more secure. The others curled up sitting and standing to show their safe and comfortable position. As the session continued, the author asked about some of the situations that would make them seek out their comfortable positions and the replies were similar, to escape the pain from physical abuse such as beating, hitting, and kicking. As the tension was obvious in their bodies, the group was redirected towards doing some physical stretches to relax.

The session ended with a feedback about how they felt during that time. The author again reiterated the confidentially aspect and acknowledged that it is difficult to see and go through the violence experienced in one's family. They were encouraged and invited to talk and share about their experiences as this was a safe group and sharing helped to understand and be aware of the violence.

Session 3

Session three started with checking in with the girls with simple breathing and stretches. The author led an activity where the girls were asked to sit as far away as possible from each other. Next, they were asked to sit all huddled together. They were then invited to share how they felt. All of them said that when they were sitting all huddled, that was the more uncomfortable of the two. The were then encouraged to again get into the huddled position standing and then take steps away from each other till they found that they were not feeling uncomfortable. All their positions were different in terms of proximity from each other. One girl stood close to the author who also took part in this exercise. Another girl stood at an arms length, while the third stood a foot away. The fourth girl went to a wall and stood there. At this point, the author explained about personal space. Uncomfortable experiences make one wary of our personal space. The girls were asked who they would invite into their personal space. Everyone said her mother. Strangers, fathers, stepfathers, brothers, uncle, and teacher were put outside their personal space.

The author did another exercise where the girls stood in parallel lines facing each other and they were asked to approach each other maintaining eye contact and when they felt that their personal space was being invaded, to say stop. The girls again had varied response timings of saying stop. The author explained that everyone has an inner voice, which tells them when it is feeling uncomfortable. It differs from one person to another and it good to know when to stay stop so that they are able to recognize and be aware of signs of perpetrators. The session ended with playing a children's game called: what is the time Mr. Wolf and a feedback. The girls shared that they learned about personal space and how to recognize and listen to their bodies. They also mentioned that they were feeling comfortable coming to the group and were enjoying the games.

Session 4

Session four was the last of the Embodiment section. The session started with a breathing exercise to relax the mind and body. This time the girls were encouraged to lead these exercises every week to gain confidence. After initial help, they managed to lead the beginning quite well. After doing simple stretches, the next activity was done to prepare the group to progress to the stage of Projection. A big chalk circle was drawn in the middle of the room and the girls were guided through an imagination. They were invited to close their eyes and imagine that the circle represented their home and or personal space. An intruder appears and tries to grab it from them. With this background scenario, the girls were encouraged to think of different strategies they would use to protect their space. They were also invited to imagine what or who the intruder would be. Each girl took turns to be in the circle. One girl said that the intruder was a dog and should scream to scare it away. One said that it was a stranger and she would not open the door and then shout for help. Another one said if the intruder were somebody known to her and tried to touch her, she would bite and kick hard. The last one said that that she would call her mother. As this was the last of the embodiment sessions, the girls were reminded that eight more sessions were left and they were given positive feedback about their participation and contribution. The girls mentioned in their feedback that even though it was difficult to talk what had happened to them, they felt relieved to share the pain. They also mentioned that all this time they thought they were the only ones who experienced such violence, but hearing the others in the group, they felt supported and less vulnerable. The also mentioned that they felt stronger emotionally and learned how to recognize abusers and trust their inner voice.

Projection Stage

As children develop more and more into the Projection stage, it is noticed they move from exploratory play where things are tasted and tested to more patterned and organized play with objects, to more dramatized play with stories. Although it has these variations, it is still projected play, i.e., it is play beyond the body and objects take on roles and meanings rather than the child (Jennings, 2007). Some Projective Techniques includes play with substances, objects, art and craft medium, etc. These activities can be incorporated using imaginary play (Jennings, 2007).

Session 1

The first Projection session began with the ritual of doing the breathing exercise led by one of the girls. The warm-up activity was a trust walk. The girls had to make eye contact to choose a partner, and then one of the partners would follow the other with closed eyes. After some time they would switch. This activity was done to develop and build up trust. By this time, girls were really relaxed and were given paper and colors to draw how they saw themselves. The drawings were that of a dark colored face, lot of utensils, a torn book, and a mass of dark paint. When they were invited to add anything to their drawings, yes came the reply. Then they added a red flower to the dark faced girl and a yellow frock, a multi colored bird near the heap of utensils, (see Figure 1 and Plate 11) a new book by the torn one and a green border surrounding the dark paint (see Figure 2 and Plate 12).

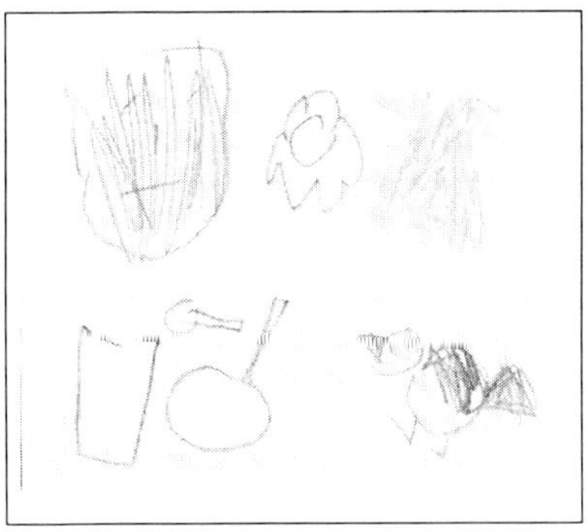

Figure 1. Multicolored Bird (see also Plate 11 in color).

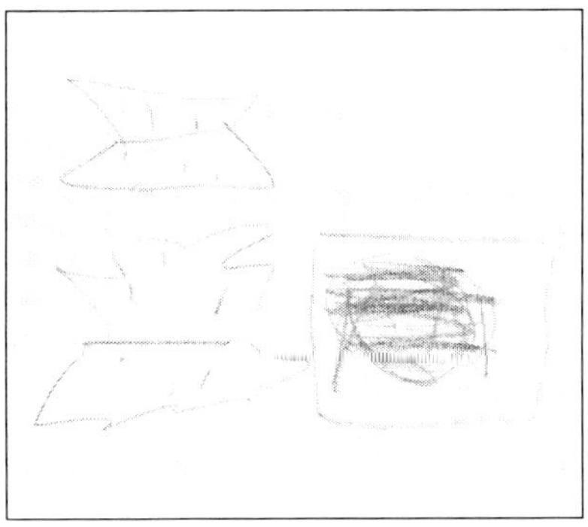

Figure 2. Torn Book (see also Plate 12 in color).

The session ended with a game of hopscotch and feedback. In the feedback, the author shared some of the positive images the girls had drawn to add to their original drawing and invited them to share their feelings on this. Some of their remarks were: *I thought I am ugly because of my black color but a red flower and nice frock made me look beautiful, I never got a chance to play its work,*

work and work but I became a bird, I did not know how to read and write but am going to school now, Now I know I can do so many things.

Session 2

Session two started with breathing exercise. This was one ritual, which was always followed. It helped them group to focus on the here and now. The warm up activity touched on expressing feelings. As the group walked around the room, they were invited to say one positive and one negative feeling and they could relate it to any person, any thing or any event. Some of the expressions were: *I like your session but hate to study. I feel sad when mothers come on visitor's day but I feel happy to go to school. I feel angry when I get punishment and feel happy when I get a star.* This activity was followed by doing a collage of cutout magazine pictures. The theme was to cut pictures of different people, objects, and actions that they liked or do not like. The group was then invited to share their creations. There was an angry male face *(my father, I hate him)*, a sick dog *(reminds me about my punishments)*, festival of colors *(I used to play with colors with my brother)*, face of a goddess *(I am sure she will punish my stepmother)*, an ice cream cone *(I love it)*, blue sky with some birds flying *(I used to fly kites in our school).* The session ended with a feedback about how metaphors help us to discuss our problems Addressing the violence that happened, from a distance helps to share it in a non threatening manner (Jones, 1996).

Session 3

Session three of Projection started with the ritualistic breathing exercise led by one of the girls. The warm up exercise chosen was to be blown up like a balloon. This activity was done with each girl having their own individual balloon or with them watching the facilitator. The author went through some of the challenges faced by the girls at home. These challenges were discussed before the activity. With every challenge, an emotion is experienced, again being identified by them. With each challenge and the corresponding emotion experienced, the author blew into the balloon, representing the metaphor of experiencing an emotion, but not knowing how to deal with it. Over a period, one last event happens and the balloon is so full of emotions that when it was let go, it flies all over the room or it may explode before this happens. The group discussed what that might look like in a child when they experience such a range of emotions over a period but do not have the strategies to manage them. The strategies discussed were that they should talk to a grown up preferably a teacher or their mother. One of the girls said that if it was difficult to talk to anyone then to scream into pillow when no one was at home. The girls acknowledged that they did not have anybody to listen to them or even believe that they were sad or angry. So often, the stress would build up and would end up in aggression or depression.

This led to the next activity of playing with objects. The girls were excited to see the assorted objects. At first, they played freely with them and seemed to enjoy the activity. As they became comfortable using them, they were invited to choose a particular object and describe the object in a different way and by giving it a meaning. They chose a scarf, a small box, a stick, and a plastic bottle respectively. The descriptions were, the scarf became a snake representing bad man, a belt used to bite some one, a headgear to save head from rain and sun. The box became a bowl full of food, a surprise gift, a suitcase to keep cloths safely. The stick became a sword protection from bad man, a sitting stool, and a fishing rod. The plastic bottle became a flute, a bad man's drink. The group ended with another game of, *What Time is it Mr. Wolf* and feedback. The girls mentioned that they felt relived to share the violence they have seen with the others and with the facilitator. Children who are exposed to violence in the home need to know that they are not alone and that the violence is not their fault (UNICEF, 2006). It was important to help the children to learn to talk about the violence with a trusted adult. When children share their feelings, it can help them feel less frightened and alone (Strauss, Gelles, & Smith, 1990). The author mentioned that the objects described and the drawings from the previous sessions would be used to build up a story in the next session and hence she had to write the descriptions down.

Session 4

Session four started with another girl leading the breathing exercise. As the group warmed up through simple stretches, the facilitator shared the descriptions of the objects and drawings from the previous sessions, encouraging the group to start building a story. After many trials and discussions, the group came up with this story: In a far away village, there lived a family consisted of a father, mother, one brother, and one sister. The mother died during her third childbirth. That child was a girl. Every body branded her as bad luck for the family. The father neglected her totally. After couple of months, he remarried and the stepmother came home. She was also indifferent towards the children. The elder sister was supposed to look after the other two. She had to discontinue her studies. She had to stay at home and do all the chores. The stepmother would often complain to the father on the evening against the elder daughter. He would drink heavily and regularly beat her with the stick or his belt. She would often spend the night without food as punishment. She was not able to tolerate this any longer and one day ran away from home. Now she is in a safe place but always feels guilty for abandoning her brother and sister. The group described the stepmother like a snake, the father was the bad man and the torn book represented dropping out from school. The red flower and yellow frock represented the safe place at the shelter home. Here the projection of personal material into roles, the use of enactment to create a transformed, changed perspective on a life situation, and the group working together in witnessing and improvising with the client combined to produce change. The piece aims to enable a psychodynamic exploration of material presented by the family. The playing and enactments results in the personal dynamics being reflected and resolved through the play and the involvement of the therapists (Jones, 1996).

The facilitator decided to use another breathing exercise to derole (Jones, 1996). The group was invited to find a comfortable spot in the room. A discussion about the importance of breathing, how it helps the body, especially when experiencing overwhelming a feeling was done. The girls were directed to inhale through the nose and exhale through their mouth, trying to blow a large bubble. Then they were invited to watch all or just one bubble, continuing to breathe deeply from their comfortable spot. In the above case, the modality sought to find a structure and language to achieve aims of changing behavioral patterns and to lean new ways of learning (Jones, 1996).

This marked the end of the Projection stage. Here it can be observed that towards the end of the Projection stage, a child's play is becoming more "dramatized" with stories and scenes being enacted from newly created stories or stories that already exist. A child is developing their own narrative structure, stories which have a beginning, middle and an end, but also they are increasing their capacity for "free-play," what would be termed as improvisation, where one starts with a topic or an object and see where it goes. This is also the transition phase to the next stage of Role Play (Jennings, 2007). During this transition, one can observe children become their own directors and the directors of others as they create plays in which they both perform and direct. They are able to exist separately with their creativity as well as being part of pair or small group (Jennings, 2007).

Role Play Stage

Dramatic play involves the child taking on roles in stories from texts or through improvisation, and involving the therapist and other things in the role: chairs draped with material, large toys and so on, can all take on roles within the scene. Children may make and wear masks, and masks need to be a part of the play therapist's equipment. It is crucial that the character and the scene and indeed the space are deroled before the session is ended (Jennings, 2007).

Sessions 1 and 2

Sessions one and two had to be combined in to two hours as the next session was a national holiday. As the session continued with the girls leading the breathing exercises, they became relaxed. After initial warm ups, the groups were invited to chose a scenario where they could imagine themselves to be helping in difficult situations. The group was told that one of them would be the director like in a cinema and direct a story. One of the girls volunteered to be the director. She sat and discussed with the group a difficult situation that they can enact. After many ideas, they settled on this improvisation. The scenario was set up in a house. One of the group members was chosen to represent a small girl and placed her farthest from the enactment space. She gave a hand drum to another girl and asked her to make loud sounds on it and stamp the ground with her feet. She labeled her as the "father." She asked the last group member to make crying sounds and she represented the "mother." As the enactment started, she asked the drummer to play as loudly as possible and the girl who was crying to cry and fall on the ground. As the enactment progressed, she brought the girl into the space and placed her in the middle of the other two "actors." She then directed her to try to stop the drummer from drumming and to stop the crying girl from falling down. This went on for some time, when suddenly, the director, grabbed the girls' hands, took her out of the action, and told her to scream for help. The director then told all the actors to stop their action and ended the enactment. The girls still in their roles seemed to belittle shaken up and it was necessary to derole themselves, the props, and the space around them. Deroling marks the closure of active work involving dramatic forms. It is important for the clients to have a clear demarcation at which try leave or disengage themselves from the dramatic space or activities. If materials such as play objects are used, this phase includes an opportunity for the clients to shift their engagement with the materials. If the group activities have taken place then the closure is a time for the group dramatic relationships to have ended (Jones, 1996).

During the feedback, the author acknowledged that the enactment was very powerful and the little girl in the story was very brave. She mentioned that the girl was trying to do the right thing for the mother, by trying to save her but she could have gotten hurt. She then asked the director why did the girl come away from the fight and why did she scream. The answer was that, the girl realized that she was too small to stop the fight but not small enough to scream for help. The author spent time developing awareness of safety issues. The girls were then asked to identify safe places to use when they were in a difficult situation. The answers were, *I will hide under the bed, I will hide in a closet, and I will run and get my neighbor.* Once the safety plans were discussed, the group was invited to play a game of Tag before ending the session.

Session 3

As session three started, the group was reminded that the next session would be end of the project and were asked what they would like to do in the last session. The group decided to enact the story they had made during the projection sessions. The rest of the session was spent in making a list of materials, props, toys, colors, and scarves that would be needed to do the enactment. The girls and the author made masks of the characters and painted background scenarios. The session ended with a reminder that the next would be the last session as well as the end of the project.

Session 4

Session four started with all the girls taking turns in leading the breathing exercise. The girls were reminded that this was the last session and if they needed to discuss or talk to any counselor after this the facilitator and others would be there in the shelter home for further support. Once the girls had done some simple stretches, they started preparing for the dramatic enactment. It was the same story that they had made in one of the previous sessions. There were six characters, so the group played more than one character and the ending was different. Instead of running away from home, all the siblings decided to punish the parents. There were difference of opinion regarding the punishment as one girl wanted the parents to die, another thought that no food for the rest of their lives would be severe enough but eventually decided to talk to the local doctor who made the parents apologize to the children and gave them enough love and affection for the rest of their lives. The enactment went well with the girls changing roles and using their props with ease. They were able to use the dramatic space with ease and were please with the ending. During processing the enactment, they said that it is easy to be revengeful and angry towards the abusers but very difficult to forgive them and seek help. Towards the end, they were then invited to listen to a piece of music and think about the positive things they had learned about themselves in these twelve sessions. The session ended with the girls choosing any medium that they liked and expressing how they felt after the project. This would be their evaluation and feedback.

Conclusion

I am not scared anymore, I am not alone anymore, I am not crying any more
I am not hitting any more, I am not going to run away anymore
I am not going to lie anymore, I am not going to be silent anymore
I am not afraid to fly anymore, I am not the battered caterpillar any more
I am the beautiful butterfly and I am free

As seen in the poem written by one of the group members at the end of the project and in these session vignettes, the Embodiment, Projection, and Role Play was found to be effective in exploring dometic violence witnessed by these children. The therapeutic play sessions provided a space to find out how these children used the various modalities to explore and express their emotions and in their own way heal themselves. They also learned to regain and redevelop healthy and trusting relationships with the adults through proactive and positive interaction.

The author would like to thank the children and staff of ABWF, the editor, and publisher of this book for giving the opportunity to share their work with a larger audience.

Terms

Deroling marks the closure of active work involving dramatic forms. It is important for the clients to have a clear demarcation at which try leave or disengage themselves from the dramatic space or activities. If materials such as play objects are used, this phase includes an opportunity for the clients to shift their engagement with the materials. If the group activities have taken place then the closure is a time for the group dramatic relationships to have ended (Jones, 1996).

Domestic Violence, under the new Protection of Women from Domestic Violence Act 2005, India, includes actual abuse or the threat of abuse whether physical, sexual, emotional or economic. This Act aims to provide for more effective protection of the rights of women guaranteed under the Constitution who are victims of violence of any kind occurring within the family and for matters connected therewith or incidental thereto.(http://wcd.nic.in/wdvact.pdf.)

Embodiment-Project-Role Play Therapy Approach (E-P-R) is a developmental paradigm, which uniquely charts the progression of dramatic play from birth to 7 years. Pioneered by Doctor Sue Jennings, a drama therapist from England, this approach is based on extended observations with babies and young children, and pregnant women, it provides a parallel progression alongside other developmental processes such as physical, cognitive, emotional and social (Jennings, 2007).

Embodiment Stage sees how the child's early experiences are manifested through bodily movement and the senses (Jennings, 2007).

Personal Space is the region surrounding each person, or that area which a person considers his domain or territory. Often if entered by another being without this being desired, it makes them feel uncomfortable. In a sense, all abusive problems are boundary and personal space problems. The abuser is intruding past your boundaries and not allowing you to get close to his or hers. Boundary problems involve both people: the abuser intrudes too far into another's space and the abused does not set limits where limits need to be set (http://en.wikipedia.org/wiki/Personal_space)

Projection Stage is the stage when the child is responding to the world beyond the body, to things outside the body. The child's responses may well be physical, for example, when a child plays with finger paint but the important point is that the paint is a substance outside the body boundaries (Jennings, 2007).

Dramatic Play, or the Role Play stage, is the culmination of the primary E-P-R stages and is usually complete by about the age of seven years. We can see a difference in the 'drama' of children at this age from the "dramatic play" of the years before. Dramatic play involves the child taking on roles in stories from texts or through improvisation, and involving the therapist and other things in the role: chairs draped with material, large toys and so on, can all take on roles within the scene (Jennings, 2007).

References

Cattanach, A. (1993). *Play therapy with abused children.* London: Jessica Kingsley, p. 47.

Cattanach, A. (1996). *Drama for people with special needs* (p. 19). London: A&C Black.

Ellam, K. (1996) The semiotics of theatre and drama. In P. Jones (Ed.), *Drama as therapy, theatre as living* (p. 113). London: Routledge.

Indian Child. (2007). Retrieved from http://www.indianchild.com/domestic_violence_in_india.htm on January 21, 2008.

Jennings, S. (2007). *Embodiment-projection-role, A developmental model for the play therapy method,* in http://www.suejennings.com

Jones, P. (1996). *Drama as therapy, theatre as living* (pp. 27, 37, 39, 113, 116, 243). London: Routledge.

Juvenile Justice Act, India. (2000). Chapter 3 in http://socialwelfare.delhigovt.nic.in/juvenile justice1.htm

National Crime Records Bureau. (2005). Ministry of Home Affairs India, Crime against women (Tables 5.1-5.4).

Strauss, M. A., Gelles, R. J., & Smith, C. (1990). *Physical violence in American families: Risk factors and adaptations to violence in 8,145 families.* New Brunswick: Transaction Publishers.
UNICEF. (2006). *United Nations Secretary-General's study on violence against children*, in www.unicef.org.
UNICEF. (2006). *Behind closed doors, the impact of domestic violence on children*, in www.unicef.org

BIOGRAPHY

Sonali Senroy (BA) is a senior counselor and a therapeutic storyteller residing in Kolkata, India. She works with children, adolescents, women, and adults at risk in her private practice. She has been working in a shelter home for rescued girl children, women, and the elderly who have been rescued after being psychically, sexually, emotionally, and socially abused, for the last four years. Sonali also teaches at various training programs both in India and abroad.

Chapter 12

"NO TIME TO SAY HELLO, GOOD-BYE" (DISNEY, W.): DRAMA THERAPY WITH CHILDREN ON AN INPATIENT PSYCHIATRIC UNIT

KRISTIN LONG and BARBARA MCKECHNIE

Introduction

In this chapter, we will examine the impact witnessing domestic violence has on children and how treatment is provided for them on a psychiatric inpatient unit. Both authors have worked in the same child and adolescent inpatient unit setting, which offers services for children ages three to seventeen who have a primary Axis I diagnosis. It is rare to find a child in this environment who has not been exposed to domestic violence, whether witnessing hostility against a parent, sibling, relative, or experiencing it directly. Like the hare in Lewis Carroll's Alice's Adventures in Wonderland (1865), the pace of the unit is rushed with sometimes no time to say hello or good-bye to the children and, most frequently, no way to know the effectiveness of treatment. However, the current trend toward shorter stay has created a revolving door form of treatment, bringing the same children back to the unit three and even four times.

Children on this unit are admitted during various stages of their traumatic experiences, some whose most recent trauma occurred only hours prior to admission; others whose negative symptoms surface years after the trauma. In the following pages, the writers will identify the impact of domestic violence on the children we treat, and illustrate, using case anecdotes, how drama therapy can be used to reduce negative symptoms that surface after domestic violence exposure. Assessment tools used in this setting will be discussed. Methods of treatment will be examined, as well as the reasons particular interventions were selected. The therapeutic milieu and hospital environment are examined to provide context to the drama therapy used for treatment. In many cases there was a commonality of stories or symptoms allowing for the creation of a composite patient to illustrate a specific point within the chapter. Consents for treatment were obtained for all the children discussed and all identifying information has been altered or combined to protect each client' identity.

Impact of Domestic Violence on Children

Returning violence for violence multiplies violence,
adding deeper darkness to a night already devoid of stars.
Martin Luther King, Jr. (1967, p. 72)

At one time, it was assumed that in domestic violence situations the primary victims were battered wives and most research on domestic violence has centered on abuse toward intimate partners. However, recent research has established that children witnessing domestic violence may also be severely impacted (Fantuzzo & Mohr, 1999). We now know that children who have been exposed to domestic violence, either directly (in same room and/or in direct sight) or indirectly (hears noises, sees effects of exposure such as broken bones, bruises, wrecked furniture) are at a greater risk for delays in social, emotional, and cognitive development (Arroyo & Eth, 1995; Harding, 2006; James, 1996; Lynn & Nisivoccia, 1996; Rossman et al., 2000). Furthermore, households in which spousal abuse exists, also show an increased risk of physical abuse being directed toward children (Rossman et al., 2000). Bessel van der Kolk (2003) reports that children are abused in these households "at a rate 1500% higher than the national average" (p. 169). Thus, it is likely that many more children are exposed to violence in their home than was previously believed (Arroyo & Eth, 1995).

Trauma experienced early in a child's life has extreme effects on the maturation of self-representation and on the functioning and development of the ego (Bolby, 1988; James, 1996; Webb, 1999; Weber, 2005). A child who has been traumatized secondary to their experience of domestic violence will likely develop some psychiatric symptoms as a result. Some researchers have divided these symptoms into two clusters, internal and external symptoms (Rossman et al., 2000). Externalizing symptoms include behaviors that are conveyed outside one's body, such as aggressive actions toward others, destruction of property, bullying, disobedience, attention deficits, and hyperactivity. These behaviors are often found in children diagnosed with Oppositional Defiant Disorder, Conduct Disorder, Disruptive Behavior Disorder, and Attention Deficit/Hyperactivity Disorder (Harding, 2006; Rossman et al., 2000). When comparing groups of children who have been exposed to domestic violence with children who have not, Arroyo and Eth (1995) found that children who have witnessed violence "have more overall externalizing problem behavior" (Jaffee, Wolfe, Wilson, & Zak, 1986) and more overall internalizing behavior.

Internalizing symptoms are observed more than externalizing symptoms in depression and anxiety disorders. Included in this category are self-mutilating gestures, isolation, and somatic complaints. Symptoms related to Post Traumatic Stress Disorder (hyperarousal, excessive reaction, withdrawal, and avoidance) may be found in both external and internal behaviors (Herman, 1997; Rothschild, 2000; van der Kolk, 1996).

The above symptoms and effects that are identified with domestic violence can be readily seen on the children admitted to an acute inpatient psychiatric unit. The admission of these children and adolescents to such a unit may immediately follow their exposure to violence, or may even happen years later. Symptoms in these children vary greatly and clinicians working in this milieu observe a range of behaviors such as isolating (secondary to depression), bullying, aggressive outbursts, self harming gestures or actions, severe anxiety, or somatic complaints.

The Child Inpatient Unit

The illness in a child is sometimes missed since it gets hidden behind the quickness and restlessness that belongs to a young life.

(Winnicott, 1954-5, p. 272)

Children must wait twenty-four hours after admission to the unit before they can receive an order from their doctor permitting them to have physical activity at the gym, which is located on another floor of the hospital building. During this time period, they are assessed by all staff members and a treatment plan is developed and implemented. The children are encouraged to contribute to this plan and are expected to work toward established goals for the duration of their hospitalization.

The average length of stay is one to two weeks and the focus for treatment, as is the norm in these settings, is on crisis intervention and stabilization, not long term solutions (Haen, 2005; Tyson & Baffour, 2004). Great effort is made to create a safe structure for the children. The hospital has onsite classrooms and instruction which allow the children to continue their education while on the unit. After school hours, the children have group therapy, where they are either separated by age, symptoms, or developmental level.

Some approaches recommended for treatment include assisting a child in identifying and labeling feelings, developing adaptive ways to express anger, fear and sadness, increasing positive interactions with peers and adults, improving ability to empathize, strengthening outside support systems, applying for additional services, boosting self-esteem and self-confidence, developing consequential thinking, discovering family roles and dynamics (Haen, 2004), and validating "wishes children have about their families" (Rossman et al., 2000, p. 110). The treatment goals focus primarily on the presenting symptoms in an attempt to stabilize the child, which is the ultimate goal for discharge. Outpatient treatment goals may be very different from inpatient treatment objectives as attachment issues intensify and children cope with the long term psychological affects the exposure to violence has on their cognitive, emotional, and personal development.

Initially many children have difficulty tolerating a group setting as they are adjusting not only to being away from family and home, but also to the structure of the unit. They may become aggressive toward staff or peers, refuse to come out of their room or isolate completely, or show signs of regression such as encopresis, thumb-sucking, or using a younger voice than usual. While these patients would benefit from more individual treatment, individual sessions are generally not realistic in this acute, crisis based setting due to time restraints, staffing, and small group sizes to ensure therapeutic environments.

Some individuals may initially find the unit more traumatizing than safe, as they witness peers being restrained, sent to the quiet room (a room designated to decease stimuli), or overhear a primal cry of anguish. Familiarity with the structure, staff support, and reassurance about the temporary status of hospitalization usually help assuage these fears.

While a detailed psychosocial and family background would help a clinician to guide her treatment, these histories are rarely available. Sometimes the children have been too recently placed with foster parents and there is little known history, or they have literally been dropped off in the emergency room of the hospital. In these instances, family secrets are still locked inside the child and clinicians must work from a position of not knowing, at least initially.

Approach to Acute Treatment

Because the abused, neglected or emotionally abused children are frequently under- or overstimulated, they lack the ability to explore, experiment, or even play. The clinician must facilitate these natural, now constricted or disorganized tendencies.

(Gil, 1991, p. 63)

Children on the unit often have tough exterior shells (Haen, 2004), or a "gorilla suit" (Crenshaw & Mordock, 2005, p. 1). This defense mechanism is very useful in homes with violence as it serves to keep others at bay. On the unit, these children present as oppositional, defiant, and are often labeled "difficult." Children without this defensive cover may attempt to attach too quickly to any adult on the unit and provide staff members with verbose accounts, accurate or not, of their past in an attempt to please or comply as a "good" boys or girls. In either case, both behaviors serve to protect the child from the impact of the trauma of witnessing domestic violence and further add to the difficulty in obtaining accurate historical information.

Beverly James (1996) defines trauma as "overwhelming, uncontrollable experiences that psychologically impact victims by creating in them feelings of helplessness, vulnerability, loss of safety, and loss of control" (p. 1). She explains that in children, a clinician may see symptoms that range from mild to severe. James (1996) recommends a specialized course of treatment, not always continuous, as most advantageous for children who have been traumatized. This is because at various developmental stages children and adults may suffer varied symptoms and require additional treatment. While James (1996) is referring to mostly outpatient and individual treatment, her proposal parallels what occurs for many chronically psychiatric child patients. Children hospitalized on inpatient units often have had multiple previous psychiatric admissions. A revolving door of treatment occurs as the same children return again and again to the hospital, or are admitted onto another unit, during their childhood, into adolescence, and their adult years.

Although James (1996) states that "a direct, active treatment approach" (p. 3) is often desired when working with these children, one does not always have this luxury on inpatient units. All too often individual treatment goals are addressed in group settings. Some children need to be approached less directly, either individually or in a group setting, to ensure they have ample ego support to tolerate group settings and to prevent their trauma from igniting reactions in others.

Therapy groups in this milieu will almost always contain children who are presenting with a range of pathologies. Patients on the unit change frequently; therefore the culture and stability of the floor depend on consistency with group leaders, time, space, and materials. Groups are arranged by age, developmental level, or diagnosis. There are times when this arrangement is not possible as the group of children on the unit present with such diversity that treatment goals must be further adapted and reduced to a common denominator. For example, groups may include children diagnosed with depression, autism or ADHD while the universal goal is to maintain personal boundaries and sharing materials. While certain drama therapy techniques can target most of the symptoms present in a group, it is certainly challenging as a clinician to facilitate therapy in this setting and provide treatment for all group members. Demanding, but it is possible! Group therapy can address goals such as maintaining safe physical boundaries, interpersonal skills, and turn taking (Haen, 2005; Lynn & Nisicoccia, 1999). Occasionally there is the opportunity to provide individual sessions for children who have the most difficulty with group modalities, often due to psychosis, autistic spectrum disorders, or antisocial tendencies. Discharge for some children may be delayed due to a lack of available foster homes, or lack of an open bed in a group home or longer term treatment center such as a state hospital, or delays transferring to a residential facility. These children are also offered individual sessions as additional support during this extended stay.

"The Play's the Thing" (Shakespeare, W. 2.2. 638-39): Touching Pain at a Safe Distance

It is by playing and only by playing that the individual child is able to be creative and use the whole personality, and it is only in being creative that the individual discovers the self.

(Winnicott, 1971, p. 53)

"Child's play, charged with suspense and conflict, is rooted in imitation and centered in transformation: the essential elements of drama/theatre" (Koste, 1995, p. xx). Drama therapy, with its use of dramatic play, storytelling, projective techniques, body work, and aesthetic distance can safely engage children who are in the midst of painful circumstances by giving them a chance to return to a place of play. Through the use of distancing, central to many methods of drama therapy, the drama therapist can help the child gain some separation from overpowering, traumatic affect states and beliefs (Landy, 1996; Weber, 2005). Landy (1986) describes the concept of distancing as a "range of closeness and separation" (p. 98). Projective techniques, such as storytelling, puppets, masks, and use of a sand tray, are often used in creating distance. While a monster puppet may be over distanced, a more realistic puppet, such as a life sized little girl, may be under-distanced for certain clients, allowing a more immediate access to his/her personal story. By initially utilizing over distancing techniques, whereby the child is encouraged to play roles and create stories or metaphors, remote from their own reality, the child begins to feel secure enough to risk and trust the therapist and engage in the healing process (Landy, 1997). Less distanced techniques can be used once the client feels safe, allowing for a more direct approach to treatment. The goal is to help the child patient have balance or to find what Landy (1986) calls a "midway point of over-distance or under-distance" (p. 100). This in-between place is known as "aesthetic distance, where catharsis can occur" (p. 100).

According to the National Association for Drama Therapy, drama therapy is the "intentional use of drama/theatre processes to achieve the therapeutic goal of symptom relief, emotional and physical integration and personal growth" (National Association of Drama Therapy, 1979). Drama therapy techniques can target the identified internalized and externalized symptoms present in most children as a result of their exposure to domestic violence. Dramatic play and theatre technique/exercises address socialization delays and also help children to develop a language, both verbal and nonverbal, to express and communicate their feelings (Emunah, 1994).

Huizinga (1950) wrote of the centrality of play in all aspects of human life and in play "the child and the poet are at home with the savage" (p. 26). Play is the language of children when words are not enough or are not yet known. Children use play to express and address their conscious and unconscious worlds. Erikson (1950) believed that play allows a child to gain mastery over traumatic situations (Huizinga, 1950; Irwin, 2005; Lynn & Nisivoccia, 1999; Terr, 1990). Winnicott (1971) informed us that "playing is itself a therapy" (p. 50). He developed the concept of "transitional objects" and explored the "me" and "not me" phenomenon central to most drama therapy work (Winnicott, 1958, 1971). Like the actor performing in a play, one takes on the persona of a character while still maintaining a sense of true self. This persona allows the child to have the strength and support of the role, which can permit the freedom of expression that might not be available without it. As Oscar Wilde so candidly wrote, "Man is least himself when he talks in his own person. Give him a mask, and he will tell you the truth" (Ellmann, 1969, p. 389).

Drama Therapy Assessments

You can discover more about a person in an hour
of play than in a year of conversation.

(Plato 427-347 B.C.)

Because every person responds to trauma in different ways, it is important to assess the effects of domestic violence on each child individually (James, 1996; Webb, 1999; Weber, 2005). This assessment occurs for each child admitted. During the first twenty-four hours, children are assessed by members of an interdisciplinary treatment team. A treatment plan is then developed and implemented. The children are encouraged to contribute to this plan by identifying their personal treatment goals and are expected to work toward them for the duration of their hospitalization.

During this assessment time, the child meets with a creative arts therapist for a group which includes the children newest to the unit. This session occurs during scheduled gym time, an off unit activity, and also includes children who have been restricted to the unit due to illness or behavior. Documentation of the creative arts therapy assessment occurs within a seventy-two-hour period, which means there are children who are discharged prior to the results being documented or the treatment plan being implemented. In individual or group sessions a variety of drama therapy assessment tools are used to engage the child in treatment on the unit and to assess for ongoing treatment needs.

Prior to conducting the assessment, children are introduced to the concept of roles and the playfulness of drama therapy. In the beginning of a group session, while children are being orientated to the therapist, the space, and one another, the clinician might say, "Raise your hand if you have ever seen a movie." Depending on the group, the therapist can continue with, "Touch your nose if you have ever seen a television show." This introduces the concept of play while assessing if the children can tolerate questions and can sit or stand next to each other without physical contact. The command can be given, "Tap your shoulders three times if you have ever seen a play on stage" in order for the therapist to assess if the children have an understanding of theater and can grasp the concept of acting and role.

Another way to introduce roles is to ask the children how they behave when they are spending time with certain other individuals. Asking if they talk or behave differently when they are with their parents versus with a friend can help them identify the different social expectations of these roles. Children can be further helped to identify the roles they may already have, such as child, brother, sister, student, friend, bully, and patient. Future roles may also be explored: teacher, doctor, fire fighter, therapist, or parent. Feeling states, such as angry, upset, excited, or scared can also be played with as emotional roles are introduced. Fantasy roles, such as a superhero, devil, king, elf, magician, or an animal can sometimes give the children a special role that can allow them to express intense feelings to which they may not otherwise have access. All these roles can help children identify special qualities they have or would like to develop as well as the accepting and understanding of disowned parts of themselves. Past and future developmental roles may also be explored, so a child can begin to experience the continuity of self. In drama therapy, a goal of health is to have a greater range of roles and the flexibility and accessibility of roles as they are needed (Landy, 1986). Each child in a drama therapy group is helped, in age appropriate language to identify what a role is and what roles they may play (or have been assigned) in his/her own life. Eventually, throughout the course of their hospitalization, their childhood, or their life they may choose to accept or not accept certain roles. As Jean Paul Sartre (1961) has stated, "We only become what we are by the radical and deep-seated refusal of that which others have made of us" (preface).

One assessment tool is a simplified version of Landy's (1997) role checklist which asks, "Who Am I?", "Who Do I Want to Be?", "Who is Blocking Me?, and "Who Can Help Me?" (Landy, 1997). Fifty-six roles are listed in each of theses four categories and the person being assessed is asked to identify which roles best answer each question. This has been adapted for older adolescents on the unit. These modified roles include artist, child, gangster, searcher, popular one, boyfriend, girlfriend, student, nerd, warrior, and survivor.

Landy's assessment was further adapted for the younger children on this unit to help them affirm and support desired aspects of themselves (what might be referred to as strength-based roles) and for them to begin to identify maladaptive traits which developed in response to the violence to which they were subject. When given the assessment individually, a child writes down responses to the following three thoughts: "I Am, I Am Not, I Wish to Be." Older children may understand that how they act in the role of a student is different from how they act in the role of a friend. For younger children this may not be as apparent. Landy's assessment can be adapted for a cognitively younger client through the use of more concrete questions, such as "I Like" versus "I Am."

A child's responses can alert the therapist to both negative and positive self-concepts the child holds, his/her coping skills, conflicts, and mood. The lack of responses or omission of specific roles can also be valuable information. For example, a child who leaves the "I Wish to Be" column blank may be communicating a lack of hope for the future. Sometimes this is clearly stated, such as in the case of Marie, a clinically depressed child, who wrote "I Wish to Be . . . dead" to complete her sentence. Other times the therapist must discuss the assessment in more detail with the child and the treatment team in an effort to understand what the child meant by the response. Tyrone, another child, wrote, "I Wish to Be . . . with my brother." Upon further discussion, Tyrone shared with the therapist that he witnessed his brother's fatal shooting from across the street.

Assessment tools like this one can help a child differentiate the self from the behavior of those who have perpetrated violence, and recognize that they are not responsible for the violence (Cattanach, 1994). Amanda, a patient who had been removed from her home just prior to admission, explored ways she was different from her abusive mother by saying, "I Want to Be . . . someone who lives in peace," and added, ". . . someone who doesn't get their children taken away." Mike, a twelve-year-old child diagnosed with conduct disorder identified with his aggressive father as a means of coping and surviving. He wrote, "I Am . . . hitting others" and "I Am . . . mad, I don't let anybody push me around." As Anna Freud (1937) first identified, when confronted with an external threat, a common defense to develop, like Mike's, is to identify with the aggressor.

Case Account–Kara

Kara, a ten-year-old, who had recently been removed from her home, was admitted to the unit after assaulting her teacher and a security guard. She was a witness, a victim, and a perpetrator of domestic violence (biting and hitting her younger sister). She completed her role assessment in the following way:

> "I Am . . . angry, a nasty girl, sometimes I am nice, I am a very pretty girl who wants to be nicer. A girl with a bad attitude, a student, a sometimes good girl, only me and not anybody else.
>
> "I Am Not . . . a bad, bad girl who makes friends with people who shoots people, a girl who smokes or swears, a girl who fights cops or makes fights for no reason.
>
> "I Want to Be . . . a good girl, a nice friend, married to a husband I don't fight with, a mother who doesn't get her children taken away, important."

This assessment allowed Kara both to express her autonomy, self-acceptance, and compassion for herself as well as the anger she felt toward her mother. In asserting that she was not her mother, Kara was able to imagine a more hopeful possibility for her future self. Through the process of letting go of a role that was assigned to her by others, that of the bad girl, Kara had a chance to develop her own sense of self. The assessment and naming the above qualities helped Kara to identify these different roles as an aspect of her self, without being the entire definition of her self. She was able to acknowledge what might be considered shadow roles and her own ambivalence by identifying herself as "a nasty girl," as well as someone who "wants to be nicer," all in the same person. Drama therapy assists children in challenging rigid belief symptoms and gives them a safe place to "try on" new roles and to play with new, more flexible life patterns.

While these role assessments are ideal for the therapist to gain specific information at the time of admission, assessment is ongoing throughout the child's hospitalization. Non-physical assessment tools allow for a more gradual entry into the embodied work of drama therapy. The assessment can lead to enactments in individual and group settings as well, with the child taking on roles or casting others in the group to play a role. When others are cast, the therapist checks with the child frequently to insure that the role is played in a manner that maintains the integrity of the child's creation.

Most children jump into physical play, although there are some "non-players," as Irwin (2005) notes. These are children who typically have extensive trauma histories, depressive symptoms, or tendencies toward dysregulation and who need increased assistance and structure.

The use of sculpting, externalizing, and concretizing one's projection can offer more structure by providing aesthetic distance greater assurance that the child has more control over his or her creation. The child can pose a group member or the therapist in a posture representative of one of these roles and give them a word or a sentence to say. As with most assessments, it is best to understand the symbolic information obtained by supplementing the drama therapy assessments with other diagnostic tools and personal histories (Irwin, 2000). Sculpting can lead into more dramatic play and scene work, creating dialogues between different roles, and encouraging flexibility and integration.

The Play Space/Transitional Space: Creating Safety

We experience life in the area of transitional phenomena,
in an exciting interweave of subjectivity and objective observation,
and in an area that is intermediate between the inner reality of the
individual and the shared reality of the world that is external to individual.
(Winnicott, 1971, p. 64)

The room that the drama therapy session takes place in may serve several purposes (dining room, class room, visiting room). The ritualized structure of the session helps create what is referred to in the theatre as suspension of disbelief by transforming the multipurpose room into a special space. The drama therapy session's warm-up facilitates movement toward what Winnicott (1971) calls the "transitional space" and what drama therapists often refer to as the play space. This is the space in between the known and unknown, bordering on subjective and objective, teetering between conscious and unconscious, moving between primary and secondary processes.

In comparing ritual and drama therapy sessions, Jennings (1987) referred to Van Gennep's "rites de passage" or "life-transition ritual" (p. 13), which breaks down the structure of ritual into three components: "separation, transition and reincorporation" (p. 13). A drama therapy session is structured with an opening or warm up (separation) which readies people for the enactment, the middle phase. Closure at the end of the session supplies containment and integration of the experience. Both ritual and drama therapy sessions serve to separate the participant from the daily and mundane activities into the transitional time where learning takes place (Jennings, 1987; Winnicott, 1971).

While the ritualized structure can provide a level of containment and security, for some children whose home is a place of danger and fear, much of the early emphasis in treatment may involve assisting them in creating their own individual sense of safety. In group settings, drama therapists can assist children in enacting affirming memories, which may provide comfort and reassurance, either through story work, drama games, or projective techniques. "Remembering how safe and secure it felt to sit in grandma's kitchen – with emphasis on the comfortable bodily sensations – may be even more important to current functioning then remembering a frightening incident. Sometimes a positive memory can help an individual resolve a difficulty without having to confront the traumatic memory that is triggering it" (Rothschild, 2000, p. 118). This is important especially in acute settings where it may be contraindicated to address extreme trauma.

In some groups, children have an opportunity to create their own planet, island, or country; a place where they are in charge and in command of their own customs, laws, and population. Once special places are created, the rest of the group members, with the child's permission, can ask questions and visit each other's created places. In one application of this exercise, adolescent girls were invited to create their own island. Group members were guided to visualize a safe place and then they were asked open ended question that allowed them to further develop it in their mind's eye. They were then given dramatic materials to recreate their safe place. Group members shared experiences, either by showing their image or by letting the group visit the safe space though improvisation. One member invited the group to a pristine beach where group members walked along the water's edge with bare feet, looking for seashells. Another group member, Sara, a fourteen-year-old girl diagnosed with Post Traumatic Stress Disorder and Borderline Personality Disorder, told the group that she would neither show her island nor take anyone there. Sara, who had been beaten so badly by her grandfather that part of her skull was crushed, told the group that no one else was permitted on her island. The group members were supportive, accepting her request, which made it possible for her to then talk about the feelings that had guided her choice. Obtaining permission is important and some children may prefer to not allow others to view their created world. Permission, in these cases, equals control, and perhaps this is the first time a child's "No" will be respected.

In another group, younger children were invited to take on the role of king, queen, or a title of their choice. This invocation is aided with costume props (crown, velvet robes, and a larger chair). In turn, group members told about their kingdom and let others ask questions. Six year old Johnny, the youngest child in the group, was last to take a turn as king. He had been selectively mute since admission, uttering only a few words. He had been recently removed from his home because of neglect and abuse and placed in foster care. He displayed little interaction with others, always staying on the periphery of the session. Johnny seemed delighted to put on the costume and brightened even more when he had the entire group's attention. However, after a few moments in the spotlight, he was still silent. As his peers become less attentive, he looked more anxious and uncomfortable. The therapist asked if Johnny would allow his peers to ask questions about his kingdom, taking pressure off of him to speak and make up something on his own. When there was no response, the therapist, pretending to speak in a foreign language, spoke in gibberish to Johnny. Johnny's anxious look was replaced with surprise. The therapist then spoke to the group members and introduced him as the Royal Highness, further explaining that the King came from a faraway land and did not speak their language, but allowed the therapist to serve as his translator.

Johnny continued to look at the therapist who again spoke to Johnny in gibberish. Johnny slowly smiled and said a few words of gibberish back. The therapist translated Johnny's gibberish and offered to translate the group's questions. With each gibberish interaction Johnny seemed more confident, speaking longer, and smiling broadly. After this group, Johnny would greet the therapist with gibberish for the remainder of his hospitalization. His experience in this group boosted his self esteem and elevated his status with his peers. His comic side was seen by others, which allowed acceptance that was not there before. He was able to have increased interpersonal experiences during his hospitalization, which led to eventual verbalization with both children and adults.

Embodied Play

. . . Mastery of the trauma is not complete unless it includes body-work that allows the child to reclaim ownership of her body and to feel a sense of respect and mastery on a basic physical level.

(James, 1996, p. 28)

It is now widely accepted that one's body is linked to both memory and affect. As van der Kolk (1996) writes: "Brain, body, and mind are inextricably linked, and it is only for heuristic reasons that we can still speak of them as if they constitute separate entities. Alternations in any one of these three will intimately affect the other two" (p. 216). Working in an embodied way allows a client to approach traumatic memory, which is stored in the body (Rothschild, 2000, van der Kolk, 1996). "To make meaning of the traumatic experience usually is not enough. Traumatized individuals need to have experiences that directly contradict the emotional helplessness and physical paralysis that accompany traumatic experiences" (van der Kolk, 2003, p. 188). Appropriate use of drama therapy techniques can provide safe access to these feelings without retraumatization. Emunah (1994) writes, "emotions and sensations lodged in the past are accessed and once again experienced in the body, but this time within the safe confines of the dramatic mode and among supportive others" (p. 122).

Case Account–Risa

Following is a case example of how physical play was used to assist Risa, a beautiful five-year-old girl who was admitted to the unit after numerous fights at school resulting in suspensions. Within minutes of arriving on the floor, she became aggressive toward staff and her peers, throwing her arms in an uncontrolled attempt to strike another. She related poorly and was unable to interact safely with her peers without an adult's constant intervention. She would scratch or bite others, demonstrating no fear of retaliation. Risa was all impulse and action. She did not seem to have the internal space for anything in between. A culture of violence was evident in her home. Following several case conferences, some of her history began to unfold. There was a dangerous combination of substance abuse and domestic violence that went back two generations. While she was never (as far as we know) physically harmed, she did witness most of the physical attacks and was verbally abused. Both of her parents were inconsistent and neglectful in their parenting. In spite of this, Risa felt connected to her father, who had been the aggressor. Risa had internalized the role of the aggressor and seemed to have no remorse for her actions.

Risa was able to tolerate only small group therapy sessions, where she was able to have more individualized attention. Group play with Risa centered on helping her develop an awareness of choice. During drama therapy sessions the command of "Stop and Go" was incorporated into the play in a variety of ways and contexts. Usually these games were in the context of dramatic play, with Risa and group members enacting stories or experiences. For example, during one group, group members were asked to fasten their seat belts as they pretended to fly to the moon. Risa, usually unable to remain seated for than a minute was able to remain seated until the group decided the rocket had landed. While seated, she was able to keep her hands to herself, not scratching or touching another child. Risa had been given the role of pilot and was busily steering and pushing imaginary controls. Walking on the moon further slowed Risa down, increasing her awareness and control of her own movements. As the weeks of her hospitalization continued, she was slowly able to increase the time between her movement and her stillness and was slowly developing increased tolerance in small group settings. In spite of this decrease in her assaultive behavior, Risa was discharged to a state psychiatric hospital for long-term treatment.

Case Account–TJ

TJ was a nine-year-old boy admitted after breaking the arm of his younger toddler-aged sister and displaying physically violent behavior toward his mother. He presented with an oddly related affect and seemed with a complete disconnect between his actions and emotions. For the first week of his admission, the staff had no history about TJ since he had been abandoned by his mother in the emergency room. He would bully the younger children on the unit. He attached quickly to any available adult and was considered clingy by others. Later, the staff learned that his mother was very young and clinically depressed.

TJ was encouraged to engage in embodied play in an effort to help him expand his range of emotional expression and modulate his affect. The drama therapist gave him permission to express emotions in group and individual sessions and assisted him in identifying the continuum of feeling states. He was allowed to be upset, sad, angry, or annoyed as long as these were explored safely. A variety of theater games and techniques were used to help TJ develop skills to identify and express feelings. One of these therapeutic games involved the use of Action Cards, cards created by the drama therapists with various activities written on them. These cards list an assortment of actions and activities people may engage in regularly, such as brushing your teeth or tying a shoe. Emotion Cards can also be added to the activities, instructing the children to perform the action from a specific feeling state. For example, in one group, when TJ had a turn, he chose one card from the first pile, on which was written, "make a phone call" (Action Card). He added a card from the second pile, which had written "anger" (Emotion Card). TJ was encouraged to act out this activity while expressing anger. In the group setting, the job of the "audience" was to guess TJ's action and feeling. While most group members were able to guess the action correctly, no one could identify what feeling he was conveying. TJ, with flat affect, mimed picking up a phone. He had no visible expression on his face. His actions were slow and unremarkable. Members guessed he was feeling bored or that he did not care. TJ was surprised that no one knew that he was expressing anger. Following the enactments, the therapist helped both TJ and the group members consider how easy it is to misinterpret another's affect. TJ shared with the group that often when he was angry, he felt that no one was seriously considering his feelings. This contributed to his verbal outbursts and aggression toward others. The group assisted him in realizing that conflicts on and off the unit frequently begin with the misreading and misinterpretation of his non-verbal expressions. In addition, anger, which may allow for one to feel powerful, is often substituted for feelings that leave on feeling more vulnerable such as sadness and shame. Research examining the correlation between "verbal ability and display of aggression" (p. 217), indicated that children with higher levels of aggression ranked low on language skills (Crenshaw & Mordock, 2005, p. 217). Helping TJ and others to accurately identify and label their feelings helps to develop and improve communication and social skills. This results in diminished conflict and increased empathetic response to others.

When working individually, TJ often chose to work with action figures, playing both hero and villain. In the early stages of play, there was little dialogue, with the action figures colliding and TJ supplying sound effects such as "BAM" and "WHACK." The therapist, serving as witness, would be given a commentary about what was happening in the battle and story. Over a period of several sessions, TJ enrolled the therapist as villain, still with little dialogue, but continued the physical aggression targeting the smallest figure. The therapist, in role, would respond to TJ's assaults in a variety of ways ("Oh no, you got me again," "You think you can stop me?" "Please don't hurt me"). All of these seem to delight TJ, and encouraged TJ to offer increased verbalizations with the actions. The play continued to have repetitive themes of TJ alone, fighting evil with little pause. After several sessions, the therapist in the role of the battered villain began to compliment TJ's hero and voiced both admiration and envy of his great skills (flying, jumping high, and seeing through walls). TJ began to befriend the villain, offering to show the therapist/villain how to fly and enlist this new friend to fight other villains. In forming an alliance with the therapist, TJ, who was frequently rejected by others because of his aggressive, bullying behavior, was able to form a positive attachment in his projective play. During the beginning of his hospitalization, TJ's participation in more interactive groups with improvisation usually resulted in conflict, primarily because of his provocative and aggressive behavior. Working with action figures gave him a chance to practice and to "develop playacting skills in the microsphere. Such play contributes more to affect modulation than does action play without structure because play actions take place in the mind and not in behavior" (Crenshaw & Mordock, 2005, p. 232).

Projective Play

As it turns out, the puppets and the dolls in
my office can be anything a child wants them to be
(Terr, 1990, p. 236)

When used in therapy, projective techniques allow the client to project wants, needs, and desires onto objects. These objects may be masks, puppets, small toys, action figures, storybook characters, or even other people. Therapists validate a child's experiences, feelings, and memories through play in third person. Winnicott (1963) and Klein (1932) explore children's relationship to play and their primary objects. In describing Klein's work, Winnicott writes:

> [T]here has been a wholesome projection of a constellation from the child's inner psychic reality so that the room and the table and the toys are subjective objects, and the child and the analyst are both there in this sample of the child's inner world. What is outside the room is outside the child. (Winnicott, 1963, p. 185)

Puppets are excellent therapy tools when working with children who have recently been traumatized because they provide distance, a protective shield of sorts, to hide behind. Puppets, unlike children, are allowed to say anything at all (James, 1996), which often gives permission for safe verbal expression. The therapist may choose to be more direct at times by using the puppets to voice children's fears and help them know that they are not alone and not to blame.

While keeping in mind the concept of distancing, it is useful to have a range of puppets from which the child can choose (Irwin, 2000). Puppets that too closely mirror the child's self, such as puppets based on human features, may be too under-distanced for the child who has been exposed to the violence of trauma against a person (Landy, 1996). All types of animal puppets, including tame and wild ones, people puppets, and fantasy puppets should also be available for the child. Aggressive feelings can be expressed in ways that are no longer harmful and hands and arms can be used playfully. Rarely in this setting would there be time for a child to create his own puppet, so a set of sturdy puppets are available. If a drama therapist is interested in having children create their own puppets, and the clinician has not been exposed to the impact art supplies may have on children's behavior, sensitivity to the materials should be explored.

Puppets and puppetry allow a client to create his/her world by having control over the stories told or over the actual manipulation of the puppet characters. At times, one can identify with the puppet and with "the meaning behind its existence as well as its resentment of and dependence on being controlled" (Weiss, 1998, pp. 220-221). Puppets can assist those clients who find it hard to connect with other humans to find a sense of relatedness (Irwin 2000; Weiss, 1998). After playing with the puppet, most children will benefit from some additional closure, such as de-roling the puppet, by either doing a drawing of the puppet or doing a ritualized good bye as a way to terminate the session (Weiss, 1998). Irwin (2000) suggests "interviewing the puppets, speaking directly to them about what happened" (p. 689) as a way to help the clinician gain more insight into the story.

Case Account–Ella

Ella was admitted after witnessing her father violently beat her mother. Quickly overwhelmed from being Ella's only caretaker, Ella's mother cut short her daughter's once long brown hair, telling Ella it was her fault because it was always getting in knots. When Ella came onto the unit, she was sullen and quiet, refusing to talk to anyone. After her third time in the drama therapy room, Ella picked up a princess puppet with long blond hair. "Rapunzel, Rapunzel," she whispered. The therapist, matching her volume, replied, "Let down your long hair." Ella, after stroking the yellow yarn, fully enrolled in the puppet character and stated in a surprised voice, "I can't. It's been all cut off!"

As the therapist witnessed, Ella handed her a much smaller witch puppet and said, "Now you play the witch. And be mean. Really nasty." Hesitantly, the therapist agreed. As Irwin (2004) writes, accepting these negative projective identifications, while emotionally tricky, are an important aspect in the child's therapy. It was clear that the therapist's shouts of, "Get out of here!" were not what her script called for, as Ella requested stronger language with a more forceful tone. With great affect, she instructed the therapist to play the role as witch, feeding her the lines, "You horrible, disgusting child! I don't know why I ever had you! Get out of my house! Leave and don't come back home ever."

Irwin (2004) discusses the importance of a child being able to express "feelings of anger and contempt" (p. 17) in play and also to recognize the element of transference that arises. Being cast in such a horrific role challenges clinicians, trained to be supportive, kind and nurturing. And yet, this replaying, with the therapist's sensitivity to moments for reparative work, certainly was in the service of Ella's developing ego. The therapist had opportunities to express out loud just how nasty that witch is, allowing Ella to realize that her story had been heard and her feelings (through the projective objects) validated. Terr (1990) describes post traumatic play as different from children's common play. "As opposed to ordinary child's play, post-traumatic play is obsessively repeated. It is grim. Furthermore, it requires a certain set of conditions in order to proceed – a certain place, a certain assortment of dolls, certain playmates, or a certain routine" (p. 239). In free play, children will take on roles of other characters spontaneously. They can play as animals, as mystical creatures, and as other humans. Post traumatic play is monotonous and can be unsafe (Crenshaw & Mordock, 2005; Gil, 1991; Terr, 1990). While Ella felt a psychological needed to play and re-play her story every time she met with the therapist, the therapist had to help Ella to keep the play in metaphor through the use of puppets. Ella's play, through her use of projective techniques, was not as traumatic as the play of some other children. Eventually she was able to add roles to her story and direct the therapist to play others as well.

Role of the Drama Therapist

The children in our care have already been abused by a harsh life, so our responsibility is not to add to that abuse.
(Cattanach, 1994, p. 67)

When working with children who have been exposed to domestic violence, the role of the therapist is to provide a safe enough therapy space for them to tell their story, to recognize their feelings, to provide ongoing support, and to begin to suggest how a story may have a different ending. This story may or may not be the actual story of his or her trauma, and depending on the child and their length of stay, efforts to obtain the truth should not be encouraged.

In order to create this safe space, the therapist must be alert to his/her own countertransference and present with a willingness to engage in ongoing supervision to explore difficult feelings aroused in this work – rescue fantasies, hate, and pity are often felt toward child clients. As Winnicott (1947) wrote, "The analyst must be prepared to bear strain without expecting the patient to know anything about what he is doing, perhaps over a long period of time. To do this he must easily be aware of his own fear and hate" (p. 198). Cattanach (1999) also views supervision as a necessity and states, "Children are especially vulnerable to the abuse of power in a therapeutic relationship and supervision can explore this dynamic to keep children as safe as possible in therapy" (p. 81). Further, Cattanach (1994) acknowledges that work with children is "very stressful for the therapist" (p. 67) and parallels the importance of supervision in providing a safe space for the therapist to explore his/her work with the therapist providing a safe space for his/her client.

Vicarious traumatization is not a rare occurrence when providing treatment and ongoing therapy is also highly recommended for a therapist working with this population. Countertransference can be a very useful tool for the therapist in finding the right combination to open the lock to a child's inner world. This self-awareness and resolution of one's own childhood issues allows the therapist to be fully present for the child, who is in need of so much, but may not always be able to directly ask for help. "The therapist must communicate a willingness to stay emotionally present to the child throughout the process of playing or dramatizing the horrendous details that haunt them" (Weber, 2004, p. 34). The therapist may be the only supportive, authentic adult the child experiences. "A feeling of being understood is an important goal of treatment" (Robbins, 1998, p. 103).

Haen (2004) describes the role of the drama therapist on an inpatient unit as having many functions. "In addition to coordinating group therapy, the author sees children individually for trauma-specific play therapy, assists with milieu management, meets with families, . . . and may play out the roles of disciplinarian, coach, supporter, surrogate family member, advocate, guide, and clinician at different points in any given day" (p. 191). A therapist working with children needs to help the child client organize fragmented thoughts, provide grounding experiences (both physically and psychologically), assist the child in targeting against dissociations and help him to feel his body in space. The therapist interprets the child's responses in effort to relay insight and meanings to the child, family, or other professional. Clarification of events and developmentally appropriate reality responses are important steps in this process (Weber, 2005).

It is important to encourage the children to explore, to create, to talk about their experiences when they are ready, and to have fun (Weber, 2005) in effort to encourage their private self to emerge. This private self, often hidden in an attempt to self protect from the violence at home, plays an important role in ego development. It is truly a gift when the therapist is allowed to be a witness to this private self, the self many children work very hard to protect and lock forever inside a Gorilla suit (Crenshaw& Mordock, 2005). For as Winnicott (1963) states, "It is a sophisticated game of hide and seek in which it is a joy to be hidden, but a disaster not to be found" (p. 186).

Terms

(These are general definitions and in no way attempt to define complex concepts in their entirety.)

Aesthetic Distancing: Emotional expression that is clarifying and relieving, a felt intelligence.
Attention Deficit/Hyperactivity Disorder: A condition that makes it hard for children to control their behavior and/or pay attention.
Autistic Spectrum Disorders: Conditions that include non-spoken communication problems, usually with socialization/empathy.
Borderline Personality Disorder: A condition marked by a persistent pattern of instable interpersonal relationships, self-image, and affects.
Concretize: To make real or specific.
Conduct Disorder: A group of behavioral and emotional problems where children have great difficulty following rules and behaving in a socially acceptable way.
Disruptive Behavior Disorders: Also called Behavior Disorders. An umbrella term that includes more specific disorders, such as *Conduct Disorder*, *Oppositional Defiance Disorder*, and *ADHD*.

Distancing: A technique used to find balance of emotional experience and expression in treatment.
Dysregulation: An emotional response that is not well modulated.
Encopresis: Fecal soiling.
Oppositional Defiant Disorder: A disorder marked by uncooperative, hostile, defiant behavior toward authority figures.
Overdistance: A state of rationality at the expense of emotional expression.
Projective Techniques: Techniques in which aspects of the person are externalized and projected out onto an object or persona such as with the use of puppets, masks, sand tray, action figures, dolls, sculpting, storytelling and theatre.
Role: A basic unit of personality containing specific qualities that provide uniqueness and coherence to that unit.
Role Training: Behavioral rehearsal.
Sculpting: Creating a living tableau with other human bodies.
Underdistance: A flooding of emotion which brings neither relief nor insight.

References

Arroyo, W., & Eth, S. (1995). Assessment following violence--witnessing trauma. In Peled, E., Jaffee P., & Edelson (Ed.), *Ending the cycle of violence: Community responses to children of battered women.* Thousand Oaks: Sage Publications.

Bolby, J. (1988). *A secure base: Parent and child attachment and healthy human development.* New York: Basic Books.

Carroll, L. (1865). *Alice's adventures in wonderland.* England: Macmillan.

Cattanach, A. (1999). Supervision in playtherapy and dramatherapy with children. In E. Tslinkas-Portman (Ed.), *Supervision and dramatherapy* (pp. 80-91). Philadelphia: Jessica Kingsley Publishers.

Cattanach, A. (1994). *Play therapy: Where the sky meets the underworld.* Bristol, PA: Jessica Kingsley Publishers.

Crenshaw, D., & Mordock, J. (2005). *A handbook of play therapy with aggressive children.* Lanham, MD: Rowman.

Disney, W. (producer), & Geronimi, C., et al. (Writer/Director). (1951). Alice in wonderland [Motion picture]. United States: Walt Disney.

Ellmann, R. (1969). *The artist as critic: Critical writings of Oscar Wilde.* New York: Random House.

Emunah, R. (1994). *Acting for real: Drama therapy process, technique and performance.* New York: Brunner/Mazel.

Erikson, E. (1950). *Childhood and society.* New York: Norton

Fantuzzo, J., & Mohr, W. (1999). Prevalence and effects of child exposure to domestic violence. *The Future of Children: Domestic Violence and Children, 9*(3), 21-32.

Freud, A. (1937). *The ego and the mechanisms of defense.* London: Hogarth Press.

Gil, E. (1991). *The healing power of play: Working with abused children.* New York: Guilford Press.

Haen, C. (2005). Group therapy in a children's inpatient psychiatric setting. In C. Haen & A. Weber (Eds.), *Clinical applications of drama therapy in child and adolescent treatment* (pp. 189-203). New York: Routledge.

Harding, A. (2006). (Reuters Health) Pediatrics *Thursday*, retrieved on August 17, 2006. From www.ucsfhealth.org/childrens/health_library/reuters/2006/08/2006 0817elin021.html.

Herman, J. (1997). *Trauma and recovery.* New York: Basic Books.

Huizinga, J. (1950). *Homo Ludens: The study of the play element in culture.* Boston: The Beacon Press.

Irwin, E. (2005). Facilitating play with non-players. In C. Haen & A. Weber (Eds.), *Clinical applications of drama therapy in child and adolescent treatment* (pp. 3-23). New York: Routledge.

Irwin, E. (2000). The use of a puppet interview to understand children. In K. Gitlin-Weiner, A. Sandgrund, & C. Schaefer (Eds.), *Play diagnosis and assessment* (pp. 682-703). New York: John Wiley & Sons, Inc.

James, B. (1996). *Treating traumatized children: New insights and creative interventions.* New York: The Free Press.

Jennings, S. (1987) Dramatherapy and groups. In S. Jennings (Ed.), *Dramatherapy: Theory and practice for teachers and clinicians* (pp. 1-18) Cambridge, MA: Brookline Books.

Klein, M. (1932). *The psychoanalysis of children.* London: Hogarth.

King, Martin Luther Jr. (1967) *Where do we go from here: Chaos or Community?* New York: Harper Row.

Koste, V. (1995). *Dramatic play in childhood.* Portsmith, NH: Heinemann.

Landy, R. (1997). Drama therapy and distancing: Reflections on theory and clinical application. *The Arts in Psychotherapy, 23*(5), 367-373.

Landy, R. (1996). *Essays in drama therapy: The double life.* Pennsylvania: Jessica Kingsley Publishers.

Landy, R. (1986). *Drama therapy: Concepts and practices.* Springfield, IL: Charles C Thomas, Publisher, Ltd.

Lynn, M., & Nisivoccia, D. (1996). Helping forgotten victims: Using activity groups with children who witness violence. In N. Webb (Ed.), *Play therapy with children in crisis: Individual, group and family treatment.* New York: Guilford Press.

National Association for Drama Therapy. (1979). Definition of drama therapy, retrieved on December 18, 2006, from www.nadt.org/about.html.

Plato (427-347 B.C.)

Robbins, A. (1998). Affect and therapeutic presence as a diagnostic indicator. In A. Robbins (Ed.), *Therapeutic presence: Bridging expression and form* (pp. 87-104). Philadelphia: Jessica Kingsley Publishers.

Rossman, B., Hughes, H., & Rosenberg, M. (2000). *Children and interparental violence: The impact of exposure.* Philadelphia: Brunner/Mazel.

Rothschild, B. (2000). *The body remembers: The psychophysiology of trauma and trauma treatment.* New York: W.W. Norton and Company.

Sartre, J. (1961). Preface to Fanon, Frantz (1961) *Wretched of the earth.* New York: Grove/Atlantic.

Shakespeare, W. *Hamlet. Shakespeare: The complete dramatic and poetic works of William Shakespeare, Red Letter Edition.* Intr. Frederick D. Losey. Philadelphia: John C. Winston Company, 1952. pp. 1000-1040.

Terr, L. (1990). *Too scared to cry.* New York: Basic Books.

Tyson, E., & Baffour, T. (2004). Arts-based strengths: A solution-focused intervention with adolescents in an acute-care psychiatric setting. *The Arts in Psychotherapy, 31*(4), 213-227.

van der Kolk, B. (2003). Post traumatic stress disorder and the nature of trauma. In M. Solomon & D. Siegel (Eds.), *Healing trauma: Attachment, mind, body and brain* (pp. 168-195). New York: W.W. Norton and Company.

van der Kolk, B. (1996). The body keeps score: Approaches to the psychobiology of post traumatic stress disorder. In B. van der Kolk, C. McFarlane, & L. Weisaeth (Eds.), *Traumatic stress: The effects of overwhelming experience on mind, body, and society* (pp. 214-241). New York: Guilford Press.

Webb, N. B. (1999). Assessment of the child in crisis. In N. Webb (Ed.), *Play therapy with children in crisis.* New York: Guilford Press.

Weber, A. M. (2005). "Don't hurt my mommy": Drama therapy for children who have witnessed severe domestic violence. In C. Haen & A. Weber (Eds.), *Clinical applications of drama therapy in child and adolescent treatment* (pp. 189-203). New York: Routledge.

Weiss, F. (1998). The field of wings: Puppetry as therapy from an object relations point of view and incorporating field psychology. In A. Robbins (Ed.), *Therapeutic presence: Bridging expression and form* (pp. 219-244). Philadelphia: Jessica Kingsley Publishers.

Winnicott, D. W. (1971). *Playing and reality.* New York: Tavistock/Routhedge.

Winnicott, D. W. (1963). Communicating and not communicating leading to a study of opposites.

Winnicott, D. W. (1954-5). The depressive position in normal emotional development. In *Through pediatrics to psychoanalysis: Collected papers* (pp. 262-273). New York: Basic Books.

Winnicott, D. W. (1947). Hate in the countertransference. In *Through pediatrics to psychoanalysis: Collected papers* (pp. 194-203). New York: Basic Books.

Biography

Barbara McKechnie, LCAT, RDT, LPC (NJ) is President of the National Association for Drama Therapy. She is a drama therapist working with children and adolescents on a psychiatric inpatient unit. Barbara has worked with child, adolescent and with adult populations with co-occurring illness (mental illness and substance abuse). Her post-graduate training includes New York University's International Trauma Studies Program. She is on the faculty at the New School teaching drama therapy courses in the Creative

Arts Therapies Certificate Program. Barbara also has additional training in psychodrama and developmental transformations. Contact Barbara at mckechnieb@earthlink.net.

Kristin Long, LCAT, RDT/BCT has facilitated groups with children and adolescents in recreational, educational, and mental health settings for over fifteen years. She is currently completing psychoanalytic training at the Institute for Expressive Analysis in New York City, where she maintains a private practice. Kristin works with children, adolescents, and adults in individual and family sessions. She also supervises mental health professionals. Contact Kristin at klongnyc@nyc.rr.com or 212-982-1065.

Chapter 13

USING DRAMA THERAPY IN DOMESTIC VIOLENCE GROUPS FOR INCARCERATED WOMEN

LIORA ABRAHAMS BROSBE

Introduction

Working with survivors of domestic violence requires flexibility, spontaneity, and a toolkit of interventions that work well with groups. The domestic violence program at Project Pride in Oakland, California primarily uses drama therapy to create a safe place for survivors to get support around their past abusive histories and commit to maintaining a life free of violence for themselves and their children. The use of drama therapy is particularly conducive to working with domestic violence survivors because the embodied process connects directly to the embodied experience of trauma (Herman, 1997). Furthermore, the experience of incarcerated women can perpetuate systems of violence, power, and control. Drama therapy is an empowering, embodied action method and most directly allows for witnessing in a therapeutic sense that can also be instrumental in breaking the cycle of violence.

Drama therapy is often geared specifically for group psychotherapy. In an age of decreased funding and an increased demand for effective short-term therapeutic alternatives, this chapter outlines an eight-week group therapy series and corresponding drama therapy interventions that accomplish institutional as well as individual treatment goals. Additionally, this chapter proposes a curriculum that combines the psychoeducational models such as: the Duluth model of wheels including power and control (Domestic Abuse Intervention Project, n.d.). Walker's (2000) cycle of violence, personal safety plans (Fazzone, Holton, & Reed, 2003), and action techniques from drama therapists Renée Emunah (1994, 2000, 2001) and David Read Johnson

(2000). My techniques are also drawn from the work of Augusto Boal (1997) in Image Theatre, Forum Theatre, and Theatre of the Oppressed. In addition to the specifics of working with domestic violence and trauma, my clinical work also examines how to incorporate clinical issues relating to domestic violence in a substance abuse treatment model and the challenges and benefits of integrating each approach.

The clients in the weekly domestic violence group are residents of Project Pride, a Mother-Infant program officially titled a Community Prisoner Mother Program (CPMP) for incarcerated women and clients court ordered to a residential drug recovery program. The group is designed to provide psychoeducational resources about domestic violence and also be a processing group for women who are survivors of domestic violence. Drama therapy provides a forum to explore past experiences and also embody possibilities for the future. The content of the groups' process is around violence against women which can range from the clients' experience of poverty, pregnancy and the medical system, the foster care system, sexual violence including rape and incest, gang violence, and the pervasive violence related to using and dealing drugs. The clients are incarcerated and the group explores, discusses, and processes the violence they experienced when they were arrested and in the prison system itself.

Client Population

Project Pride is the residential treatment division of East Bay Community Recovery Project in Oakland, California. There are two different populations of women that live at Project Pride. One group is women from the State of California Department of Corrections and Rehabilitation (CDCR). These state inmates come to Project Pride to participate in a CDCR Community Prisoner Mother Program also called a Mother-Infant Care program or (Legal Services for Prisoners with Children, n.d.; Pierson, 2003). Mothers are reunited with their children under the age of nine, and pregnant inmates come to give birth and subsequently bond with their child outside of prison. Inmates with more than one child under the age of nine must make a choice of which child comes to live with them. Often, they choose the youngest child, so as to develop a strong attachment at some of the more sensitive stages of development such as infancy through toddlerhood. Women from the prison system serve the final months or years of their sentence at Project Pride while living with their children. Working with incarcerated women around issues of violence and trauma provides an opportunity to examine relevant examples from the clients' experiences in the prison system.

Also living at Project Pride are "perinatal" clients who come into residential substance abuse treatment because they are court ordered, mandated through Child Protective Services (CPS), or receive a community referral. The majority of the perinatal residents come to live at Project Pride as a result of CPS involvement due to drug use or as an alternative to serving county jail time for crimes involving drugs. The crimes committed among the prison inmates are also predominately related to drug use or sales. The primary drug of choice of the women is methamphetamine; however, heroin and crack cocaine are also common. The intersection of recovery from substance dependence and recovery from trauma is the crux of where the treatment lies. Both the perinatal and CDCR clients live in the communal residential setting structured around a therapeutic community (DeLeon, 2000).

Group Structure

The series typically includes 8-10 sessions. Each session is once a week for ninety minutes. The amount of sessions largely depends on the programming structure of other groups, holidays or factors that might contribute to a more successful program, such as a group of participants with an upcoming parole date. The first session of each series is open, the entire house is welcome to attend, and the following sessions are closed to new members until the next series begins anew. Any client who completes the series is welcome to continue in the next series, and in many cases women will continue for multiple series. Using drama therapy aids in keeping the material fresh and eliciting new responses from group members, even when clients have already participated in a series. There is an average of six clients in each group with a range between four to ten clients. Attendance can vary based on illness, child care, and a client's parole date.

The racial and ethnic makeup of the group resembles that of the entire house with about 50% white and 50% women of color, including Asian American and Native American women. Although in the house, 25% of the residents are African American and 25% are Latina, the participation of African-American clients is sporadic and inconsistent. I attribute this to the racial tension in the house. While the white women tend to come and consistently attend the group, African American clients may choose not to come if there are white women in the group. The initial distrust or resistance to attending the group may also be based on my race as a white therapist. I have attempted interventions to recruit African-American women into the group, and the most successful circumstances have been with clients without children in the house and waiting for placement (usually CPS is involved and the children are with family members or foster care). This leads me to believe that in addition to the racial tension in the house, African-American women experience both cultural and personal obstacles to delegating their children during the group.

The clients in the group are mostly in their mid twenties but range from age 19-48. The sexual orientation of the group members is primarily heterosexual, and although in one-on-one discussions with me a client may disclose that they are in or have been in same-sex relationships, there have been only a handful of members who openly identify as bi-sexual or gay. The lack of out homosexual clients is largely due to institutional and internalized homophobia and heterosexism. This dynamic is replicated in the demographics of the entire house, where a bi-sexual or lesbian may be out on some level; yet, the women are not officially out about their sexual orientation for multiple reasons. Since every resident is a mother, this gives them credibility as heterosexual women when living and interacting with homophobic residents or staff.

The group is a voluntary evening group, although some residents are mandated to attend the group by their CPS worker. Encouraging clients to attend the group on a voluntary basis reduces resistance, encourages accountability, and creates an atmosphere of willingness to learn, rather than forcing women to examine their relationships when they are not ready. Because the group is voluntary, the women often come to group willing to share past experiences in violent relationships, as well as situations that are very present in their current lives. As a result, the challenges the women face in the program, including separation from their family and children, loneliness, grief, cravings for drugs, body image, and conflicts with residents and staff are a frequent source of processing and sharing in the group. Often the clients come with frustrations and anger about dynamics between other residents "on the floor" and also the dynamic with staff. When issues come up that are not explicitly related to domestic violence, I will often ask them to explore how this relates the structure of power and control. This has been a delicate balance in the sense of professionalism, appearing united with the other staff to avoid splitting, and also having empathy for the concerns of the clients.

Working with clients in a residential in-patient setting provides an opportunity to facilitate self-reflection and examination while the client is physically removed from their communities and, by extension, violent relationships. The advantage to working with inmates in the prison system is that the women are by definition supervised and contained so that they are physically safe from their abusive partners. This does not mean they do not have contact via the phone and mail, but often this form of contact can spark deep personal inquiry in a relatively safe environment. As the therapist, I am constantly aware of the complexity of addressing themes of institutional power, including racism and sexism, from within the prison system. It is crucial to understand that clinical work around domestic violence does not happen in a vacuum. One of the many clinical challenges I face at Project Pride is to identify the therapeutic implications of doing domestic violence work within an inherently racist system that also exemplifies the dynamic of power and control.

Group Guidelines and Standards

Group guidelines are a central part of the therapeutic community model (DeLeon, 2000). Beyond the established rules for each group and the residential community (which does include confidentiality), during the first session I ask the women to create a list of group agreements that would create a safe group environment. I often add to their list my own requirements about being on time and committed to the group. I type up the agreements, and on the following week each client signs a copy of the agreements as their commitment to the agreements and participation in the group.

The two rules that I require as the facilitator is that there are no children allowed in the group and group confidentiality. Not allowing children in the group is complicated since Project Pride is a program for mothers and their children. The overall programming is geared toward facilitating family reunification, clean and sober living, providing a supportive atmosphere to learn, and develop positive parenting skills. Most groups held at Project Pride allow infants to attend, and often changing diapers, bottle-feeding, and fussy babies are incorporated into the dynamic of the session. The special parameter of not allowing children in this group incorporates two important lessons that is the basis for the rule; to practice the skill of securing childcare and to set clear boundaries for what material is inappropriate for children. Once a woman paroles, child care may be a financial stress, but the emotional stress of finding childcare is one of the most challenging aspects of living at Project Pride. When a resident must delegate her child the process often triggers an entire range of emotions including trust, guilt, fear, anger, and anxiety. The delegation of a child involves asking another resident to be responsible for the child during the 90-minute group. In the best case scenario, two residents that have a respectful and trusting relationship can rely on each other for consistent support including child care. In the worst case, other clients may choose to deliberately sabotage a client's participation in optional groups and refuse to support the client by watching their child.

My standards for clients honoring confidentiality is that if I learn of any group member talking about what is discussed in the group with other residents, I will ask them to leave the group. I make very clear the limits to confidentiality and my duty to report in specific cases, and state how both the strict enforcement of confidentiality and the professional limits of such are about safety. Although this is largely about the structure and expectations of the group members, it introduces the theme of safety as a central clinical element that will be a theme throughout the group.

Establishing during the first session my zero tolerance policy for talking about what is shared in the sessions outside the group is one of the ways I have found the group to be so successful. Many clients report that they do not share in other processing groups because it is common for other residents to retaliate and use information shared in groups against each other, whether it is undermining child care or direct verbal abuse. The daily life at Project Pride involves childcare, roommate relationships, and communal responsibilities which are all affected by the process in the groups and vice versa. By creating a safe, confidential environment during the domestic violence group, members of the group continue to support one another during their interactions within the community.

Theoretical Orientation

Drama therapy is the primary modality I use in the group. I also incorporate visual arts techniques including collage and a group poetry technique (Emunah, 1994). Within the field of drama therapy, there are a variety of theories with corresponding interventions that I use in my groups. Pioneer of the field of drama therapy, Renée Emunah (1994), developed the extensive Integrative Five-Phase Model which sets the foundation for the group therapy, using techniques that build safety, trust, group cohesion, and creative expression. I also use methods from Developmental Transformations (Johnson, 2000) that further facilitate spontaneity and free play. In an institution that often limits the client's ability to imagine, explore, and discover alternative possibilities to violence and criminal behavior, drama therapy provides an appropriate opportunity for clients to do just that.

In addition to drama therapy, my therapeutic framework is primarily influenced by feminist theory (Herman, 1997; O'Toole & Schiffman, 1997; Stark & Flitcraft, 1998) that very much resembles Lenore Walker's survivor therapy (Walker, 2000). Relational psychology (Jordan, Kaplan, Miller, Stiver & Surrey, 1991; Miller & Stiver, 1997) has also provided me with a strong foundation in which to explore relationships between group members and their relationship with me as their therapist. Relational psychology also allows me to provide the women with whom I work the opportunity to build relationships that incorporate trust and empathy in an institution that is impersonal and deemphasizes the basic humanity of inmates. Feminist theory incorporates the importance of power dynamics, systems of oppression, patriarchy, and empowerment of women to create a tapestry of complex, inter-woven issues, and challenges.

The writing of Paul Kivel (2002) and bell hooks (1997) on racism and social justice inform the therapeutic attention I give to race, class, sexuality as well as immigrant status. As a professor of psychology and prolific writer on issues of race and class, Shamita Das Dasgupta (1998) makes these important connections between cultural diversity and domestic violence. Although the Cultural Context Model designed by domestic violence experts, Rhea Almeida and Tracy Durkin (1999), is primarily designed for couples, Almeida and Durkin point out the negligence in ignoring race, culture, class, and religion in treatment models of domestic violence. Their article calls for consciousness raising that inspires and empowers therapists to look beyond normative models of power and control (Almeida & Durkin, 1999). Impacted by these writings, I do not see a woman in my group simply as a woman who has survived abuse at the hands of a partner, maybe a parent, and now certainly multiple institutions, but I also acknowledge how other systems of oppression may be at play.

Neil Websdale (2005) explores the intersection of domestic violence for incarcerated African American women who have lived in poverty. Websdale's study echoes many of the sentiments of my clients regarding the conflict of calling the police to intervening in a battering incident when drugs are involved or if one or both partners are in violation of parole conditions. It often becomes the lesser of two evils, to take the abuse when police intervention could risk arrest for illegal behavior resulting in the children being taken away or a loss of family income. The correlation between drug use and domestic violence will be discussed later in this chapter. Overall, the experiences of the clients in my group are shaped by ethnicity, race, socio-economic status, sexuality, and overall cultural background, and therefore attention to diversity of every kind must be paid.

The structure of the group is psychoeducational, in giving the women concrete tools to use when they parole. The group is also a therapeutic space in which to process past traumatic experiences. The goal is not to get the women to leave their partners or cut off connection. Many have complex relationships with their partners through children. Often substance abuse was a large part of their relationship and may have been deeply interconnected with the criminal behavior and violence in the relationship. The programmatic emphasis at Project Pride on recovery from addiction and leaving a criminal lifestyle can ultimately help a client see the parallels between her lifestyle of substance abuse and criminal behavior to the violence in her intimate relationships. However, the focus of the group on domestic violence underscores that the dynamics of power and control can exist in sober, clean, and crime-free relationships, and cultivates the awareness of warning signs or red flags of potential abusive relationships, regardless of the presence of drugs.

The term *violence against women* is more consistent with my theoretical framework as well as the experiences of the client population. Violence, rape, abuse as a result of prostitution, drug use and sales, Child Protective Services involvement as a result of their neglectful and abusive parenting, and the experiences of being in the prison system do not fit the label of "domestic violence" when much of the trauma is located far from the sphere of domestic life. It is crucial to recognize how semantics influence policy and politics (Kurz, 1998). However, for the purpose of this discussion and placing it in the context of this book, I will use the words domestic violence and violence against women interchangeably.

Drama Therapy

Drama therapy is an ideal therapeutic modality as an embodied form that can go beyond verbal processing. Bessel van der Kolk (1994, 1996) has provided the field of trauma with important insights on the physiological impact of trauma. Daniel Wiener (2001) further makes a case for action based therapies by using van der Kolk's work, claiming that embodiment is fundamental to the healing process: ". . . experiential therapies may have the potential to shift traumatic experience in cases in which verbal ones [therapies] cannot" (Wiener, 2001, p. xiii). A leader in the field of drama therapy, David Read Johnson (1987) describes his work with combat veterans and how creative arts therapies can be instrumental in diagnosis and treatment. Linda Winn (1994), a drama therapist who has worked with Post Traumatic Stress Disorder, writes that group dynamics and support are crucial in drama therapy work with trauma survivors. Drama therapy also incorporates the process of witnessing and being witnessed by one another in the group setting. The very nature of the trauma of domestic violence is perpetuated because domestic violence is saturated with experiences of denial, minimization, and societal blaming of the victim. This can also be internalized by the survivors, so that the fundamental experience of being seen can be transformative. Another central tenet of drama therapy is that it facilitates the capacity for empathy for self and others (Emunah, 1994; Volkas, 2002). Developing the skill of having empathy for self lays a foundation to legitimize survivors of domestic violence feelings of anger, grief, and fear about the abuse so that healing can take place.

David Read Johnson's (2000) later work with Developmental Transformations has influenced moments in the group when free play became the focus of the drama. Often the group would collectively decide to take an idea, an experience, or particularly a perpetrator and throw it out the window. Together we gather in mime that which we no longer wish to have in our group space and heave it out the window and look below, and it inevitably falls and crashes the windshield of the director's car parked below. Using this aspect of Developmental Transformations, we make space for our processing and creativity through playful action using imagination and spontaneity.

Using theater with incarcerated individuals and groups has long reaching and important applications. Current examples of this work in the San Francisco Bay Area are The Soapstone Theater Company (Gordon, 2005) and The Medea Project led by Rhodessa Jones (n.d.). Additionally, the film, *Shakespeare Behind Bars* (Spitzmiller, 2005) documents the use of theater with male inmates. Although there are inherent therapeutic implications of using theater in the prison system, few drama therapists have documented the work in published form. The exception is that of John Bergman (2000), the founder of Geese Theatre Company USA, a performance-based drama therapy project in prisons. Bergman's chapter in *Current Approaches to Drama Therapy* (Johnson, 2000), about therapeutic communities in prisons speaks to the importance of including the staff in an institutional-wide program that incorporates drama therapy. Drama therapy's versatility and ability to foster empathy enable it to serve as a modality well suited for prisons and therapeutic communities alike.

The Integrative Five-Phase Model

Renée Emunah (1994) outlines five phases that provide a structure as well as a progression for a therapist to guide clients toward self-exploration and discovery. Emunah (1994) describes the five phases as the following: "While elements of all five conceptual sources are evident in each phrase, each source is most correspondent to a particular phase. Phase One is most influenced by dramatic play, Phase Two by theatre, Phase Three by role play, Phase Four by psychodrama, and Phase Five given by dramatic ritual" (p. 34). The Integrative Five-Phase model has a progression that can work to develop group cohesion.

Marty Mulkey (2004) wrote about his clinical work with male survivors of rape and The Integrative Five-Phase Model used alongside Judith Herman's (1997) stages of recovery. Mulkey (2004) describes in details the overlap between the trauma of the assault as well as the aftermath of shame or consequences of disclosure for the victim. In addition, Mulkey uses the Integrative Five-Phase Model as the basis for the treatment and also incorporates Herman's theoretical framework to focus on safety, grieving, and reconnection. Mulkey's work with trauma outlines how Emunah's model, alongside other action methods and trauma focused work, can achieve important steps in working with survivors of sexual violence.

Beginning of the Series

The beginning of the domestic violence group series primarily focuses on Phase One and Two. The techniques I use in the beginning of the series, and often as warm-up or check-in in the beginning of each session, are taken directly from Emunah's (1994) work. These processes are particularly effective, as they directly meet my goals of establishing safety and trust in the group. Emunah writes, "During Phase One, trust begins to develop-trust in one's own capacities, trust between group members, and trust in the therapist. Acceptance of self and others, a growing connectedness between group members, and group cohesion are central features of a successful group process" (Emunah, 1994, p. 35). While I follow Emunah's Five Phases, she also states that "the early phases remain present even as a group progresses to later phases" (Emunah, 2000, p. 72). By using play, spontaneity, and action based techniques, "a nonthreatening, playful environment is established," which is central to creating a group dynamic where the painful and often traumatic material can be explored (Emunah, 2000, p. 73). I have also found that by introducing playful activities designed to reduce inhibitions, clients' resistance is also largely minimized as they enjoy themselves with the other group members.

Many of the interventions and techniques I use in Phase One and Two are from Emunah's *Acting for Real* (1994). Some of these activities include "party with secret roles" (p. 163). A variation that I created is called "celebrity mixer," where each group member has a sign on their back (that they can't see) stating who they are. The celebrities include Oprah Winfrey, Wonder Woman, Bart Simpson, Madonna, and even some staff at Project Pride. Women mingle, and by interacting they try to figure out their character using the hints the other people give them to inform their guess. This can lead into a game where one person leaves the room and returns as a celebrity that the group has determined. Through our interactions they have to guess who they are. Often, a client (and sometimes myself) is enrolled as President George Bush and the group has a playful time expressing their views on politics, the war in Iraq, and funding for social programs.

Other interventions that involve role playing, guessing, and group involvement are "group mood" (Emunah, 1994, p. 148) and, a consistent favorite of the clients, "congratulations" (Emunah, 1994, p. 211). Clients will return to the room and try to guess why they are being congratulated by the group. Clients have been congratulated on graduating high school, quitting smoking, or winning the lottery, to name a few. I often encourage the women to come up with the role for the person out of the room but will add my input if necessary. I have found that when I volunteer to leave the room, I can get a good sense of group projections onto me when I return. For example, I have returned to the group to discover I am being congratulated on being pregnant. Taking their cues, I complain about my body aches and morning sickness. The women are delighted that, even in fantasy, I could share their collective experience of motherhood.

Adam Blatner (2000), a psychiatrist and psychodramatist, has written extensively on the applications of play and group action methods. He describes sociometry as a psychodramatic technique that helps a group explore "interpersonal relationships" (Blatner, 2000, p. 252). Blatner also outlines how psychodrama, in general, can facilitate therapeutic factors attributed to Irving Yalom (1995). Among these therapeutic factors, I see sociometry as central to the development of universality and group cohesion within the group. I primarily use three sociometric exercises, and one of them has three variations. Often in the first group I will use one of three variations of "step into the middle if. . . ." One way that works well in groups of five or more clients is to have a circle of chairs with one chair missing, so one member of the group is left standing in the middle. I often begin it by being the one standing in the middle, saying something that is true for myself and asking that whoever shares that quality or experience has to get up and move to another seat. Getting up and moving can be challenging for some of the pregnant group members, but everybody tends to participate. This can also present an issue for the therapist in terms of disclosure, because ultimately not moving is also disclosure. I begin by stating that I will participate but may choose to move only on certain rounds. I often do not move on themes of inter-personal violence such as rape, incest or physical abuse, or topics of drug use. When I am in the center, and in the beginning of the round, I give statements that might have to do with my favorite food, movie star, tattoos, or music preference. This models professional boundaries but also demonstrates for the clients that they do not have to self-disclose intimate details of their lives, particularly in the first group.

A variation of this that I developed works well with fewer clients. It looks very much like mother may I with one client at one end of the room and the rest of the group at the other end, facing each other. The leader says statements that are true for her. I might suggest alternating between sharing about her personal life and also her experience with violence. For each statement that the other group members have in common with the leader, they take a step forward. Regardless of which of the leader's statements are true for other group members, there is always one person that shares multiple things in common with the leader. When a group member reaches the other end, she becomes the leader. I might comment, asking the group to notice when the entire group steps forward together, having all acknowledging that a statement about violence or motherhood is true for them.

The final variation is the women form a circle and silently step in and back when they have experienced a statement that I give. This can also be done in a line with participants stepping toward the facilitator as in the previous exercise. I give examples ranging from ethnic, cultural, and religious identity. I intentionally name races that may not be present, asking the group to notice who does and does not step forward. I might progress to statements about being a mother, having abortions, or miscarriages. I increase the intensity of the statements to include violence such as rape, having a gun pulled on you, being hit, having your teeth knocked out, if you have ever hit another person. This exercise is better done in the 2nd session or at the end of the first session once ground rules and safety guidelines have been established.

Spectograms (Blatner, 2000) are a well known psychodramatic technique and I often use them in the 2nd or 3rd session to both better inform me of where the group is emotionally and also to introduce some basic themes of the group to the clients. Some examples include: What kind of relationship do you expect your children to have with their father; no contact on one end, full parenting relationship on the other. Another example is for clients to place themselves in relation to the degree of violence (emotional, physical, and sexual) that was present in your family of origin. I might phrase it as one end is for people that identify with the statement "in my family growing up there was never any yelling, pushing, hitting, screaming, or violence of any kind." The other end of the spectrogram would be for those that identified that in their family growing up there was always "yelling, pushing, hitting, screaming, or violence of any kind."

In most spectograms, a few group members go to each extreme. This often identifies some of the splitting that clients do as well as their black and white thinking. Most often, however, the majority of the clients gravitate toward the center. Often spectograms initiate important discussions about how to protect your children from a violent parent who may still be involved in drugs or illegal activity. Questions are raised about how appropriate it is to cut off contact with your child's father and whether it is ultimately better to have a negative (violent or actively using drugs) father figure than no father at all. Many of the women were raised with no father present, and this spectrogram can trigger some important realizations about intergenerational cycles of violence, abandonment, and choices the women make based on their own upbringing. This can also provide an opportunity to discuss the importance of modeling partnerships that are not violent for the sake of the children. We also brainstorm where a woman in recovery on parole might find positive (male) role models for their children if they are committed to parenting without the child's father.

I have also developed a process that I call "the questions box," which facilitates action methods as the group progresses through the Five Phases. It is simply a cube Kleenex box with a sock attached to the top (this inevitably inspires giggles and curiosity when first introduced to the clients). Inside are strips of paper with typed questions and instructions for actions. In Phases One and Two, a client might pull a prompt from the box that asks her to pretend she is a U.S. Presidential candidate and the action is to give us a 30-second campaign speech. Clients have a chance to role-play and also communicate to the group about their values and views on social policy. Some are less action oriented but still involve a degree of sharing. For example, "tell us about a woman whom you admire and share with the group ways that you have those qualities or are working towards developing them." As the group progresses, I replace the slips of paper with prompts and actions that are related to what the group is exploring and is also relative to the phase of the group, such as role plays or psychodramatic enactments.

Additional processes that Emunah (1994) developed that I have found to be very successful in the beginning of the series are theatre based games used in Phase Two. Clients enjoy and demonstrate spontaneity and creativity in games such as "guess where we are" (Emunah, 1994, p. 179) with the progression of watching, waiting, and then doing which often the leads into "join the scene" (Emunah, 1994, p. 204). I provide the scenes which can range from watching a boxing match to waiting at a doctor's office and doing laundry at the laundromat, all activities with which the women are very familiar. I often divide the group into teams and have each team guess the other's action. In the beginning of the series, we might also do "emotional greetings" (Emunah, 1994, p. 150), "newspaper" (Emunah, 1994, p. 201) or "true and false statements" (Emunah, 1994, p. 238).

In one group we began a trial scene and the women chose to prosecute a shark puppet that I had as a projective technique to provide aesthetic distancing (Landy, 1983, 1994). The group members spontaneously created the trial scene similar to the court trial that Emunah outlines (Emunah, 1994, p. 206). The scene evolved as clients switched roles from judge to jury to attorneys. All of the women have extensive experience with the court system, and this allowed a way to play out some of the challenges and anxieties they face in the court room. By the end of the scene, the shark was found guilty for, quite appropriately, beating his girlfriend.

Check-in and Closing of a Session

I do not have a standard check-in at the beginning of each group. This choice was made in part by advice from Abigail Leeder, the previous domestic violence group facilitator who is also a drama therapist (personal communication, April 22, 2005) and from my experience in other groups where a verbal check-in does not necessarily create a positive environment for self-reflection. A check-in for the group might be in the form of a warm-up that may include a self-sculpt for how the client is feeling in that moment, creating a newspaper headline for their state of mind, or a simple rose and thorn statement where a client could say the thorn (the challenge) in their life since the last group as well as the rose (the positive). Sometimes if a client really expresses the need to share something with the group–perhaps an outcome from a court date with CPS or a situation in the house that resulted in disciplinary action – I will have them share and try, if possible, to move it into action. This might be in the form of the client "directing" a scene or sculpting other clients to represent their feelings. I sometimes do a variation of TV interviews (Emunah, 1994, p. 202). I welcome the client onto the "Liora Brosbe Show" where I interview the client and also take questions or comments from the rest of the group immediately enrolled as the in-studio audience. This is often a playful way to get feedback from the group and also give the client a chance to share what is present for them.

At the closing of every group, we do the same ritual. I learned this from my professor and mentor, Armand Volkas, as he used it as a psychodramatic closing to classes he taught at California Institute of Integral Studies (personal communication, September 1, 2004). The women form a circle with their hands, everyone the same hand, usually the right. We form a fist with the hand, but insert our thumb into the fist of the person next to us creating a well of enclosed, intertwined hands. As closure, and depending on the material explored in the group, I will direct the women with a prompt. Often, I ask them to drop into the "well" something that they are going to leave behind in the group and something they will take with them. A variation is to ask each participant to share a word that reflects their experience of the group process during that session.

A common closing is that I ask the clients to share what they will do after group to take care of themselves. This closing ritual is important to me as well as to the clients when I can also reflect with the group how to model and commit to my own practice of self-care. It is common for therapists working with survivors of trauma to feel helpless, anxious, and impacted by witnessing the clients' stories and experiences (Cunningham, 2004; Herman, 1997). A simple phone call to a loved one or a bubble bath the evening after a group allows me to create an intentional space to counter the effects of vicarious traumatization. Clients name activities such as reading bedtime stories to children, reading The Bible, and writing a letter as their commitment to self-care. This also helps me to notice who might need some extra attention or support after the group; I can notify the evening staff of any potentially vulnerable clients. Afterwards, I might follow-up with a client that I think may need to chat one on one, or get help with caring for their child after the group.

Middle of the Series

The middle of the series continues to use drama therapy, primarily with Emunah's (1994) Phases Three and Four. Much of the group is structured around psychoeducational materials that focus on dynamics of power and control (Domestic Abuse Intervention Project, n.d.) and the "three-stage cycle" of violence (Walker, 2000, p. 63). At this stage, the group has achieved a level of trust and safety so that the clients can learn about domestic violence but also make relevant and clear connections to their own lives. I often introduce the wheel that includes culture and institutions in order to explore the idea that, as Shamita Das Dasgupta (1998) writes, "The individual abuser and the victim do not operate in a vacuum; rather, they are nested within the supportive circles of social institutions and culture" (p. 211). Sometimes we explore this wheel with role play or frozen tableaus between teacher and student or police officer and a person getting a ticket. In each scene, I ask who has the power. I have also shown images from magazines and asked the women what they see in each image. Together we try to incorporate the messages from pop culture into the overall picture of the wheel. This creates a foundation for the clients to examine and form an awareness of the pervasive structures of power and control.

Despite the limitations of the prison system, incarcerated women often bring with them a diversity of cultural heritage that, when honored and respected, can be applied as a valuable tool in their recovery from addiction and violence. Given the opportunity to examine their own relationship to institutional, cultural, and personal structures of power and control, clients discover a new language to relate to generations of abuse and trauma (Dasgupta, 1998). And yet, this also poses a challenge for me as the therapist to be constantly aware of personal bias, countertransference, prejudice, as well as internalized oppression.

I introduce the Domestic Abuse Intervention Project's wheel of power and control in action using subtle processes. One technique I developed is an enlarged power and control wheel with an arrow that clients spin and share based on where the arrow lands on the wheel. Another way is to take masking tape and create a big wheel on the floor of the group room. We sit around the wheel and I ask clients to read each section that I have typed up in large print. In another series, I posted the same pages with the sections of the wheel around the room. Together the group imagined where we would travel and how we would get to a place where we could explore more deeply the dynamics of domestic violence. The group formed an imaginative journey in a bus and we made our way around the room, stopping at each destination. With each process, I ask the women if they can relate or have experiences that they would like to share after we read each section of the wheel. This process is about containing and introducing eight very concrete elements of power and control.

I have been consistently touched and moved by the depth and vulnerability the women bring to their exploration of power and control. In one particularly small session with three clients, we decorated a box with images from magazines that represented domestic violence. Each client then took small multi-colored pieces of paper that I had cut in small triangles to resemble the pieces of the power and control wheel. The women wrote down experiences they had that fit the sections of the wheel. They shared, if they wanted, and then we put all the pieces into our decorated box. It was a simple embodiment of containing all the memories that the wheel can inspire, and also a creative way of sharing their trauma. The box remains in my office, a powerful reminder of the work to honor and heal the realities of abusive relationships. Collage is the best way I have found for clients to express their relationship to the wheel. I often take an entire session where I ask clients to work in silence to create any form of collage to represent their relationship to the wheel of power and control.

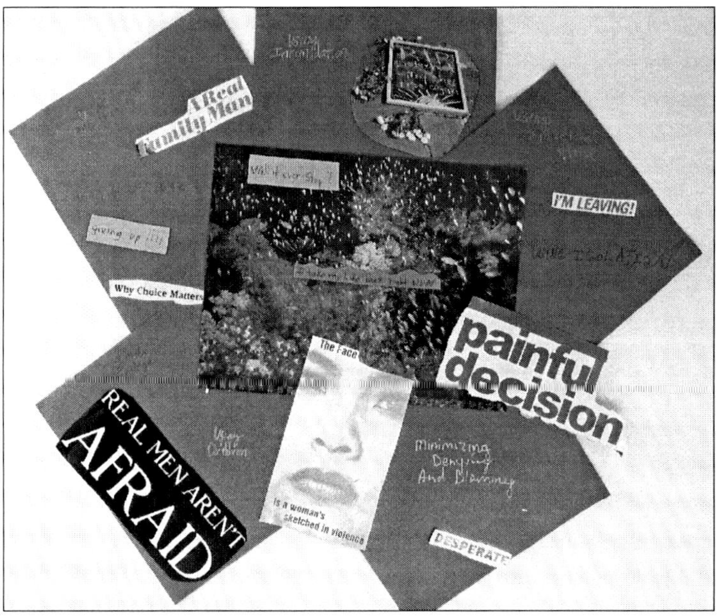

Figure 1: Sample Collage from Power and Control Wheel (see also Plate 13 in color).

Some women are very literal, dividing their page into eight sections with titles. Other clients have a more non-linear approach with multiple images that inspire them based on their reaction to the wheel. Figure 1 is a client's collage that is divided and labeled with the sections of the wheel of the power and control. The images she selected represent her experience in an abusive relationship. In the center is an image of a tropical coral reef over which she placed a phrase that she wrote: "I take my life back right NOW."

I provide the women with art and collage materials that include magazines, old calendars, gel pens, pastels, colored pencils, and other arts and crafts items such as Cool Foam® sheets. I have a diverse collection of magazines that include *National Geographic* and parenting magazines. I also make a point of having magazines, postcards, or calendars that represents racial diversity. It is challenging to achieve that solely with magazines, as the women of color in the media often represent the cultural bias and racist messages of society. The images of women of all races can be problematic mainly because body image is a huge issue for the clients as many of them struggle with physical changes related to post-partum weight gain and recovery from addiction.

Despite the body image issues that many of the clients present, I find sculpting to be a very useful form of exploring images, emotions, or messages from society. Linda Winn also uses sculpting to get "an indication of where people are at that moment" (Winn, 1994, p. 24). Emunah describes a "self-sculptures" process that is an effective form of self-revelation used in Phase Four (Emunah, 1994, p. 211). Sculpting can also be applied to some of the psychoeducational topics, including the cycle of violence with clients sculpting the stages of tension, acute explosion, and honeymoon (Walker, 2000).

In one session, I used a combination of Emunah's (1994) sculpting process and the work of Augusto Boal (1997). Boal's work with non-actors provides concrete descriptions and scenarios in which to work with this population. I set up three chairs and asked clients to sculpt "the family" (Boal, 1997, p. 169). This quickly evolved into family members using drugs. Each sculptor gave her statues lines and in some sculpts each character came to life as in Emunah's (1994) work in stage three of self-sculptures (p. 212). The family sculpts also evolved into parole sculpts when clients sculpted their future with a clean and sober family. With sculpting dynamics of addiction or violence, it is important to close the process with a sculpt or embodiment that contains an element of hope or future projection, as in Emunah's process of "sculpting a scene" (Emunah, 1994, p. 157).

Once there is a significant level of trust in the group and the clients are experienced with role play and self-revelation, I introduce the drama therapy phone. The telephone technique used during Phase Four provides an outlet for communicating deep personal truths (Emunah, 1994, pp. 185-189). Clients enact phone calls to communicate with children on the outside, past partners, or even future parole officers. In general, clients often struggle with the process of doubling, so I frequently take a more active role as director during telephone conversations that would call for a double or line repetitions.

Residential treatment including the Community Prisoner Mother Program through the CDCR can be very isolated from the broader community. I have exposed the group to different ways of turning a personal experience into activism or healing. This is a fundamental step in empowerment for many of the clients. One program is the Silent Witness Initiative (Hagberg & Bardwell, 1992). In a smaller group of four clients, we watched a video about the project and the march on Washington, D.C., available from their website, www.silentwitness.net. The women were moved by the stories of the founders and survivors. Together we created a project to honor their experiences of survival. I used *The Silent Witness Story* (Hagberg & Bardwell, 1992) as a resource for the clients to re-create their own unique versions of the witnesses. Each woman had her body traced on butcher paper and selected a pastel color to paint the silhouette (not the traditional red of the Witnesses). Again, tracing the body created anxiety and responses to body image and proved to be a powerful process in and of itself. It is the custom of the Silent Witness to display the date and details of the murder for each Witness that represents an actual woman in the community who was murdered by an intimate partner. Instead, each woman in the group created her own shield that stated the date she got out of the relationship and how she had survived. We called these survivor witnesses. The women decided to include one cutout (drawn freehand, not traced) that would be red and represent "the victim" who did not escape the relationship and remind them that domestic violence can be deadly.

I have also received clearance to take the women out of the facility to an art exhibit or performance around themes of violence against women or incarceration. These outings have been moving experiences where the women connect with the broader art community and often see their experiences reflected in the pieces. I also try to have an open house for the group to invite their case managers, staff, other clients to have some refreshments and have the women share some of their experiences and artwork from the group. This often gives clients a chance to share their success in the group with other service providers and can inspire other clients to join the next series.

Intersection of Substance Abuse and Domestic Violence

The majority of clients in the domestic violence group make the connection between their substance abuse and the violence in their relationships. This correlation between domestic violence and substance abuse is documented in the literature addressing both domestic violence and substance abuse treatment (Fazzone, Holton, & Reed, 2003; Walker, 2000). I often use O'Neil's (1996) "Power and control model for women's substance abuse" to introduce the complexities and specifics of domestic violence in relationships where drug abuse is also a factor. One of my challenges is to honor the role drugs play in abusive relationships without making absolute parallels between addiction and violence. For many of the clients, the use of drugs is equated with their experience of abuse. I do validate the clients' experiences that drug use can increase the risk of abuse, violence, and chaos in the women's lives and that addiction can intensify jealous, impulsive, and manipulative behaviors that are also characteristics of violent relationships. However, it is crucial to distinguish for the clients that the presence of drugs and alcohol does not mean there will definitely be violence, and violence can occur in sober relationships where drugs and alcohol are not a part of the dynamic. It is my goal to help the clients view substance abuse as a component of the abusive relationship but try to avoid viewing the violence as a direct result of drug use.

To communicate the nuances of addiction and violence, it is essential to get back to the basics of recognizing the presence of power and control in the relationship and how it contributes to the violence. While it is definitely possible to identify controlling behaviors as a result of substance abuse, clients also learn to recognize dynamics of power and control that are present during periods of sobriety. Narcotics Anonymous and therapeutic communities often utilize slogans to make a point about certain messages. I have introduced one such slogan to emphasize that often the dynamics of power and control may be present whether either person in the relationship is using. The slogan, "using is the excuse for abusing" helps the clients try to notice controlling behavior that would be present without drugs. It also can be an added incentive to remain sober, as clients identify that their thinking patterns and behavior are overall more healthy, safety oriented, and honest when not trapped in their addiction.

End of the Series

The structure of the last two sessions of the series focuses on commitments to non-violent alternatives, safety planning, and closure of the series. I require that each client fill out a Personalized Safety Plan (Fazzone, Holton, & Reed, 2003) before they receive their formal certificate of completion. The certificate of completion is valued by each client, as it is used with other group certificates to present to parole officers, social workers, and judges to demonstrate successful participation in programming at Project Pride. This is the only homework I give in the group. I also use it as a form of measurement for how a client has integrated the information from the group in order to make a viable safety plan when they leave. This is required for women who have already taken steps to not return to violent partners and serves as a commitment to their safety and the safety of their children.

The topic of children is explicitly explored at this point in the group, with the two wheels of "Equality" and "Nurturing Children" (Domestic Abuse Intervention Project, n.d.). Using the concepts in previous sessions, clients can make parallels to their own experiences and how it impacts their children and their role as parents. Some processes have included drama therapy phone calls to their children or making a collective scrapbook. Together we act out in mime, sharing photos from their memories of happy and nurturing moments with their children. I also hand out blank versions of the wheel where the clients can fill in their own commitments to their selves and to their children to create a life free from violence. For example, a client might write in the section for "Economic Abuse" a commitment to getting a bank account, a job, or maintaining her own financial independence.

One process I use toward the end of the series is "Group Poem" (Emunah, 1994, p. 237). The prompts I use for the group poem are "When I look back . . ." and "Today I feel. . . ." Clients complete the prompt and we pass the paper around and each person gets their paper back with a completed poem, each line written by a member of the group. We share our poems, I collect them, and the following week I distribute all of the poems together printed on elegant paper. One group poem evoked tears from many of the clients when the original 'author' read it out loud:

When I look back I see all the things that were way out of whack.
So lets move forward and never look back.
When I look inside I find a love that will never end
I pray for the healing of hurts I hope to mend
Please help me father.
Take back broken promises and start over again.

The poem can serve as a transitional object, each line a gift from a member of the group. Clients have also remarked on the spiritual and magical nature of the process. Although different women contribute to the poem in sequence, it can make sense and speak directly to the heart of the person who wrote the first line.

The last group focuses on processes in Phase Five in different forms of sharing, sometimes talking about what we learned, or doing role plays based on different scenarios that the women might face. In pairs, I hand out index cards with a scene such as: You see one another in ten years, and one of you confides in the other that you are in an abusive relationship. The other reminds them of what you learned in the domestic violence group at Project Pride ten years earlier. Other scenes are about resolving an argument with a partner in a non-violent fashion or dealing with your child hitting another child. This last scene can bring up feelings of guilt for exposing children to violence and the deep beliefs that children should be taught how to defend themselves.

The end of the last session includes blank certificates for women to write their own accomplishment for the group and each group member signs it below (Emunah, 1994, p. 246). I present each woman with the certificate and we applaud the accomplishment for which she chooses to be honored. I also serve sparkling apple cider and we toast to each other and remember times from the group (Emunah, 1994, p. 245). Groups often toast to each other, to a member who might have an upcoming parole date, as well as to themes of independence, strength, their children, and their future. Group members are invited back, and often many return to participate in another series. This speaks to the importance of the relationships formed in the group. The group clearly offers clients a unique opportunity to share, grow, and be vulnerable in a safe environment.

Conclusion

I am consistently surprised when clients share experiences and conditions of their life in the state prison and county jail system. Pregnancy, labor and delivery, and separation from family beginning with their arrest are frequently a deep source of trauma, often perpetuating the trauma that the women have experienced in their families, relationships, and communities. I want to help end this cycle of institutional violence by using creativity, action methods, and relational connections in my groups and with my clients. I can do this as I keep myself grounded through self-care, including my own spiritual practice and process in my own therapy.

Working toward justice and healing in an inherently unjust institution is exhausting, limiting, and often disheartening. Nevertheless, I strongly believe in self-expression and in the fundamental human right not to be harmed by another. I see my clients as my teachers, as women who, while they were denied the right to safety and love in the past, can receive support and care in my groups. I know that the conditions of their lives and communities set them on a track where sexism, racism, and poverty were often present to lead to choices of crime and substance abuse. I do not idealize their behavior or lifestyle, but I do not hold them as the only ones accountable for the failings of society. Therefore, I enter each session as their therapist, but also as a social activist who is ultimately attempting to do just work in an unjust system.

In this chapter, I have provided a window into the reality of how creative arts, specifically drama therapy, are used with marginalized populations. Incarcerated women and women in recovery from substance abuse are often survivors of domestic violence and require a therapeutic approach that holds the complexity of their treatment needs. Together with my reflections and experiences as a therapist and practical examples of therapeutic interventions that shape my work, I hope to give you a sense of what this work looks like. Furthermore, these outlines of processes represent how I integrate the various influences on my work in order to reach my treatment goals in a safe space for my clients. I encourage you to discover your own touchstones and to be curious in order to further explore the depth of working with domestic violence in action, play, and group therapy.

Terms

Consciousness raising is a process that was fundamental to the women's liberation movement in the U.S. during the 1970s. Consciousness raising attempts to mobilize groups of people from seeing their personal oppression in isolation toward the broader societal implications. Ultimately, the goal is to create a group with greater knowledge and a developed commitment toward political action in regards to the specific issue.

"**Developmental Transformations** utilizes an improvisational embodied encounter in the playspace between the therapist and client in order to treat disorders of embodiment, encounter, and play" (Johnson, 2000, p. 455).

Doubling is a psychodramatic technique that provides support and coaching to a protagonist so that they may explore deeper levels of their enactment. The double, who can be a group member or the leader, may stand behind or to the side of the participant and "expresses unexpressed thoughts and feelings of an enactor in order to maximize the feelings expressed by the enactor, through verbal and nonverbal gestures" (Johnson, 2000, p. 455).

The Duluth Model was developed in 1981 and includes the Domestic Abuse Intervention Project (DAIP). The Duluth Model uses a framework in which a variety of community-based programs work collectively to effectively address issues related to domestic violence including law enforcement, the court system, and human service providers. The DAIP has developed a comprehensive Wheel Gallery that can provide a visual and concrete model in which to examine domestic violence.

Sexism, in the context of this chapter, is the dynamic in which women have less power than men. This systemic oppression exists on a societal, institutional and interpersonal level.

Sociometry is a psychodramatic technique to discover commonalities and differences that exist between members in a group. It can also be used to investigate interpersonal dynamics between group participants.
Spectogram is a psychodramatic process in which participants collectively and physically place themselves on a continuum of extremes based on their relationship to, experience with, or feelings about a given topic.

References

Almeida, R. V., & Durkin, T. (1999). The cultural context model: Therapy for couples with-domestic violence. *Journal of Marital and Family Therapy, 25*(3), 313-324.

Bergman, J. (2000). Creating new cultures: Using drama therapy to build therapeutic communities in prisons. In D. R. Johnson & P. Lewis (Eds.), *Current approaches to drama therapy* (pp. 303-330). Springfield, IL: Charles C Thomas, Publisher, Ltd.

Blatner, A. (2000). *Foundations of psychodrama* (4th ed.). New York: Springer Publishing Company.

Boal, A. (1997). *Games for actors and non-actors* (A. Jackson, Trans.). New York: Routledge.

Cunningham, M. (2004). Avoiding vicarious traumatization: Support, spirituality and self-care. In N. B. Webb (Ed.), *Mass trauma and violence: Helping families and children cope* (pp. 327-346). New York: Guilford Press.

Dasgupta, S. D. (1998). Women's realities: Defining violence against women by immigration, race, and class. In R. K. Bergen (Ed.), *Issues in intimate violence* (pp. 209-219). Thousand Oaks, CA: Sage.

DeLeon, G. (2000). *The therapeutic community: Theory, model, and method.* New York: Springer Publishing Company.

Domestic Abuse Intervention Project. (n.d.). "Wheel Gallery" Retrieved August 24, 2006 from http://www.duluth-model.org/documents/wheelshandout.pdf

Emunah, R. (1994). *Acting for real: Drama therapy process, technique, and performance.* Philadelphia: Brunner/Mazel, Inc.

Emunah, R. (2000). The integrative five phase model of drama therapy. In D. R. Johnson & P. Lewis (Eds.), *Current approaches to drama therapy* (pp. 70-86). Springfield, IL: Charles C Thomas, Publisher, Ltd.

Emunah, R. (2001). Drama therapy in action. In D. J. Wiener (Ed.), *Beyond talk therapy: Using movement and expressive techniques in clinical practice* (pp. 99-123). Washington, D.C.: American Psychological Association.

Fazzone, P. A., Holton, J. K., & Reed, B. G. (Eds.). (2003). *Substance abuse treatment and domestic violence.* [Center for Substance Abuse Treatment, Treatment Improvement Protocol (TIP) Series No. 25]. Rockville, MD: U.S. Department of Health and Human Services.

Gordon, J. (2005, August). *Playing with violence: The work of Soapstone Theater Company.* Paper presented at the National Association of Drama Therapy Annual Conference, Portland, OR.

Hagberg, J. & Bardwell, C. (1992). *The silent witness story: Speaking out against domestic violence.* St. Paul, MN: Minnesota Women's Consortium.

Herman, J. L. (1997). *Trauma and recovery.* New York: Basic Books.

hooks, b. (1996). *Killing rage: ending racism.* New York: Owl Books.

hooks, b. (1997). Violence in intimate relationships: A feminist perspective. In L. L. O'Toole & J. R Schiffman (Eds.), *Gender violence: Interdisciplinary perspectives* (pp. 279-284). New York: New York University Press.

Johnson, D. R. (1987). The role of the creative arts therapies in the diagnosis and treatment of psychological trauma. *The Arts in Psychotherapy, 14*, 7-13.

Johnson, D. R. (2000). Developmental Transformations: Toward the body as presence. In D. R. Johnson & P. Lewis (Eds.), *Current approaches to drama therapy* (pp. 87-110). Springfield, IL: Charles C Thomas, Publisher, Ltd.

Jordan, J. V., Kaplan, A., Miller, J. B., Stiver, I. P., & Surrey, J. L. (1991). *Women's growth in connection.* New York: Guilford Press.

Jordan, J. V. (Ed.). (1997). *Women's growth in diversity.* New York: Guilford Press.

Kivel, P. (2002). *Uprooting racism: How white people can work for racial justice.* Gabriola Island, BC: New Society.

Kurz, D. (1998). Old problems and new directions in the study of violence against women. In R. K. Bergen (Ed.), *Issues in intimate violence* (pp. 197-208). Thousand Oaks, CA: Sage.

Landy, R. J. (1983). The use of distancing in drama therapy. *The Arts in Psychotherapy, 10*(3), 175-185.

Landy, R. J. (1994). *Drama therapy: Concepts, theories and practices* (2nd ed.). Springfield, IL: Charles C Thomas, Publisher, Ltd.

Legal Services for Prisoners with Children. (n.d.). *Mother infant care program.* Retrieved April 8, 2007, from http://www.prisonerswithchildren.org/issues/pwcmic.htm

Miller, J. B., & Stiver, I. P. (1997). *The healing connection.* Boston: Beacon Press.

Mulkey, M. (2004). Recreating masculinity: Drama therapy with male survivors of sexual assault. *The Arts in Psychotherapy, 31*, 19-28.

O'Neil, M. T. (1996). "Power and control model for women's substance abuse." Retrieved January 23, 2007 from http://www.ncdsv.org/images/WomensSubAbusewheelNOSHADING.pdf

O'Toole, L. L., & Schiffman, J. R. (Eds.). (1997). *Gender violence: Interdisciplinary perspectives.* New York: University Press.

Pierson, C. (2003, Spring). Legal corner: Community based programs for mothers. *The Fire Inside, 24.* Retrieved from http://www.womenprisoners.org/fire/000115.html

Spitzmiller, J. (Producer), & Rogerson, H. (Director). (2005). *Shakespeare behind bars* [Motion picture]. Philomath Films.

Stark, E., & Flitcraft, A. (1998). Women and children at risk: A feminist perspective on child abuse. In R. K. Bergen (Ed.), *Issues in intimate violence* (pp. 25-41). Thousand Oaks, CA: Sage.

van der Kolk, B. A. (1994). The body keeps the score: Memory and the emerging psychobiology of post traumatic stress. *Harvard Review of Psychiatry, 1*, pp. 253-265. Retrieved April 8, 2007 from, http://www.trauma-pages.com/a/vanderk4.php

van der Kolk, B. A., McFarlane, A. C., & Weisaeth, L. (Eds.). (1996). *Traumatic stress: The effects of overwhelming experience on mind, body, and society.* New York: Guilford Press.

Volkas, A. (2003, Winter/Spring). *"Keynote address."* Dramascope-the newsletter of the NADT. 6-9.

Walker, L. (2000). *Abused women and survivor therapy: A practical guide for the psychotherapist.* Washington, D.C.: American Psychological Association.

Websdale, N. (2005). Nashville: Domestic violence and incarcerated women in poor black neighborhoods. In N. J. Sokoloff (Ed.), *Domestic violence at the margins: Readings at the intersections of race, class, gender & culture.* NJ: Rutgers University.

Wiener, D.J. (Ed.). (2001). *Beyond talk therapy: Using movement and expressive techniques in clinical practice.* Washington, DC: American Psychological Association.

Winn, L. (1994). *Post traumatic stress disorder and dramatherapy.* London: Jessica Kingsley Publishers.

Yalom, I. D. (1995). *The theory and practice of group psychotherapy* (4th ed.). New York: Basic Books.

Biography

Liora Abrahams Brosbe, MA was introduced to the therapeutic use of theater at Kid Street Theater, an after school program for at-risk youth in Northern California. Ms. Abrahams Brosbe continued her work with adult and children survivors of DV in Baltimore, MD with Active Coalition for Transitional Services, Inc. (ACTS) and House of Ruth. During her undergraduate work at Goucher College in Psychology and Sociology, Ms. Abrahams Brosbe conceived, produced and directed a performance/workshop senior thesis examining the correlation between witnesses of domestic violence and the theatrical audience. While pursuing a Masters in drama therapy at California Institute of Integral Studies, Ms. Abrahams Brosbe completed her clinical practicum at Project Pride, a residential treatment program for incarcerated women and their children. As part of her internship, she developed a comprehensive domestic violence program using predominately drama therapy interventions and techniques. Ms. Abrahams Brosbe currently serves as a MFT intern using drama therapy in the San Francisco Bay Area.

Chapter 14

DRAMA THERAPY AS TREATMENT FOR SURVIVORS OF DOMESTIC VIOLENCE

DEBORAH K. PIERCE

Introduction

You may know someone like Rachel. She's a bright, articulate young woman with two small children, who would never have described herself as a victim of domestic violence-until the night her husband pulled a knife on her and threatened her life. When she told him she was going to call the police, he ripped all the phones out of the wall. Months later, after Rachel got out and got help, she said that she did not consider herself a "victim," because "Victims are dead people, and I'm not dead! Besides," she said, "He never hit me" (Anonymous Survivor, 2004).

In this chapter, I will explain how drama therapy can work as an effective treatment modality for women who are survivors of domestic violence. Women account for 85% of the victims of intimate partner violence, according to the Bureau of Justice statistics (2003). Since I work with women, I use feminine pronouns to refer to the clients. I will describe some of the drama therapy techniques I have used to help clients to recognize losses, express emotions, be heard and supported by their peers, and reclaim a sense of dignity and autonomy. I will also explain how I incorporated domestic violence resource materials in the creative work, such as the power and control wheel, developed by the Domestic Abuse Intervention Project in Duluth Minnesota (1985), and information from Lundy Bancroft's (2002) book, *Why Does He Do That?* The power and control wheel is a chart which depicts the control tactics used by abusers. These resources validated my clients' experiences and gave us a place to start in creating dramatic ritual and dialogue, as well as strategies to practice when coping with the tactics of abusers. Finally, I will describe the play, *Rule of Thumb*, which I developed in my work with clients, and explain how theatre and drama can be used as a training tool for advocates, counselors, and other professionals working in the field of domestic violence.

Drama Therapy and a Theoretical Context for Working with Survivors

The National Association for Drama Therapy (NADT) defines drama therapy as "the intentional use of drama and/or theater processes to achieve therapeutic goals" (NADT brochure, n.d.). Drama and theatre processes could include acting or role-playing, script writing or story-telling, theatre games, dramatic ritual, improvisation, mask work, or many other forms of dramatic play, performance, or therapeutic theatre. Drama therapy draws perspective from many different psychological theories. It is rooted in humanistic psychology in that it taps into the individual's ability to grow, change, and discover her own potential. In her book, *Acting for Real*, Renée Emunah (1994), founder of the Drama Therapy program at California Institute of Integral Studies, states, "One of the primary relationships between humanistic psychology and drama therapy is that dramatic enactment can create a bridge between human limitations and human aspirations, between who we are and whom we hope to become. . . . Drama therapy draws upon the human capability of influencing one's behaviors and modifying one's life script-a tenet of humanistic philosophy" (p. 27). Drama therapy also incorporates aspects of psychoanalysis and cognitive-behavioral therapy in that it allows for the discovery of the unconscious, wounded, or hidden aspects of the self (Emunah, 1994), but it also helps clients to discover or re-assess the logic of their faulty or distorted thinking (Burns, 1999). Drama therapy especially helps clients to rehearse changes in their behavior.

While drama therapy with survivors draws upon several well-established psychological theories, it must also take into account that a survivor's *learned helplessness* (Seligman, 1998) and feelings of inadequacy stem directly from living under the threat of abuse, and that threat is very real. Psychological theories that fail to recognize the influence of violence and outside control over a victim's life will not help because they don't take in the whole picture. Survivors do not, nor do any of us, live in a vacuum.

Women who are survivors of domestic violence often blame themselves for what has happened to them. In my experience working with survivors, I have noticed that they often minimize the effects of the abuse, internalize the shaming voice of their abusers, and they are often socially isolated to an extreme. It is important to remember that while a victim of abuse may have many issues of her own, her main problem is *outside* of herself: a perpetrator of abuse who seeks to control and dominate her life. Our goal as therapists must therefore be to *empower* survivors. In other words, to give back to them a sense of authority over their own lives. Survivors often do not understand the dynamics of power and control that underlie physical and emotional abuse, which is one of the reasons it takes so long for them to move on with their lives. Victims may spend years living in fear, isolation, anger, resentment, and shame. They need to understand that they are not to blame for the crimes someone else has committed against them.

Drama is a powerful therapeutic modality for these women because it can help them to recognize what has really happened to them. Story sharing and drama can help survivors to more realistically assess their own physical and emotional safety, and it helps to reduce their sense of isolation. It provides a safe place and a format to help them explore, identify, and express their losses, their feelings, thoughts, needs, and their values. Drama therapy can help survivors to regain a sense of dignity by validating their experiences, and it can help them to practice the next steps of their recovery, including preparing for trial, or setting limits with children or other family members. It can also be fun. One of the elements most lacking in the lives of survivors is humor, and the opportunity to laugh. Later in the chapter, I will explain how drama therapy can be used to address the specific problems that typically confront a survivor of domestic violence.

General Overview and Structure of Drama Therapy

Drama therapy has its roots in Greek Theatre and developed in modern times as an outgrowth of group psychotherapy. Jacob Moreno is considered to be the founder of the current drama therapy movement (Johnson, 2000). Moreno started the first group psychotherapy session in Vienna in 1913 and he later developed the first psychodrama and sociodrama groups, from which other forms of drama therapy have emerged (Sternberg & Garcia, 2000). Today, there are numerous variations, methods, styles, and approaches to drama therapy including psychodrama, sociodrama, Playback Theatre (Fox, 1999), Life Stories Process (Rubin, 2007), Developmental Transformations (Johnson, 2000), Narradrama (Dunne, 2000), the Role Method (Landy, 1993), the Integrative Model for Drama Therapy (Emunah, 1994), ritual drama, and Augusto Boal's Theatre of the Oppressed (Boal, 1979) to name a few. *Current Approaches in Drama Therapy*, edited by Doctors Penny Lewis and David Read Johnson, documents sixteen of the most widely used methods of drama therapy practiced in the United States and Canada and the theoretical context for each method (Lewis & Johnson, 2000).

For the sake of simplicity, in this chapter I will describe drama therapy work as it falls into two categories: drama and theatre. *Drama* is process-oriented and involves the clients themselves taking part in the activity. *Theatre* is performance-oriented and involves a presentation for an audience. Both of these styles, process/drama and performance/theatre are beneficial, though they are very different in structure and purpose. In a drama session the therapeutic goal is to help the participants. In therapeutic theatre, the goal is to reach the audience, or to make a connection between the audience and the story tellers through the actors. In my work with survivors, I have used both forms. I have used drama and story-telling in group for the benefit of the survivors, and I have adapted those stories for performance, to reach audience members at risk and to help train service professionals who work with them.

A process-oriented drama therapy session may include story-telling, artwork, puppetry, theatre games, role-playing, role-doubling, re-enactment with alternative endings, simulated conflicts, mask work, past and future projections, status games, dramatic ritual, or affirmations. Each session is unique and driven by the specific needs and goals of the clients, but a typical drama therapy format with clients as players would include five steps: (1) a check in time, (2) a warm-up activity, (3) a dramatic enactment or story sharing with the group as the main focus of the session, (4) a discussion period, and (5) a closing activity (Bailey, 2000). Some therapists, such as Landy (1994) and Blatner (1996), have condensed these into three steps: (1) a warm-up which includes checking in, (2) an enactment, and (3) closure, which includes discussion or integration. The warm-up components of a session are important because it takes time for the clients to get comfortable with the process, the content, and each other. The overall structure and pacing of the session can help ease them into doing the deeper work. Emunah (1994) states: "A higher degree of structure alleviates anxiety and diminishes resistance . . . facilitates interaction, and paradoxically releases spontaneity and creativity" (p. 36). The discussion period helps the clients to process and assimilate the work, and the closing activity helps them to complete the work emotionally and prepare to leave the session (Blatner, 1996).

Aspects of drama therapy can also be introduced in group work without engaging in a full enactment as part of the session. Theatre games, ritual, or other dramatic elements may be used to help clients in numerous aspects of their emotional recovery. In a survivor's support group, I added elements of drama, games, and rituals to enhance the clients' sense of inclusion and to reinforce concepts that the group members were struggling with. For example, by adding vocal re-enactment and improvisation to a discussion of the power and control wheel (Domestic House Intervetion Project, 1985), clients were quickly able to identify and dramatically represent the control tactics their partners had used against them. When we discussed Lundy Bancroft's (2002) book *Why Does He Do That*, the clients were quick to identify their partners' archetypes (from chapter four "types of abusive men"). These descriptions lent themselves easily into dramatic representations of the clients' abusers, and their work inspired some of the masks I later developed for the play. We also used line repetition, affirmations, and scripted responses to problems which added humor and boundary-setting skills to situations they otherwise found difficult. These games and rituals are common elements of drama therapy which enhanced the group without having them go into a full dramatic enactment. In her integrative approach to drama therapy, Emunah (1994) would identify this dramatic play aspect as phase one of drama therapy work. She further suggests that some groups are better served by staying in this first phase of drama, which helps clients to develop group cohesion, trust, spontaneity, creativity, and ego-strength: in other words, confidence and self-esteem (Emunah, 1994). These are the treatment goals for most survivors.

Theatre as an aspect of drama therapy, also called therapeutic theatre (Lewis, 2000), is performance-oriented and involves a presentation for an audience. The performance may be done either by the clients or by actors, and the audience may consist of only one other person. Some drama therapists view theatre performance as a goal or the culmination of a series of drama therapy sessions, as suggested by Renee Emunah's integrative five phase model, described in her book (Emunah, 1994). Others use performance itself as the means by which to reach therapeutic goals, such as Playback Theatre (Fox, 1999), Theatre of the Oppressed (Boal, 1979), or in my own work with our training performance, *Rule of Thumb* (Pierce, 2004).

As part of my work with survivors, I wrote and directed a play based on their true stories. The play, *Rule of Thumb* (2004), was written at the request of the survivors and with their explicit written consent. By creating composite characters which incorporated multiple stories, and by using actors to portray the characters, survivors were able to have their stories heard in public and to reach out to other women at risk, without compromising their anonymity or their safety. "Rachel" is one of the composite characters in the play. Her character is based on the true stories and experiences of several clients. As a character, she embodies and expresses the truth of many survivors. Later in this chapter, I will describe in more detail the process I used to solicit the stories and develop the script, and how the script is being used as an outreach tool to help women who are still in abusive relationships, and as a training tool for professionals who work with survivors.

What Drama Therapy Does and Why it Works Well with Survivors

Drama therapy is effective because it involves a whole-body approach to therapy (Pierce, 2003). Since drama normally involves physical movement as well as sound or dialogue, the body and the mind are both engaged in the therapeutic/learning process. This approach works faster and the skills developed are easier to retain than in traditional "talk" therapies because it incorporates all of the learning styles simultaneously: visual, auditory, and kinesthetic. Drama therapy also incorporates all of the other arts–music, dance, poetry, and visual arts. Furthermore, according to the *Learning Pyramid*, people remember 5% of what they hear, 10% of what they read and 75% of what they do (National Training Laboratories, n.d.). Working in a group context also makes drama therapy effective. According to Jacobs, Masson, and Harvill (1998) in their textbook on group counseling, "Groups replicate real-life situations better than one-to-one counseling" (p. 5). Drama therapy can also provide emotional distance from the issue being addressed (Landy, 1994). By observing stories being enacted, the client can see the bigger picture and put events into context and perspective. This aspect of drama therapy is especially helpful in working with survivors of trauma or abuse.

Dramatic enactment helps people to practice skills they want to use in real-life. Status games, developed by Keith Johnstone (1979), can help clients to develop a repertoire of responses or 'power' levels to play when interacting with others. As Doctor Leticia Nieto explains in the March 2006 edition of *Colors NW magazine*, "High-status behavior is marked by a dominant or assertive posture. . . . Low status behavior is marked by a submissive or passive posture" (p. 30). I use status games to help clients to present themselves with more confidence and assertiveness, and to help people in positions of authority to develop rapport. Drama therapy can help people learn to manage difficult situations with more finesse, but it cannot remove a threat or danger imposed by someone who is determined to cause harm to a client. It can, however, help the client to recognize that threat, and help her to plan and practice safety procedures, much like a fire drill.

Creating a safe space to practice is essential for drama therapy work, and particularly more so for survivors of domestic violence. Groups should meet at a neutral, undisclosed location, preferably near other businesses. This is especially true in rural areas, where a victim's car may be known by many members of the community who could report the victim's whereabouts to her partner (NiCarthy, 2005). Within the group emotional safety is created by establishing ground rules for confidentiality, group integrity, and behavior. In a drama session, clients are free to speak and behave *differently* than normal. The space serves as a safe container for their feelings and a laboratory for discovery. Drama allows clients to explore and express emotions, and to practice new behaviors and interactive strategies. For safety reasons, it is also important for the therapist to make a distinction between drama that is used as a rehearsal process, and drama that is used for catharsis (Emunah, 1994). What a victim would *like* to say to or about her abuser, and what she *should* say or do, may be quite different. As an example, in one session we held a mock trial in order to give one of the clients her "day in court." In her actual lawsuit, the case was settled out of court and she felt somewhat disappointed that she had not been able to have her say. So we staged a mock trial with other group members playing the roles of judge, attorneys, jury, even the victim's ex-partner, and we allowed the client to have her "day in court." The mock trial was very cathartic for the client, but was quite different from a group session where a client would rehearse what she might say in a real trial. In the former, the client could say whatever she wanted to say. In the latter, she would want to rehearse appropriate courtroom attitude, language, and procedure.

Survivors face numerous problems in leaving an abusive relationship, reclaiming authority over their lives, and recovering from the effects of living with domestic violence. In the next section, I will describe how drama therapy can address specific problems for survivors. These problems include safety, identifying the problem, loss of the self, duration of recovery, fear, and isolation.

How Drama Therapy Can Address Specific Problems for Survivors

Safety

Safety is the number one concern for survivors. A woman is most at risk when she decides to leave the relationship (Websdale, 1999). Drama therapy can help clients to rehearse safety procedures and strategies, including role-playing or practicing what she may need to do or say or in different circumstances. For example, what to say to the teachers at her children's school if she has a protection order that they need to enforce.

Identifying the Problem

Cultural myths and a lack of understanding about domestic violence may make *identifying the problem* the most difficult aspect of this issue. Non-physical symptoms of abuse are often disregarded by survivors, therapists, and doctors. Many survivors do not identify themselves as victims of domestic violence because of the stereotypical thinking that is so common in our culture. "I didn't think I was being abused because he never hit me" (Anonymous Survivor, 2004). This is a typical statement for survivors, and one I have heard many times from my clients and audience members. Christine Millican (2003), a social worker and community advocate who works with survivors, explains that it is possible to address *safety* issues with a client before the client fully understands or identifies the nature of the problem, but recognizing and naming the problem of abuse is a huge step in the client's emotional recovery (Millican, 2003). Theatre and drama can increase a woman's safety by helping her to recognize abusive behaviors that she may have experienced, but not taken seriously. The theatre project I designed, based on true stories, demonstrates some of the power and control tactics that abusers use to dominate their partners. These tactics range from manipulation to physical violence. Watching scenes from the play can help women to recognize and assess their own stories, and can help therapists, advocates, and doctors learn to identify the problem as well.

Loss of the Self and Duration of Recovery

Part of the challenge for victims in identifying or naming the problem is that abusers *minimize* the effects of abuse (Domestic Abuse Intervention Project, 1985), and victims, especially long-term victims, have often internalized the voice and perspective of their abuser. Victims are simply used to accepting the blame (see Appendix). A victim is disempowered through emotional abuse, threats, put downs, verbal abuse, crazy-making, and physical assaults (Bancroft, 2002). She may not see herself as a victim of abuse, or she may deny or avoid facing the problem out of fear, or magical thinking, and she may hope it will all just go away. Drama therapy can help victims to regain a stronger sense of themselves in a number of ways. Theatre games can help them to explore and express their values and re-discover their sense of humor, and a sense of safety in connection to others. Role-playing can empower victims by helping them to prepare for job interviews, or to rehearse interactions with other family members. Status games can help them to *express* confidence and assertiveness, and improvisation can help them to think quickly on their feet. These are the skills which foster self-esteem and self-respect.

Separation and recovery from living with an abuser can take a very long time. Many of the women I worked with were still in the process of separating from their abusive partners, or were still living with them. There are many reasons why it takes a woman so long to leave: fear of harm to herself or the children or pets, financial dependency, religious beliefs about marriage and/or commitment, and inertia stemming directly from the long term effects of abuse, to name a few. A simulation game called *In Her Shoes*, developed by the Washington State Coalition Against Domestic Violence (2004), uses role-playing cards and scenarios to help people learn how hard it can be for survivors to "just leave." By walking "in her shoes," or in role, participants can quickly discover that leaving an abusive relationship is a very complex and dangerous process.

When a woman has been living with verbal, emotional, or sexual abuse for a long time, her self-esteem is eroded like an eraser on a pencil–down to nothing. When a woman internalizes the message that she is worthless, stupid, ugly, and incapable of doing anything right, she is crippled emotionally. Women who live with abusers may be heroic in what they can achieve within the home: doing all of the cooking, cleaning, shopping, and caring for the children or family business–but they may also hold the belief that they are not capable of surviving outside the relationship. Some of my clients were just beginning to name the abuse they had been through, even after being divorced for several years. Unfortunately, the abuse and control issues continued for them in terms of custody battles, parenting plans, and other courtroom dramas. Drama therapy can help improve recovery time for survivors, because it gets right to the point. Within a dramatic enactment, numerous problems or aspects of problems can be viewed, addressed, or recognized at once. As Robert Landy, director of the drama therapy program at New York University says: "Unlike talk therapy, drama therapy gets there really fast" (NADT brochure, n.d.).

Fear, Isolation, and Other Problems

Survivors have many reasons to feel afraid, and they feel fear in many aspects of their lives, on many levels. They may fear bodily harm, injury, or death, they may fear for the safety of their children, pets, other family members, or even for the safety of their abusers. They may fear retribution from their abuser for speaking to anyone outside the family, let alone what the repercussions might be if they attempt to get a protection order or a restraining order. Along with fear they may feel ashamed, guilty, or frustrated by the responses they have had from others when they have asked for help. They may feel afraid of the responses of the police officers. In rural areas where people know each other well, survivors have to worry about being seen asking for help, in case their abuser hears about it through the local grapevine (NiCarthy, 2005). They may also fear that no one will believe them.

Some of the survivors I worked with also expressed *a lack* of fear of their abusers, even when the abuser had a history of being violent with them (Anonymous Survivor, 2003). These survivors may simply refuse to be intimidated by their abuser. Although a bold attitude may make it easier for a survivor to move forward with her life, it does not necessarily reduce her risk factor. If an abuser decides that his scare tactics are no longer working, he may decide to up the ante with more violence.

Drama therapy can address fear and other emotional issues through techniques such as group mirroring, story-telling, and re-enactment. These techniques utilize peer support, and can help survivors to identify and evaluate risk factors in their lives, with some emotional distance. Emotions can also be depicted through art or mask work, movement, sound, or other group forms, such as sociodrama (Sternberg & Garcia, 2000), group sculptures or frozen tableaus.

One of the ways in which abusers maintain power and control over their victims is by limiting her contact with others (Covering Domestic Violence, 2002). Social isolation is one of most common experiences shared by survivors. Telling and showing stories, through drama and theatre, can help survivors to realize that they are not alone. This is one of the most significant factors in a survivor's recovery.

There are many other problems facing survivors which drama therapy may be able to help alleviate, if not resolve. Drama therapy cannot solve financial problems, but it can help clients to rehearse strategies of self-care. Drama therapy can help clients to prepare for trial or for interactions with the police or other authorities or family members by having them practice respectful assertiveness and scripted responses. Drama can help clients to rehearse the words they need to say until the words come naturally. As I will explain next, drama therapy can also be used to train police officers, judges, attorneys, counselors, and doctors.

Educating Audiences about Domestic Violence through Therapeutic Theatre

One of the main projects in my work with survivors was to create a play based on the experiences of the survivors I worked with. The play is entitled *Rule of Thumb*, and as of this writing, it has been on tour in western Washington for the past three years (2004–2007). The title comes from an old British Common Law, which stated that while it was permissible for a man to beat his wife, he could not use anything to beat her with that was bigger around than his thumb. The common law was cited by a judge in Mississippi when a case came to trial in 1824 (*Calvin Bradley vs. State of Mississippi*, 1824). According to the old customs, since the wife was considered property of the husband, he must be allowed to "correct" her behavior by applying physical discipline–in other words, violence. The "rule of thumb" condition supposedly prevented a man from going overboard in a "disciplinary" assault upon his wife.

My purpose in writing and producing the play was twofold: to reach out to women at risk to help them to recognize the power and control tactics of abusers, and to give a voice to the survivors I worked with, allowing them to share their stories with an audience without jeopardizing their anonymity or their safety. Though my initial goal was to reach women at risk, it soon became apparent that if I wanted to assist survivors and their children, then I also needed to reach counselors, judges, attorneys, police officers, and other service providers to help train *them* to identify these same patterns of abuse.

How the Play Came About

From 2003 to 2005, I worked as an advocate, drama therapist, and support group facilitator with a group of domestic violence survivors. This was a group of women, ages 25–82. At one of the meetings, I was listening to the women in the group describe a time when they had told their abusers that they were hurting them. Five out of eight of them described an almost identical dialogue they had had. In each case, the abuser had minimized the pain or hurt he was inflicting, with a phrase such as "Oh, please, this isn't hurting you!" As we went around the room, and I realized how many of them had heard almost the same exact words, I thought to myself: "Oh my God–it's a script!" About two minutes later, one of the women said: "We have got to get the word out to other women and let them know what this abuse is really all about." I said, "I can make that happen."

Collecting the Stories

I spoke to the women in the group over the next few weeks about my idea for creating a script. The script was to be used as an educational, and outreach project on domestic violence. I invited the women to share parts of their stories to be included in the script. Then, with their explicit permission and written consent, I led those women who chose to participate or share their stories through a long drama therapy session to elicit the specific stories that I would use to create the script. We started off by playing a theatre game as a warm-up activity.

We played a game I call "Hand it back/take it back" (adapted from Akeyo Onoe, 2000). The game starts out by having the clients sit or stand in a circle. One person starts off as "it," and using a wand or some other prop to pass to the next person, they identify and verbalize something negative that they were "handed" by their abuser, and they "hand it back" by passing it to someone in the circle. That person receives the wand by saying "thank-you." For example, the person with the wand might say "I'm handing back all of your credit card debt that you left for me" or "I'm handing back to you all of the ugly names you called me." The receiver says "thank-you" and then becomes "it," repeating the process with whatever it is they want to hand back. After a few rounds of handing it back I switch the game to "take it back." This time the person who is "it" takes the wand from whoever had it last, saying something like: "I'm taking back my mother's necklace that you stole from me" or "I'm taking back all the hours of sleep I lost when you terrified me" or even "I'm taking back my confidence in myself."

After our warm-up, we moved into a writing session. We moved into another room and sat around a large table. I set out paper and pens, and began posing questions for them to answer. I would pose a question and have each of them write down their responses. Some of the questions were inspired directly by the group. For example, I included as a fill-in-the-blank question: When I told him he was hurting me, he said: __________. This was the initial impetus for the play, and it was the working title for several months. Other questions that I included were about how the relationship had started, when it began to change, why they did not recognize it as abuse, funny experiences they had had, and what they would say if they could warn other women about their partner. After they had written their responses to four or five questions, I had them read them aloud and share their responses. Then I would pose four or five more questions, and we repeated the process several times.

This part of the process was very powerful, because a lot of the details of their individual stories came out, which many of them had not shared before. Since so many of them had had experiences that were similar, I knew that we were finding the common threads of violence and oppression, and that these were stories that audiences would also relate to because they were universal. This was a bridging moment in the therapy process, because in this particular moment I had to be aware of what my clients in the room needed to process, and also what the audience might need to process after hearing and watching these stories unfold.

After we finished these writing sessions, we did some closing activities. Moving back into another room we formed a circle and I asked them each to share something they had learned that day. Then I also invited them to share something they appreciated about someone else in the group. This closing process helped to ensure that everyone felt complete and finished with our work for the present moment, it validated the depth of their experiences and their bravery in sharing these stories, and by making a formal ritual of closure, it helped to prepare them to go back out into the world.

Designing the Show and Writing the Script

I took the raw material, created five characters and wove the stories together. My idea for the script was to have the characters be members of a support group reaching out to the audience. Since this was to become a training and outreach piece, I wanted to include important factual data in the script and in the program. Structurally, it is a theatre piece without walls.

Rule of Thumb is a "portable" theatre service project. There is no stage set, only five chairs and a box of props. *Rule of Thumb* can be and has been taken into board rooms, conference rooms, classrooms, churches, and even into private homes. We have also presented it in theatre spaces. The bigger the space, however, the more need for technical theatre, such as lighting. We have focused on playing for small audiences because it is a very intimate show. The actors talk directly to the audience, with whom they also make eye contact. This is easier if the audience is sitting four or five feet away, and not in a theatre auditorium.

This structure of this project is very much in keeping with the vision of Jacob Moreno, the founder of modern drama therapy. "Moreno believed that there should be interaction between audience and actors. Further, he believed that the theatre was lifeless because it did not explore issues that were of vital importance to the general public" (Sternberg & Garcia, 2000, p. 197). The characters talk directly to the audience throughout the play and the audience is invited to speak with the actors directly after the play, in a post-play discussion. From the very beginning of the play the audience is invited into the stories. In her opening monologue, the character Rachel tells them:

Rachel: We are members of a small, rural community, but tonight we are sharing our stories with you, as though you were members of *our* community, *our* circle of support. You could be, perhaps. Even though our backgrounds, our culture, or our lifestyles may be different from yours, our stories may seem very familiar to you. If you find these stories troubling because something similar has happened to you, we invite you to call you local domestic violence agency after the program and talk to someone. Don't be ashamed. We are all in this together (Pierce, 2004).

In addition to addressing the audience as members of a support group, I wanted to demonstrate visually and symbolically some of the emotionally manipulative tactics abusers use to maintain power in the relationship. One of the play's strongest features is the introduction of the twist game:

Rachel: It's the TWIST game! (Spinning in a circle with Sheila) I was late coming home from work one night, and when I walked in the door he said:

Sheila: (as Rachel's ex-husband): I know you're having an affair! Who is it?

Rachel: Nothing I could say would appease him. I found out later that HE was the one having an affair!
Sheila: Twist!
Rachel: He just twisted it all around!
Cathy: (spinning in a circle with Ann): He started screaming at me one day.
Ann: (as Cathy's husband): I know you're wasting all of our money! What do you do with it all?
Cathy: What do you mean, what did I do with it? I paid the bills! I bought groceries. (to the audience) A week later I found out he'd gone out and bought a boat. A BOAT!
Rachel: Twist! (Pierce, 2004).

The twist game demonstrates how abusers accuse their victims of the very behaviors they are doing themselves. This is important to demonstrate because being put on the defensive is very confusing to the victim. The victim spends time and energy trying to defend herself, when the reality is that by accusing her, the perpetrator throws her entirely off scent. Abusers are masters at manipulation and mind games, and the twist game is only one of their tactics. Other control tactics are also demonstrated in the play.

Reaching the Audience

Rule of Thumb is an example of therapeutic theatre. It combines training materials with story-telling, and by doing so it gives audience members a deeper insight into the problems faced by survivors of domestic violence, and the attitudes of superiority, domination, and control exhibited by abusers. A copy of the power and control wheel (Duluth, 1985), is included in the program to reinforce the issues demonstrated in the play. Phone numbers and websites for local and national domestic violence hotlines are also listed in the program, and additional comments from the audience are collected after the post-play discussion.

Audiences of all kinds; men, women, advocates, attorneys, police officers, and therapists have responded well to this play. It has sparked lively discussions about gender and religious issues, legal and financial issues, power dynamics, treatment programs, and the need for more community education, funding, and professional training about domestic violence.

Prevalence of Domestic Violence and the Need for Adequate Training

A research report dated July 2000 showed that an estimated 7.7 million intimate partner assaults are perpetrated in the United States annually

(Tjaden & Thoennes, 2000). The report described the findings from the National Violence Against Women Survey, which was jointly sponsored by the National Institute of Justice and the Center for Disease Control. This estimate does not include violence against children or acts of violence in society at large such as road rage or armed robbery. Despite the prevalence of domestic violence in our society, most therapists and doctors are not adequately trained to deal with this issue. Doctors and counselors are trained to address physical and emotional problems within the client or patient herself. However, the main threat to a survivor's physical, mental, and emotional well being, and to her very *life*, comes from someone outside of herself. Her *safety* should be their number one concern.

> When I was living with my abusive ex-husband many years ago, I was just exhausted all of the time from living under the stress. So I went to the doctor to see if they could help me, and they ran blood tests. Guess what? There was nothing wrong with my blood. They told me "You're the picture of health, on paper" and they sent me home. They didn't even send me to a mental health clinic for counseling–it didn't get that far. But if they had, the counselors would have probably given me an anti-depressant. It wasn't my blood, and a pill wouldn't have cured me. It was domestic violence. (Anonymous Survivor, 2006)

Doctors, counselors, and other service providers need basic training in domestic violence in order to identify the psychological patterns of abuse as well as the physical symptoms. They need a deeper understanding of the power and control issues driving domestic violence in order assess the risk factors, provide treatment, or make appropriate referrals for their clients and their families. Drama therapy and therapeutic theatre can help to train service providers by demonstrating the power and control games as well as the legal, financial, religious, and safety issues that survivors are up against. Therapeutic theatre is extremely effective as a training tool, because it reaches audiences on an emotional level as well as a cognitive level. By demonstrating the psychological games, manipulation, verbal and emotional abuse, threats and other patterns of abuse that survivors contend with, audiences are quick to grasp the context of domestic abuse for their clients and their families.

Conclusion

Drama therapy is an effective treatment modality for survivors of domestic violence because it involves a whole-body approach to learning and therapy which increases the ability of the clients to learn, rehearse, and remember new skills and behaviors. Drama therapy works faster than traditional talk therapies, because it incorporates all learning styles simultaneously. By incorporating a client-centered approach to drama therapy, survivors are empowered to make their own choices, which they are seldom allowed to do in abusive relationships. Drama therapy can help survivors to present themselves more effectively, and to reclaim a sense of dignity and self-respect. Theatre is also a powerful tool for training counselors and other professionals about domestic violence because it brings perspective and emotional context to the issue.

If we are to stop domestic violence, we have to recognize what is driving it. Mental illness does not cause domestic violence, but mental *attitudes* do, particularly those of entitlement and superiority (Bancroft, 2002). These attitudes are at the heart of oppression. Therapeutic theatre can illuminate the attitudes driving domestic violence so that audiences can identify them.

Rachel is a character in the play, *Rule of Thumb.* She is a composite character who embodies the experience of many survivors of domestic violence. Like many women, Rachel did not recognize the patterns of domestic violence until her life was threatened. When people see these stories come to life they begin to recognize themselves. In this way, the performance itself is therapeutic, because recognizing a problem is the first step to solving the problem. For some of our audience members, seeing the performance was like looking in the mirror.

Terms

Affirmations are positive, affirming statements about oneself or another person, spoken or received with the intention of focusing on that person's best qualities.

DAIP is the Domestic Abuse Intervention Project in Duluth, Minnesota. It is a community-based program for intervention in domestic abuse cases.

Developmental transformations are embodied improvisational encounters in the playspace between the client and the therapist designed to treat the client's ability to play and be fully present, interactively.

Distorted thinking is any form of negative thinking that causes a person to feel worse about herself, another person, or an experience than the situation warrants.

Drama is an experiential, process-oriented activity consisting of games, scenes, role-playing, or other exercises designed to help the participants work on personal or social issues, and which involve the clients themselves taking part in or contributing to the activity.

Dramatic ritual is the use of ceremony, or ceremonial elements, to help clients to symbolically transform aspects of their lives, or to acknowledge, or celebrate significant changes, or choices they have made in their lives.

Dramatic rituals can be simple activities used in group work, such as a regular closing activity, or they can be more elaborate forms of ritual drama.
Drama therapy is the intentional use of drama and/or theatre processes to achieve therapeutic goals.
Group sculptures are living statues set in place like a picture by a group member who is creating the picture. The act of 'sculpting', deciding and directing how the other group members are to stand or sit, is a significant part of the therapeutic process.
Integrative model is a developmental model of drama therapy, developed by Renee Emunah, which suggests that drama therapy as a course of treatment progresses through five phases, from simple dramatic play to deeper levels of scenework, role play, psychodrama, and dramatic ritual.
Learned helplessness is the defeated, giving-up response that follows from a belief that nothing you do will matter.
Life Stories Process developed by Sheila Rubin, is the process of creating and performing solo self-revelatory performances. The stories are true, usually deeply personal, stories of the clients, which are performed by the clients for an audience. Life stories incorporate the aesthetic challenges of theatre as part of the therapeutic process, for which the audience serves as a witness.
Line repetition is the repetition of a line or phrase by different members of a group to either emphasize or examine its meaning, or to add an element of group cohesion to a story.
Magical thinking is discounting, denying, or minimizing a problem in the hopes that it will "magically" disappear.
Mask work is the creation or use of masks to represent different aspects of the self, or different emotions, different characters, animals, deities, qualities, ideals, or institutions.
Mirroring and group mirroring are theatre games which involve group members physically and/or emotionally mirroring each other, either to learn observation skills, or so that the other person can see herself reflected back. Group mirroring involves several players mirroring the actions or emotions of one other player.
NADT is the National Association for Drama Therapy.
Narradrama is an approach to drama therapy which takes into account the client's personal and preferred stories, and works with the client to create alternative stories for her life.
Past and future projections are the improvised enactments of a person or a character's projected past or future. These enactments can be frozen as tableaus, discussed, adjusted, and replayed, depending on the goal of the session.
Playback Theatre is a performance-oriented form of drama therapy which takes stories from the audience and plays them back for them, using professional actors trained in the playback method.

Psychodrama is a deep action method in which people enact scenes from their own lives, dreams, or fantasies in order to explore and express feelings, gain insight, or practice new or more satisfying behaviors.
Ritual drama is the creation of sacred dramatic rites of passage and ceremonies to help support the client through developmental stages or create a sense of balance and healing for the client.
Role doubling is the use of an additional player or players to support, or double, the thoughts and emotions of a character in a dramatic enactment. The role double stands near the other actor, with a hand on her shoulder, and may suggest lines for the character.
Role method is a drama therapy method used to help clients access and/or work more effectively with one or more of the roles they play in life. Role method is based on role theory, which suggests that we each have a repertoire of roles which we play in life, consciously or unconsciously.
Role playing is the enactment of roles by a member or members of the group, in order to explore different aspects of a role or problem, or in order to find alternative ways of solving a role related problem.
Rule of Thumb is a one-act touring play about domestic violence. The expression "rule of thumb" came from British Common Law, which allowed a man to beat his wife in order to control her, as long as he did not use anything to beat her with that was bigger around than his thumb.
Scripted responses are the planned, if not written, responses a client may choose to say in response to a difficult situation.
Simulated conflicts are dramatized conflict scenarios using scripted dialogue or improvisation, designed to help group members rehearse behaviors they can use in real life.
Sociodrama is an action method in which individuals enact an agreed upon social situation spontaneously for the purpose of defining or exploring a problem that group members would like to address.
Status games are games and activities which help clients to identify and explore their status levels within the context of a group or dyad. Status levels are determined by postures and behaviors which vary from culture to culture and to some degree from group to group.
Tableaus are frozen sculptures which depict a snapshot in a story, or a series of snapshots. Tableaus can be choreographed by either the story-teller or by the group.
Theatre games are dramatic exercises which were developed to improve actor's focus, spontaneity, and believability, and which are used in drama therapy most often as warm-up activities to prepare group members for deeper work.
Theatre of the Oppressed is one of several models of social activist theatre developed by Augusto Boal, in which a member of the audience is chosen to

act out a problem faced by a disenfranchised group. An improvisational format is used to explore and discuss the problem, and members of the audience become the participants in the drama. While Theatre of the Oppressed is considered social activist theatre and not drama therapy, drama therapists borrow heavily from its format.

Theatre, or therapeutic theatre as an aspect of drama therapy is performance-oriented, and involves a presentation for an audience.

WSCADV is the Washington State Coalition Against Domestic Violence.

Appendix–The Power and Control Wheel

The Power and Control Wheel, below, was developed by battered women in Duluth who had been abused by their male partners and were attending women's education groups sponsored by the women's shelter. While there are women who use violence against men, and there are men and women in same-sex relationships who use violence, this wheel is meant specifically to illustrate men's abusive behaviors toward women. The Power and Control wheel is used here with permission from the Domestic Abuse Intervention Project. (Reproduced by permission of DOMESTIC ABUSE INTERVENTION PROJECT, 202 E. Superior Street, Duluth, MN 55802, 218-722-2781, www.duluth-model.org.)

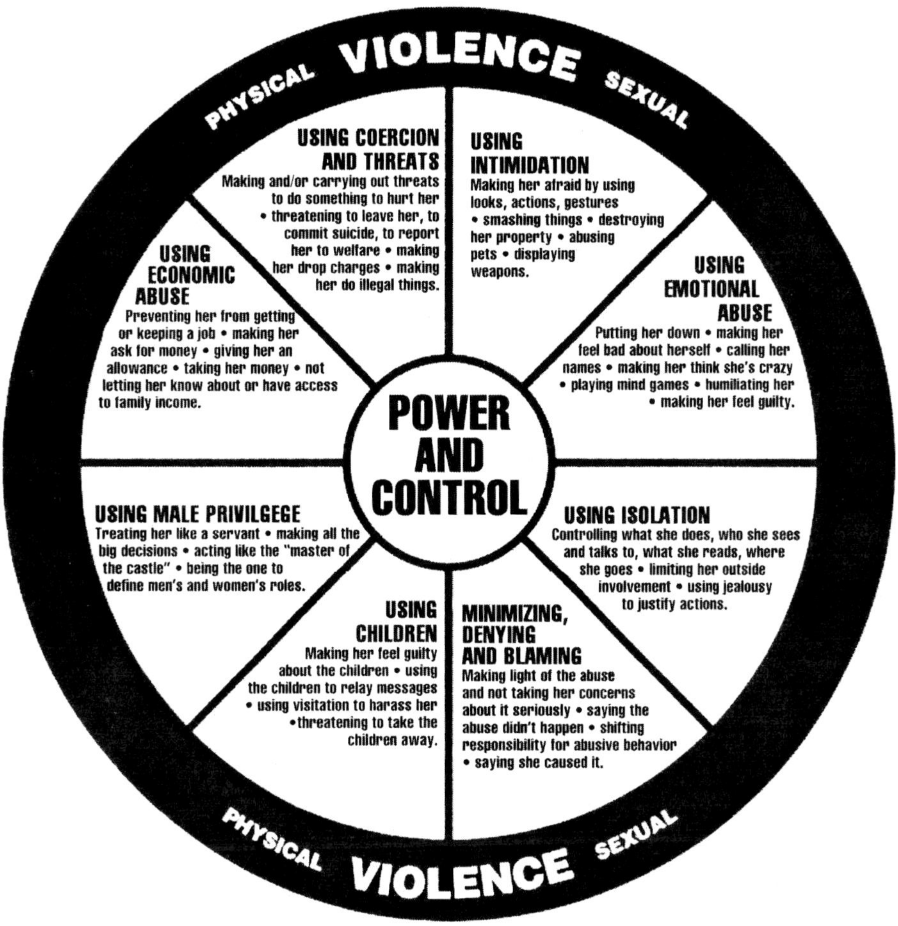

References

Anonymous Survivor. (2003). Personal interview. Vashon, WA.

Anonymous Survivor. (2004). Support group for women: Drama Therapy session. Vashon, WA: Island Domestic Violence Outreach Services.

Anonymous Survivor. (2006). Personal interview. Vashon, WA.

Bailey, S. (2000). Personal interview and class content from Principles of Drama Therapy. Manhattan, KS: Kansas State University.

Bancroft, L. (2002). *Why does he do that: Inside the minds of angry and controlling men.* New York: Berkley.

Blatner, A. (1996). *Acting-In: Practical applications of psychodramatic method* (3rd ed.). New York: Springer Publishing.

Boal, A. (1979). *Theater of the oppressed.* New York: Urizen.

Bradley v. State of Mississippi, 1 Morr. St. Cas. 20, Walker 156 (1824; December).

Bureau of Justice Statistics Crime Data Brief. (2003, February). *Intimate partner violence, 1993-2001.* Washington, D.C.: U.S. Department of Justice.

Burns, D. (1999). *The feeling good handbook* (Rev. ed.). New York: Plume.

Covering domestic violence: A guide for journalists and other media professionals. (2002). Olympia, WA: Washington State Coalition Against Domestic Violence.

Domestic Abuse Intervention Project. (1985). *Power and control wheel.* Duluth, MN: Author.

Drama therapy. [Brochure] (n.d.). Pittsford, NY: National Association for Drama Therapy.

Dunne, P. (2000). Narradrama: A narrative approach to drama therapy. In P. Lewis and D. R. Johnson (Eds.), *Current approaches in drama therapy* (pp. 111-128). Springfield, IL: Charles C Thomas, Publisher, Ltd.

Emunah, R. (1994). *Acting for real: Drama therapy process, technique, and performance.* New York: Brunner/Mazel, Inc.

Fox, J. (1999). What is playback theatre? In J. Fox & H. Dauber (Eds.), Gathering voices: *Essays on playback theatre* (p. 7). New Paltz, NY: Tusitala Publishing.

In her shoes: Living with domestic violence (Economic Justice Edition). [Role playing game] (2004). Olympia, WA: Washington State Coalition Against Domestic Violence.

Jacobs, E., Masson, R., & Harvill, R. (1998). *Group counseling: Strategies and skills* (3rd ed.). Pacific Grove, CA: Brooks/Cole Publishing Company.

Johnson, D. R. (2000). The history and development of the field of drama therapy in the United States and Canada. In P. Lewis and D. R. Johnson (Eds.), *Current approaches in drama therapy* (p. 5). Springfield, IL: Charles C Thomas, Publisher, Ltd.

Johnson, D. R. (2000). Developmental transformations: Toward the body as presence. In P. Lewis & D. R. Johnson (Eds.), *Current approaches in drama therapy* (p. 87). Springfield, IL: Charles C Thomas, Publisher, Ltd.

Johnstone, K. (1979). *Impro: Improvisation and the theatre.* New York: Theatre Arts Books.

Landy, R. (1993). *Persona and performance: The meaning of role in drama, therapy, and everyday life.* New York: Guilford Press.

The learning pyramid. [Graph]. (n.d.). Alexandria, VA: National Training Laboratories Institute for Applied Behavioral Science.

Lewis, P. (2000). Toward a body of knowledge in drama therapy. In P. Lewis & D. R. Johnson (Eds.), *Current approaches in drama therapy* (p. 446). Springfield, IL: Charles C Thomas, Publisher, Ltd.

Lewis, P., & Johnson, D. R. (2000). *Current approaches in drama therapy.* Springfield, IL: Charles C Thomas, Publisher, Ltd.

Millican, C. (2006). Personal interview. Vashon, WA.

National Association for Drama Therapy. [Brochure]. Pittsford, NY. (www.nadt.org).
Nieto, L., & Boyer, M. (2006, March). Understanding oppression: Strategies in addressing power and privilege. Colors, NW. 30-33.
NiCarthy, G. (2005, January). Rural women: Culture, domestic violence and activism. *King County Coalition Against Domestic Violence E-newsletter.*
Onoe, A. (2000). Class presentation and personal interview. Manhattan, KS: Kansas State University.
Pierce, D. (2004). *Rule of thumb* [Play]. Vashon, WA: Lighthouse Theatre.
Power and control wheel. [Pie chart]. (1985). Duluth, MN: Domestic Abuse Intervention Project.
Rubin, S. (2007). Self-revelatory performance. In A. Blatner (Ed.), *Interactive and improvisational drama: Varieties of applied theater and performance* (pp. 250-259). Lincoln, NE: iUniverse, Inc.
Seligman, M. (1998). *Learned optomisim, How to change your mind and your life.* New York: Pocket Books.
Sternberg, P., & Garcia, A. (2000). Sociodrama. In P. Lewis & D. R. Johnson (Eds.), *Current approaches in drama therapy* (p. 197). Springfield, IL: Charles C Thomas, Publisher, Ltd.
The learning pyramid (n.d.). Alexandria, VA: National Training Laboratories Institute for Applied Behavioral Science.
Tjaden, P., & Thoennes, N. (2000). *Extent, nature, and consequences of intimate partner violence: Findings from the National Violence Against Women Survey.* National Institute of Justice and the Center for Disease Control.
Websdale, N. (1999). *Washington State domestic violence fatality review project: Understanding domestic homicide.* Boston: Northeastern University Press.

Biography

Deb Pierce is a Registered Drama Therapist and Board Certified Trainer with the National Association for Drama Therapy. She has a Master's degree in theatre from Kansas State University. Deb is the founder and artistic director of Lighthouse Theatre, a non-profit theatre based on drama therapy principles. She has written and directed theatre for over twenty years. In 1988 Deb won the Jerome Johanning Playwriting award for her one-act play, *The Elopement.* In 1992 she founded the Pierce County Playwright's Festival in Tacoma, WA. She has used drama therapy in her work with psychiatric patients, sex offenders, women in prison, adolescents in a treatment center, and survivors of domestic violence. In her work with survivors she co-led a support group, provided client advocacy, and offered drama therapy. She wrote and directed *Rule of Thumb*, (2004), as an outgrowth of her work with survivors. It is offered as a training piece on domestic violence and an introduction to therapeutic theatre. *Rule of Thumb* has been on tour for the past three years (2004–2007) in Western Washington. Her private practice in drama therapy and training is called Stages of Healing.

Chapter 15

MA MÈRE ET MOI: CREATIVE ARTS IN A GROUP TREATMENT FOR MOTHERS AND THEIR CHILDREN

ATHENA P. MADAN

Introduction

Ma mère et moi ("My mom and me") is a twelve-week group therapy programme at a Francophone community health clinic in southwest Ontario for children and their mothers who have experienced woman abuse in their homes. The group meets once weekly for one and a half hours for therapeutic activity and discussion. Facilitated by three co-facilitators, the group is conducted on two levels: In dyads, within the larger context of the group, and in subgroups, according to age/peer group.

This chapter outlines specific programme objectives with review of applications, considerations, and rationale in planning and facilitating group work using drama and art as modalities of treatment for abused mothers and their children. Following material generated specifically from one series of sessions with preadolescent girls aged 11–13, I will discuss intervention wherein both mother and child may explore and establish a framework for greater attunement and reconnection within their relationship as it has been affected by conjugal violence. Specifically, I will discuss Harvey's Family Dynamic Play (Harvey, 1983, 1990, 1994a, 1994b, 1997, 2000) approach in working with a mother-preadolescent aged dyad.

DOMESTIC VIOLENCE IN CANADA AND IN THE NIAGARA REGION

Statistically, one in three Canadians report being victims of a domestic violence incident per year, with one-third of these having children or youth present as witnesses (Canadian Centre for Justice Statistics, 2001). While statistically the Western and prairie provinces have higher incidents of domestic violence per capita, Ontario has the highest number of reported violent incidents against women and children (Federal-Provincial-Territorial Ministers Responsible for the Status of Women, 2002): 25 female deaths per year due to domestic homicide, and 39% of domestic violence incidents with child and youth present as witnesses (Statistics Canada, 2005; and 2006, respectively). In the cases where violence ended in death, a known history of family violence was documented in 6 out of every 10 cases (Federal-Provincial-Territorial Ministers Responsible for the Status of Women, 2002). Table 1 details the breakdown of specific types of violence children and youth were reported to have witnessed in the home.

Table 1. Types and Incidence of Domestic Violence, Reported in the Past Five Years

Type of domestic violence (reported)	Incidence (Canada)	Incidence (Ontario)	Incidence (Niagara)
Pushing, grabbing, or shoving	86%	81%	56%
Threatening to hit	65%	65%	62%
Throwing something	43%	44%	47%
Slapping	50%	40%	N/A
Hitting with something	22%	23%	N/A
Choking	25%	20%	21%
Sexual assault	29%	20%	18%
Using / threatening to use a gun or a knife	16%	13%	19%

Source: Statistics Canada, 2005; Niagara Regional Police Service, 2005.

Of nearly 8,850 reported cases of family violence within a subset of 122 police departments across Canada similar to the Niagara Regional district (Statistics Canada, 2005), male parents were the primary accused against children and youth, representing 70% of the accused perpetrators of all reported incidents of physical assault. In instances (11%) where a person other than the spouse was reported harmed or threatened, 44% of these were children under the age of 15. Reporting a 30% to 40% overlap between children who witness wife assault and children who experience direct physical abuse themselves, Statistics Canada (2005) noted no urban or rural difference in these trends for domestic violence.

Group Design

Focus Research

Ma mère et moi was developed without precedent in the region. Its content, instruction and design were informed by two strands of research: (a) Practical content, or current approaches in violence prevention and intervention programmes seen in Ontario and Québec, and (b) Theoretical content, or objective guidelines in collaboration with focussed needs assessment in similar-profile communities. We discovered many community violence prevention programs implementing various arts-in-community-based approaches, but funding in these project-driven initiatives often fell short of robust evaluation and were largely unreplicated besides. Further, with the exception of a few studies on child abuse, there was relatively little epidemiological French research about group intervention and programming for youth victims of domestic violence. Even less documentation was available on mother-child concurrent programming. Particular attention was thus paid to programmes that had been evaluated, to approaches seen replicated across communities, and to programmes whose objectives were supplemented with transparent and documented focus research.

Our focus research for *Ma mère et moi* was held in consultation format between colleagues working in individual follow-up and transitional support programmes, and with client mothers whose children were attached to mental health services for witnesses of violence. We also consulted publication findings from other needs assessments conducted in Franco-Ontarian communities (Gauthier, 1998/1999), and guidelines established in group violence prevention and follow-up programmes (Baker & Cunningham, 2005; Berman & Jiwini, 2001; Jiwini et al., 1999). These consultations yielded the following recommendations:

- Groups are best conducted as a team/co-facilitator effort, with a multidisciplinary approach;
- Fatherhood should be valued as equally as motherhood is respected;
- Facilitators should not undertake any mother-specific roles in the group (such as changing diapers, feeding food, or disciplinary action, if necessary);
- Youth participation should not be gender-specific (i.e., if an adolescent male is part of subset, sustained efforts should be made to include his participation);

- Group members that are vulnerable should be given sustained opportunity to speak, balanced with the need for equal consideration within the group;
- Group work should be adapted to include components, perspectives, languages and traditions specific to the different cultural/ethnic representations within the group;
- Socialisation and promotion of non-violent values (egalitarian behaviour, the right to be different, the right to not participate) should be promoted;
- Participants should be consulted in the planning and implementation of their group activities;
- Programmes should use tools that reach its participants; and
- All forms of violence should be addressed.

The following were recommendations and practical needs specific to our clientele:

- Group efforts should contain additional and sustained efforts to preserve participants' anonymity, with space for different cultural perspectives;
- Support for transportation and car seats;
- Childcare for children under 3 years old; and
- Snacks. Many of the families came to group directly following work or after-school programmes and had insufficient time or resources to check in or eat together following their day.

Clientele (Population Considerations)

Children in violent homes are generally characterised (Jaffe, Wolfe, & Wilson, 1990) by the following: higher levels of insecurity, anxiety, fear, and hypervigilance (Health Canada, 1996); a lack of proper role model and identification for maturity in peer relationships; and an assumption that violence is the norm (Boyd & Klingbeil, 1984). They are also found to display, regardless of behavioural strategy (i.e., internalising vs. externalising behaviour), social isolation and emotional distance (Bancroft & Silverman, 2002) accompanied with poor self-esteem, sadness, depression, and impulsivity, with higher levels of aggression or passivity (Osofsky, 1998). These children display statistically lower levels of cognition and attention to task, as well as lower tolerance for frustration.

Table 2 indicates the potential impact of violence across five different stages of child development (Baker & Cunningham, 2004; Carlson, 2000). These considerations informed our facilitation and treatment plans for the various child subgroups. Children witnessing violence in their homes are more likely to exhibit difficulties across all five developmental measures. In particular, they are more than twice as likely to be physically aggressive, to bully or be bullied, to commit delinquent acts against property, and to display indirect (object- or self-related) aggression (Canadian Centre for Justice Studies, 2001).

The potential impact of violence on preadolescent-aged youth is discussed separately in Table 3. Relatively little research has been collected for the Preadolescent age specifically, though extrapolated information from current literature and analyses (Bair-Merrit, Blackstone, & Feudtner, 2006; Baker & Cunningham, 2005; Canadian Centre for Justice Statistics, 2001; Carlson, 2000; Fondation pour l'enfance, 2000; Fortin, 2005; Statistics Canada, 2005, 2006) indicates a cluster of characteristics specific to this age / level of development. Table 3 outlines these characteristics, as they develop normally and as they are seen affected by violence in the home, with their subsequent implications for intervention and follow-up. *Ma mère et moi* intervention and group plans are designed using these developmental considerations.

Table 2.
Potential Development Impact of Exposure to Domestic Violence

Aspect of development	Infants / Toddlers (0-3 years)	Preschoolers (4-6 years)	Latency (7-9 years)	Adolescent (14-18 years)
Behavioural	-Fussiness -Inability to be soothed	-Demanding -Whiny, clinging -Regression -Aggression -Low frustration tolerance -Inability to self-soothe / inappropriate self-soothing behaviors -Difficulty with self-regulation -Hyperactivity	-Aggression -Conduct problems -Opposition / defiance, or parentification -Preoccupation with violent or morbid themes -Inattention to task -Hyperactivity	-Dating violence -Delinquency -Running away -Promiscuity -Parentification / Controlling-caretaking -Self-harm -Substance abuse -Impulsivity
Emotional	-Ambivalence in attachment -Anxiety in attachment	-Fear, anxiety, sadness -Negative affect	-Fear, anxiety -Depression -Guilt, shame -Anger	-Anxiety -Depression -Suicidality
Physical	-Distress -Problems eating -Problems sleeping -Easily agitated	-Highly active -Hypervigilance -Stomachaches	-Highly active	-Anxiety -May try to use size to intimidate
Cognitive	-Inability to understand or follow simple directions -Avoidance in attachment	-Limited ability to understand or follow simple directions -Task compulsion	-Low academic performance -Pro-violent attitudes -Low task completion	-Pro-violent attitudes
Social		-Trouble interacting with peers, adults -Ambivalence in relationships	-Social withdrawal -Inability to develop mutually negotiated states -Fewer and lower quality peer relationships	-Violent dating relationships -Ambivalence / intensity in relationships

Sources: B. E. Carlson, 2000; and L. Baker & A. Cunningham, 2004.

Table 3.
Potential Impact of Exposure to Domestic Violence on Preadolescents (Age 10-13 Years) and Their Implications for Group Intervention

Aspect of development	Normal key indicators	*Possible impact of DV*		Intervention Considerations
Behavioural	-Increased sense of self and autonomy from family	-Dating violence -Delinquency -Truancy / Running away -Promiscuity -Parentification / Controlling-caretaking in attachment -Eating disorders	-Preoccupation with violent or morbid themes -Substance abuse -Self-harm -Social withdrawal / inappropriate attention-seeking / risk-taking behaviours	-Psychoeducation -Freedom of expression -Identification of emotions -Acceptance of emotions -Restructuring for age-appropriate responsibility
Emotional	-Self-worth more strongly linked to view of physical attractiveness	-Low self-esteem -Depression -Suicidality -Image-management activities (body piercing, tattoos) -Disconnect	-Fear of intimacy / abusing / being abused -Insecurity -Self-worth linked to positions of power -Emotional invincibility or hopelessness	-Create opportunities for peer support and acceptance -Examine unconditional vs. conditional acceptance -Examine body image -Acceptance of emotions -Links to community resources -Fostering of reconnection and security in attachment
Physical	-Emotional and hormonal changes	-Avoidance of or overt confrontation -May try to intimidate		-Psychoeducation -Caregiver support -Links to community resources
Cognitive	-Increased capacity for abstract reasoning and broader world view	-Pro-violent attitudes -Inflexible thinking -Inattention to task		-Psychoeducation -Support at school informed by knowledge of family adversities

Social	-Increased influence by media -Increased peer group influence and desire for acceptance -Increased value on peer intimacy and relationship skills	-Inability to develop mutually negotiated states -Fewer and lower quality peer relationships -Ambivalence in relationships -Shame -Secrecy -Social withdrawal -Fear of abusing / being abused in relationships	-May avoid intimacy / seek intimacy prematurely -Possibly more influenced by negative media messages re: violent behaviour, gender role stereotypes -High-risk behaviour to impress peers, achieve social power	-Psychoeducation -Communication skills in negotiation, assertion and compromise -Encouragement in developing talents, creativity -Examination of roles -Examination of power in relationships -Media influence & appropriate self-expectations -Create opportunities for peer support and acceptance

Additional considerations for the Mothers' group included the following emotional reactions reported (Statistics Canada, 2005) towards domestic violence: being upset, confused or frustrated because of the violence (37%); anger (37%); fear: (30%); hurt or disappointed (25%); and depression or anxiety (21%). Also reported were feelings of lower self-esteem (17%), hyper-vigilance (16%), having sleeping problems (16%), being ashamed or feeling guilty (10%), being afraid for their children (9%), being more self-reliant (8%), and having problems relating to members of the opposite sex (8%). Six per cent of women reported being "not much affected" by their experience of violence in the home (Statistics Canada, 2005, p. 22).

Participants (Assignment Profile)

The Niagara community, south of Toronto, includes three medium density cities, four medium density towns, and eight small density rural townships. The population totals 424,347 with seasonal fluctuation in some communities due to migrant workers, summer festivals, cottage tourists, and construction (Niagara Regional Police Service, 2006). Situated in the Niagara region is one of the nation's busiest border crossings and three waterfront shorelines.

Specific to the Franco-Ontarian population, there are four main cultural groups. They comprise: (a) those that have been born and raised in Niagara across the Franco-Ontarian generations; (b) those that relocate from Québec; (c) those that immigrate here from the Francophone diaspora; and, (d) those that seek asylum or refuge in the region from their respective French-speaking country of origin. The latter two groups comprise ethnicity and representation from Europe, North and Sub-Saharan Africa, the Caribbean, and Southeast Asia. While the majority of the Centre's programmes serve clients in the former two categories, the *Ma mère et moi* programme serves clients from all four.

Immigrant and refugee women in abusive relationships (where abusive relationships were reported, Canadian Centre for Justice Statistics, 2001) indicate higher levels of isolation, loneliness, fear, and economic dependence than women who did not hold immigrant or refugee status. These women tended to stay in or return to abusive relationships due to their isolation, lack of economic resources, a lack of access to employment, and language barriers. Further, fear of deportation and fear of police authority were barriers for these women to report their experience of violence. In this session, one-half of women held immigrant or refugee status. In the children's groups, two out of every three participants were siblings.

Facilitation

As the *Ma mère et moi* programme requires that the mother no longer lives with the violent partner, the children were no longer directly witnessing or experiencing situations of conjugal violence. But the indirect experiences were ongoing: emotional and behavioural consequences of the violence itself; divided loyalties associated with visitation, or guilt about not wanting contact with the father; the stigmatisation in a small community about being "different" or being from a "divided and inharmonious family." In some instances, the threat of fear and punishment was also still physically felt; in others, there were multiple losses resulting from leaving the country, cultures, and families of origin. Tension, anxiety, conflict, and stress were very much present and day-to-day realities in these youth's lives. As such, group planning's primary consideration included fostering a caring, supportive, safe, and fun environment, where equity is strongly encouraged and non-violence is literally a factor in play.

Objectives and considerations specific to the Niagara region and clientele included food and transportation support. As noted, many of the families came to group directly following work or after-school programmes. Eating together helped facilitate check-in time; it also helped facilitate belonging, create cohesion and establish a comfortable, natural intimacy. Further, with the age range of the child and youth participants, and given that the group is held during the week, giving food supported the mothers in their efforts to attend and engage in the group process.

Group format was divided. We met all together for the first twenty-five minutes. This time allowed check-in with activity and discussion about events and feelings about the week. On a more practical level, this format also allowed participants to arrive knowing what to expect in the group process, and without fear of interrupting their peers. Following this time we divided into respective age groups to address age-appropriate concerns through to the end of the hour and a half session. This format further allowed us to measure (see Ainsworth, Blehar, Waters, & Wall, 1978, for separation and reunion assessment) the quality of attachment and connection between family members as the group advanced. The group met once a week for ten weeks.

Group facilitation was designed within a Creative Arts approach as described here in Figure 1: six (Brooke, 2006; Jones, 2005) separate but interrelated modalities, collectively sharing interconnected principles, tools, and considerations underpinning the intentional use of arts in / arts as therapy process. Group exercises I will describe specific to this series' session refer to art, dance-movement, drama, and play modalities, with theoretical influences extending from dramatic and improvised play (Harvey, 1983, 1987, 1990, 1994a, 1994b, 1997, 2000).

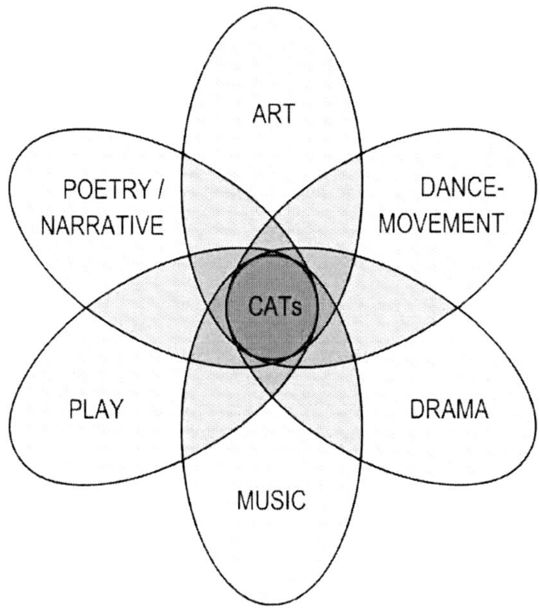

Figure 1. Modality interrelationships of the Creative Arts Therapies.

Group Method: Dramatic and Improvised Play in Dramatherapy

Dramatic and improvised play have been used for clinical applications since the 1930s. The processes of play have been analysed with regards to social development (Ward, 1930), psychosocial development (Erikson, 1950), intellectual development (Piaget, 1962), language acquisition (Garvey, 1977/1990), and psychological maturity and development (Klein, 1955; Winnicott, 1953, 1971). For educationalists, play is a way of testing, exploring, learning about, and making sense of the self in relation to the environment (Axline, 1964; Ward, 1957; Way, 1967). For cognitive psychologists, play is a way specific to children in assimilating information from, and accommodating their experiences of and into, the world (Piaget, 1962). For psychoanalysts, play is considered in children and youth to be the equivalent of verbal free association in adults (Klein, 1955), and houses the origins of creativity (Winnicott, 1971). For the drama therapist, with both children and adults, play is used as improvisation to help to create meaning, explore difficulties, foster spontaneous response, and achieve therapeutic change (Jones, 1996; Moreno, 1985).

Improvised play as used by drama therapists has the following eight applications: (1) as a way to explore and learn about reality (Cattanach, 1994;

Irwin, 2000); (2) as a way to explore and learn about what is hoped for (Grainger, 1996); (3) as having symbolic relationships to life experience (Anderson-Warren & Grainger, 2000; Jung, 1966); (4) as providing structure and distance within which to experience, or experiment with, rules, boundaries, and alternate realities (Boal, 1995; Moreno, 1985); (5) as means of understanding, confronting, and coping with difficult or traumatic experience (Boal, 1995; Irwin, 2000; Jones, 1996; Moreno, 1985); (6) as reflection of and catalyst for individual cognitive, social, and emotional development (Emunah, 1994); (7) as involving both simple and complex components of spontaneity (Jones, 1996; Moreno, 1985); and (8) as a way of free and open recreation and enjoyment (Harvey, 2000; Jones, 1996).

Within the frame for *Ma mère et moi*, improvised play is also used to foster communication, cooperation, and interrelationship within groups/dyads allowing immediacy for individual family members to project recreated dynamics and habitual roles within the larger context of the group. Improvisational drama also creates opportunity to experiment with alternate roles and rehearse alternate ways of "being" in the world, and to "create courage . . . and strengthen hope" individually (Anderson-Warren & Grainger, 2000, p. 53; Erikson, 1950, p. 215).

Dramatic and Improvised Play with Preadolescents

Improvisation with preadolescents is naturally effective in generating group process: participants are close enough to being children that they remember how to play (Johnstone, 1994), though without condescending to rules governing the play structure that are no longer age-appropriate. A dynamic of trust is inherent in the improvised play process, giving advantage and structure to learning, talking, and processing among peers about peer relationships (Johnstone, 1999; Slade, 1954; Spolin, 1963), the key developmental marker for this particular age group. Further, for this age group and for teenagers specifically, improv is simply fun.

Improvised play was considered an appropriate framework for domestic violence treatment as core components of play include examining and negotiating power, control, equality, oppression, and collective action in and across relationship. Improvised play was further implemented to build self-confidence and encourage expression at an age where participants are negotiating inhibition and vulnerability with identity construction and self-expression. These contexts are specifically and intentionally applied within an approach (Harvey, 1983, 1990, 1994a, 1994b, 1997, 2000) called Family Dynamic Play.

Family Dynamic Play

Family dynamic play uses movement, art, drama, improvisation, and storytelling creatively and systematically to address and transform family roles, and positively reconnect a family dynamic affected by trauma. The central concepts of this creative arts approach are rooted in embodied drama, improvised play, and clinical applications of attachment and systems theories (see Harvey, 2000 to discuss further applications using dance and video expression in case work). Overall, the primary goal of Family Dynamic Play intervention is to help each individual within the family to develop a greater feeling of security with and around each other (Harvey, 2000), so as to re-experience affiliation and affirmation in the recreation of intimate, trusting, and physically safe relationships. Family interactive patterns, themes, and metaphors are explored through the play improvisation for individuals within the family to regain their "naturally occurring creativity in everyday life" (Harvey, 2000, p. 380); further, for individuals to identify and resolve their respective roles and patterns contributing to the interrelational difficulties. Family members can rediscover meaning and connection in relationships that are mutually enjoyable and safe. As they interact in creative activity in close physical proximity and mutually negotiated states in play, a more positive, emotionally trusting, and bodily-felt atmosphere of safety and security develops.

The following general ideas form the theoretical base of Family Dynamic Play (Harvey, 1983, 1987, 1990, 1994a, 1994b, 1997, 2000):

1. Play both reflects and helps produce the quality of emotional life and attachment in the family to the degree that the individual members have space, trust, and motivation to engage in positive mutual emotional experience.
2. Dysfunctional family dynamics develop from an imbalanced position of power in the creation of family roles, and with the family's collective loss of ability to play.
3. Intervention attempts to help families discover or renew their play potential, so as to be more creative in solving problems and recreating new roles.
4. Intervention attempts to help individuals in families renew, repair, and resolve relationships that have become stuck in conflictual patterns, and stuck with an imbalance of power in the creation of roles.

Family Dynamic Play in Context

For the participants in *Ma mère et moi*, process and assessment was applied to activity in dyads as well as activity within the different subgroups. The implications of violence on a preadolescent and the applications of improvisational play for the development of coping and autonomy have been previously mentioned. For the mothers, group support provides opportunity for growth in the following four ways: (1) to spend time in mutual enjoyable activity; (2) to learn and rebuild internal resources specific to conflict and affirmation; (3) to obtain feedback and mutual support regarding their relationships; and, (4) to develop social alliances and strength with other women where they might otherwise feel isolated and powerless. For children and youth, group treatment provides the following four opportunities: (1) a neutral space to reconnect with their mothers; (2) a safe space to reconnect with themselves; (3) a space to play with other families who have lived through similar experience; and (4) an opportunity to learn age-appropriate expectation and responsibility within a supportive, non-judgmental and nurturing environment.

Goals of Treatment

Following are the facilitation objectives for *Ma mère et moi*:

1. Foster and increase attachment (positive mutual experience) and attunement between dyads, and recreate a physical sense of safety in relationships;
2. Break communication barriers (cultural, systemic, familial) and isolation in talking about violence in a safe place;
3. Modify behaviour, where appropriate;
4. Generate safety planning, while decreasing shame and victimisation;
5. Examine roles and boundaries in the family and learn that these need not be rigid or demeaning;
6. Break the cycle of violence by examining power and control in conflict, and expression in healthy intimacy;
7. Teach that we all make choices about whether or not we are violent or whether we respect other people and their views;
8. Understand the impact of violence in the family, the self, and on self-development;
9. Identify and normalise feelings surrounding lived experience of violence, and express these feelings in healthy and appropriate ways; and,
10. Facilitate or create an emotional sense of belonging in the group in a place where participants can share emotional intimacy in the group process.

Additional key considerations for facilitation in the preadolescent group included an increased sense of self and autonomy; allowance for anger and emotional lability; the desire to be different balanced with an increased desire for acceptance and groupthink; learning potential for leadership; and preoccupation with issues related to intimacy and interrelating. Additional key planning aspects considered mother's group facilitation included age-appropriate parenting; examination of internal and external coping mechanisms; examination of age-appropriate responsibility; and modeling of own emotions around children and youth.

Therapeutic Process

Within the framework of Family Dynamic Play, there are four general phases describing the flow of the therapeutic process in group work: Evaluation, Improvisation, Interaction, and Regeneration (see Harvey, 2000 for complete reference and review of the four phases). Within the larger circumference of Emunah's (1994) three-phase division of the therapy process that is generally considered standard in case study presentation, *Evaluation* and *Improvisation* would fall under to the Beginning-Middle phases of therapy; *Interaction* would fall under the Middle-End phase of therapy; and *Regeneration* falls under the End phase of the therapy process (see Figure 2).

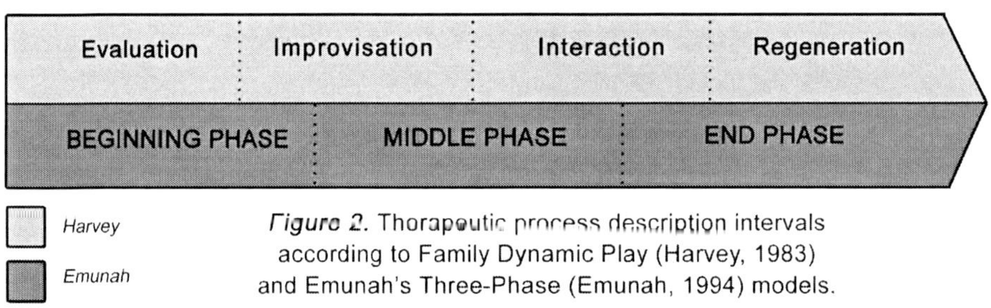

Figure 2. Therapeutic process description intervals according to Family Dynamic Play (Harvey, 1983) and Emunah's Three-Phase (Emunah, 1994) models.

Evaluation

In this phase, the verbal interview is supplemented with play activities to identify emotional and behavioural concerns, and clinical history of attachment, loss, separation, and trauma. Play activities can facilitate observation of family interaction and dynamic patterns through verbal, corporal, physical, emotional, affective, and artistic forms of expression. In this phase, the therapist generally participates as necessary to initiate or encourage flow in the activity. This serves to recreate existing connection and establish point of departure for future activity.

Improvisation

The main objective in this phase is to facilitate family members in enjoyably improvising together, for the development of co-operative and collaborative skills. The therapist introduces activities and improvisational ideas to facilitate a growth of "mutual curiosity" (Harvey, 2000, p. 302) and positive experience. The role of therapist becomes one of a more actively involved observer, modelling change, suggesting variation, and reflecting participation to the family members, using spontaneous metaphor and improvisation to facilitate more mutual play.

Interaction

The objective in this phase is to identify the basic theme(s), process, and/or emotional content that underlie the family in interaction. Symbolic activities are created, or built upon from previous activities, and unpacked so as to develop individual and collective meaning. The therapist is still an active observer, with ideas to facilitate more mutual play as specific areas of conflict and misattunement are identified. Towards the end of this phase, the therapist's role becomes less active. Instead, the therapist spends more time helping plan new activities extending outside the family therapy space.

Regeneration

In this phase, the family members use their own collaborative and cooperative ideas to generate positive corrective play. The therapist provides more encouragement than direct intervention at this point, as the family now has, ideally, their own insight and strategy to define and recreate their own interactive dynamic. Termination is also addressed in this phase.

Assessment and Evaluation of Family Dynamic Play

Harvey's main assessment tool throughout the dramatherapy process using Family Dynamic Play is the qualitative observation of the elements *Flow, Energy,* and *Form* (see Figure 3). In observing *Flow*, the therapist focuses on the play process more than the actual content that is played out: How, by whom, and when the mutual play is both initiated and stopped; demonstrated bodily level of ease or rigidity in play; freedom or inhibition of movement and expression. Examples of ebbs (breaks) in the flow include change in direction or rules of play, shift in emotional states, periods of rest or injury, sudden impulses or verbalised outbursts, and non-participation.

It is optimal to maintain an equal balance of Energy and Form so that improvisation can proceed in flow. *Energy* refers to the impulse of expression, generally physical in nature, with motivation to back it up and ideas to propel it forward. *Form* is the structure behind the impulse: Rules, plans, and directions to focus its acted expression. Figure 3 simplifies the interactive balance between these two factors: Insufficiency of energy results in loss of movement, while an excess of it results in loss of focus; an excess of form results in alienation, while its insufficiency results in ennui. The therapist sensitively and unobtrusively encourages or harnesses both elements as improvisation is played out, and as appropriate to the improvisation at hand. In most instances, the balance is best achieved with semi-directed activities, as the therapist models an improvised form of expression until the family members feel comfortable and competent embodying the process themselves. Any play without optimal Flow can be assessed using the outside four quadrants, and has the potential to address the roles family individuals hold in instances of dysfunction, disconnect, or disequilibrium.

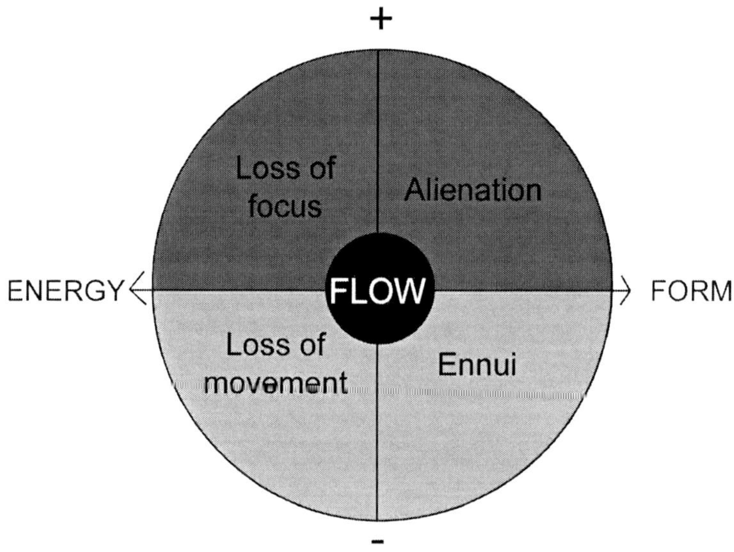

Figure 3. The interactive balance between Energy and Form in assessing dramatic improvisation in Family Dynamic Play (Harvey, 1990, 1994a, 1994b, 2000).

Other observation methods for assessing the content of dramatic/improvised play include the Expressive Inventory (Jones, 1996), Landy's (1990) role analysis, the Sutton Smith-Lazier (1981) Scale of Dramatic Involvement, and the creative-expressive model for personal and social change (Anderson-Warren & Grainger, 2000). It is important to note that methods of qualitative analyses (examining participation, involvement, means of expression and theme development) of dramatic play are difficult to standardise, as they will differ in emphasis according to the individual participants. Generally, in evaluating and assessing the process of dramatic/improvised play, *what* is specifically assessed and evaluated is secondary to *how* the dramatic process is played out.

Ma mère et moi: Group Outline

The *Ma mère et moi* group series is divided into twelve weeks. The first and last weeks are for mothers only, for a total of ten group-facilitated sessions. There is always some deviation according to the special interests, developmental considerations, and ages of the participants, but overall the group follows a particular and concurrent series of objectives. The following outline applies to and is modified specifically for the preadolescent-age group:

Prior to group. Entrance interview/evaluation–Mothers only

Week one. Introduction: Mothers only
Introduction to group format, objectives
Introduction to other mothers & child/youth facilitators

Week two. "Getting to know you"
Contract and ground rules
Icebreakers
Snack at break for respective groups
Spectogram activities
Collective group drawings

Week three. "Safety planning"
Vigilance vs. hyper-vigilance
Snack in groups
Internet safety
Basic self-defence techniques

Week four. "Family: Defining domestic violence and abuse"
Myths and facts about domestic violence
Dimensions of abuse: Emotional, physical, psychological, sexual
Power and control wheels/responsibility for violence

Snack in groups
Cycle, Warning signs and behavioural indicators of abuse

Week five. "Feelings"
Snack together
All feelings are OK
Healthy and harmful expression of feelings
When mediation is not a responsibility
How/When the victim becomes oppressor

Week six. "Anger in conflict"
Snack together
Anxiety reduction techniques
Tools for healthy expressions of anger
Anger and depression

Week seven. "Relationships"
Snack together
Responsibility in violence
Gender roles/stereotypes
Qualities
Relating to others (passive/aggressive/assertive/passive aggressive)
Community resources

Week eight. "Coping mechanisms"
Snack together
Cope, not mope
Personality preferences
Violence and addictions
Healthy coping mechanisms
Support systems

Week nine. "Me in the world"
Qualities
Self-esteem
Body image
Snack in groups

Week ten. Preparation for closing activity
Improv
Snack in groups

Week eleven. Termination and closing activity
Snack at close

Week twelve. Exit interview: Mothers only

A Case Example: Group Beginning Phase

Sylvie is the mother of two twin girls, Simone and Sophie, age 13. While Sylvie had received ongoing individual transitional support at the Centre, this was the twins' first therapeutic contact. In the mother's group, Sylvie attends with four other mothers. There are nine children/youth attending the series' session in total; Simone and Sophie attend their respective age group with two other girls.

Sylvie had experienced abuse of each type consistently from her ex-husband of 14 years, the twins' biological father, but with more frequent episodes during the past five years. Sylvie reports the twins had also been victims of physical abuse, usually alcohol-related, from their father, until she decided to leave him at the onset of their physical maturity and development. There has been no contact with the father since Sylvie moved with the twins into their one-bedroom apartment rental a little over year ago. Still quite afraid of contact, Sylvie is especially interested in the anti-bullying/assertiveness training/self-defense aspects of the group, for both her and the twins. Sylvie says the twins had input in and were prepared for the move, and rarely ask now about their father.

Simone and Sophie had changed schools the year previous. Sylvie reports Simone has received school disciplinary measures at this new school for bullying. She also reports Simone has been intimidated and bullied by other students. By contrast, Sophie's teachers report she has seemed to adjust well, interacting and involved with peers who are "popular" in her class. Sylvie also notes Sophie's marks have been considerably lower than her usual average. In the past year, Simone has gained 10 pounds and Sophie has lost three. Both are actively involved on the school's girl basketball team. Sophie also has joined drama.

Development of Themes

The first week of group, we all introduced ourselves, the children introduced their ages, and the facilitators introduced how the group would be structured. We divided back into families to establish simple contract rules that were important for the rest of the group (for example, "No bare feet in group"), upon which the rest of the group discusses any qualifying changes

("Except when boots have made socks wet or if the socks smell") and eventually agrees on a suitable phrasing ("Please wear shoes"). All the rules were written on a door-sized piece of paper on the wall. To facilitate a timely discussion, we had some rules already established, and specified our time limitation. Following this collective agreement, each individual member signed their approval with a multicoloured handprint, as designed with colours of paint of their choice. Through the process, the group facilitators were able to circulate equally among families, observe patterns and levels of participation/cooperation within each unit, and encourage all members in giving their own participatory voice. We also wanted to provide, however briefly, the group members opportunity to see a team function as leadership with open discussion, equal roles, and transparently shared responsibility.

Group Interaction

In the individual groups, the mothers were drawn to a particular metaphor representing their objectives: that of a butterfly struggling, after metamorphosis, to break free of a cocoon. Both individually and collectively, they felt that the logistics of their marital separation were completed; having established some sense of routine, assessed what were realistic components of their day-to-day lives, and "taken charge" of what they wanted in their new lives and the lives of their children, they were ready to "break free" from the fear that had held them in the past. In the preteen girls' group, the youngest member of the group seemed to spark rebuff towards Simone (incidentally the oldest member of the group), choosing her last in the initial opening activity and refusing to look at Simone when it was Simone's turn to share in the circle.

This allowed for some immediate dramatic exercises in rotating pairs on what respect, equality, and disrespect physically looked like, embodying the feelings that accompanied each dynamic as equally as its opposite. I gave two stipulations to the game: That every person's idea is incorporated, and that every person gives at least three ideas. The girls responded with immediacy, providing very insightful feedback into the non-verbal components of relating to others, and did not lack ideas in creating alternative outcomes. As each pair took turns dissecting, exaggerating, and modifying the non-verbal components of the other pair's interactions, specific comments pertaining to eye contact, posture, and shoulder position were all laughed at and openly discussed. I was struck at the collective malleability in play, the pointed hilarity of their exaggerated ideas, and the immediacy in which we were able to discuss group issues without casting people in unyielding roles.

While the girls did not disclose their own personal experiences with how they had come to feel the feelings they had discussed, this projective work acknowledged that there was a certain amount of kinship and understanding about feeling. I felt like we had jumped to a group "norming" phase abnormally quickly–having reached such flow in activity and reciprocity in play–though perhaps the girls were so used to conflict that they were either accustomed to working around it regardless, or relieved to be finally talking about how it affected them. This was not a question I chose to address. At the end of this session one, the girls gave each other hugs in their favourite most exaggerated and awkward of postures.

Mid-Session of the Series: Progress in Therapy

Continuation of Themes

About the third week in, during one of our weekly planning meetings, my colleague who facilitated the women's group brought a poem she had come across that connected with the women's butterfly metaphor. It spoke of a child who helped a butterfly struggle free from its cocoon but watched with tears as, a few feet after it could take flight, it fell unable to the ground. The child's parent in the poem explained that the butterfly's freedom from the cocoon was something only the butterfly itself could facilitate, as it was in the act of struggling that gave the butterfly strength to open its wings (poem in J. Ouimette, 2005, p. 10).

Discussion surrounding the emotional significance this poem held evolved into an activity idea for the Dramatic Play portion of the group: The handprints that had been generated the first session could be cut out and attached together at the thumbs, forming butterflies. Each family member's individual handprint could constitute one individual butterfly wing (each butterfly could be comprised of two, or four, different handprints, as desired). Following this, the collective family butterfly scene could be decorated in whatever setting the family chose. We prepared construction paper for the backing with the idea that participants could be as creative as they wanted with the backgrounds.

This ended up being an enjoyable activity for the group members across ages. Given that we were using construction paper and safety-scissors, we were surprised to discover almost all the participants scurrying to finish some fairly elaborate butterfly scenes at the end of our 25-minute activity time plan. During the activity, we were able to continue circulating equally amongst families, observing patterns and levels of participation/cooperation within each unit, with time to observe the general dynamic and roles in task completion: who initiated, controlled, or followed the activity; who responded to this initiation or control; whose ideas were given and encouraged and whose ideas were not listened to.

With Simone, Sophie, and Simone, we noticed that all three were collectively focussed on the work, with communication flowing collectively and largely non-verbally. This is not to say that direct communication was lacking, or that the girls were not habitually silent. It seemed simply that the activity absorbed their attention to focus their energies at hand. During the construction of the background scenes, Sylvie would, for example, cut out a flower and lay it on the paper, to which Simone would pick up and attach a leaf, and then Sophie would glue it somewhere on the paper. This interaction pattern was shared across all three individuals. Most "decisions" about what would go where seemed to be shared collectively, until each twin glued something somewhere they later changed their minds about; following which the task of gluing was deferred to Mom. The collective theme flowed very flowery and light, with sweeps of wind and sky spirals denoting upwards, circular patterns of movement; the butterflies (one big and somewhat lopsided, with three handprint wings; the other small, dainty and pink, cut out of construction paper) gathered together toward the top right hand corner of the frame. The work reflected a point of departure marked with movement, cohesion, and hope, and a not uncertain amount of personal journey.

Sharing their butterfly scenes also took some time, as each dyad/family was quite proud of their work. We decided collectively to laminate the pieces, and as it turned out that most families ended up having made enough background scenes for each of the younger children to have one, the women decided they would use them as placemats. From this group forward, the butterfly placemats (promptly laminated for the week following) became a staple for our snack.

Group Interaction

In the pre-teen group, the girls really enjoyed Spectogram activities. This type of activity used the floor space around the room as a barometer of sorts for measuring preferences, and each individual found her respective place according to the preference at hand. I had introduced this activity in groups seven and eight, while reviewing qualities and coping mechanisms. This activity was introduced again in the ninth, with a twist.

I had the girls chose specific qualities (we had a list) and write them on a piece of paper, which I said I would read aloud, twice. The first time they would find their space according to how they felt they embodied this quality. The second time they would find their space according to how they felt they wanted to embody it. Particular attention was to be noted of other members in the group, and following the second read, those members on the desired "end" of the spectrum would respectively call out lines, thoughts, or feelings that could help each individual across to the point they felt they were able to reach towards the desired end of the spectrum. I gave the following two stipulations: First, that if there were more than one person with a ways to go, that we would encourage one member's journcy at a time; second, that we come up with an 'end signal' to indicate when a journey was completed and when the rest of the group could stop their calling out their lines, so that if a member did not need to want to advance to the extreme (high-low) end of the spectrum, this was all right. The girls chose a raising of both arms straight above their heads with a vocal "Yay!" as their end-signal.

"Brave[ry]" was a quality where, in session seven, the girls had found themselves all at about the same point two-thirds the way down the spectrum. They had spontaneously huddled together, pretending to be afraid and needing "protection" from the frightening surroundings. The girls used this same point of departure in session nine. When asked where they would like to be on the brave spectrum, Sophie pointed towards the high end of the room; the others followed suit.

I asked them what sorts of phrases they might be able to tell themselves to help them advance to the desired end. One of the girls said, *"J'ai rien à dire–j'n'suis pas brave"* ("I have nothing to say–I'm not brave"), to which someone else asked, *"Comment veux-tu que je le fasse?"* ("How do you want me–How am I expected to do that?"). I handed over the Hat of Qualities, saying they could choose a phrase informed by the quality they picked out of the Hat. Phrases that ensued: Intelligent (this was Sophie): *"Je connais l'auto-defense!/*I know self-defense!" Confidence: *"Mais quoi qu'en soit-il, pour que j'ai peur?/*What am I afraid of, anyway?" Strong (this was Simone): *"Je m'en tirerai/*This I will survive." Each phrase precipitated an exaggerated, swaggering Hat-drawn-quality walk across the remainder of the spectrum to the high end of the room.

End Phase of the Therapy Process

Termination of Themes

The last group with all the participants had a special closing end activity together, of a participatory nature. Each group would bring something to present to or facilitate with the others. The girls wanted to facilitate an exercise. Though they did not want to recapture with the group at large what they had created as "theirs," they did want to share a piece of their fun. After closing exercises such as "Fortunately/Unfortunately," an Awards Ceremony where all the material generated from the group was returned, followed by the individual members' acceptance speech of the awards, the attention was redirected to the rest of the time with the larger group. The girls addressed what they wanted and how they would go about creating it. Considering the amount of time there would be (about ten minutes) and the number of younger children present, they decided they would facilitate Miming Gifts to the rest of the other families. They rehearsed giving the exercise directions, quickly assigned families, and started gesture-brainstorming rather specific gifts (red high-heeled shoes, pepperoni pizza, all the vanilla wafer cookies at Wal-Mart) to individual and collective family group members. We rehearsed by giving gifts to ourselves. The youngest group member offered hugs to all the girls in closing; Sophie serenaded each person a portion of Christina Aguilera's "Beautiful"; and Simone gave a piece of her heart in her palm.

The mothers had literal gifts to give. Sylvie actually did bring pepperoni pizza, and another mother brought traditional jewellery for everyone from her country of origin. In the flurry of group activity and sharing of gifts, my colleagues and I had a rather frantic and brief consultation: Gifts? While we explained that gifts were not expected of the mothers and that as therapists we did not generally accept them, we reconsidered these tokens, as they were gifts for and from the collective. The beaded bracelet I received is hanging on my office bulletin board.

Summary

"Results" of Therapy: Conclusion and Recommendations

The course of therapy designed in Ma mère et moi seemed to have provided Sylvie space to plan life in contexts of desires and hopes balanced with bills and limitations of time, instead of vigilance, fear, and worry in reaction to the violence she had endured. While her life was still a series of stressors, she did report she felt relieved to have pressures that were predictable and practical ones, learning to manage life on her own terms, designed by what she wanted, with her own consequences.

While disconnect was not present in her relationships with her daughters prior to the group, she did gain insight into her daughters' feelings specific to the violence, and was able to safely express and deal with the anger surrounding being a victim of domestic violence. Discussion (as reported by the women's group facilitator) in the Mom's portion of the group seemed to help foster awareness as to how her future attitudes toward fighting and conflict, as well as her expressions and responses in them, could help recreate behavioural blueprints for Simone and Simone, who were also probably struggling with learning some of the same tools. Group intervention in the girls' group for the twins helped foster strength and courage in expression and self-knowledge, in enjoyable and non-threatening ways. The twins expressed feeling "good" about having space where they could leave what they were used to carrying about with them everywhere else.

Limitations of this Group Focus and Future Considerations

The exit interviews with the mothers provided opportunity for us to give feedback about children's overall processes and observations. It also provided the mother an opportunity to give feedback about pieces of the programme she felt were helpful, and pieces she would like to see further addressed. While there were evaluations the mothers did fill out the last session of their group meeting, we found it helpful to have one-to-one meetings where needs could be more personally identified, and where the mothers could have opportunity to ask questions.

Overall, mothers were satisfied with the outcome of the group, suggesting only that the group could be accessible to more mothers, and that they very much felt the limitations of time. Future efforts could include a follow-up group, not necessarily for purposes of refreshing the psycho-educational components of the first group, but to therapeutically process anger, fear, and disappointment that was still often felt residually. Sylvie indicated that for the pre-teen group, she would have liked to see components specifically addressing verbal intimidation in addition to the physical. This is a valuable comment that we have since included in our group plans. We have also planned additional follow-up therapy group series (six weeks) for mothers.

One key limitation with the girls' group was that for this age, and for that of the teens, semi-directed activity was difficult to consistently follow. The girls had relevant collective ideas and personal interests, plus they had participated in anti-violence programmes (offered by the Centre staff) at their schools. Using a client-led approach to follow topic objective outline, however general, took some negotiation. I found that the best way to facilitate this negotiation was to be as prepared and transparent as possible with the objective outline, encouraging opportunity for input and opinion. This was best generated the week before.

Creative Arts Therapies in Intervention with Domestic Violence

While improvised and Family Dynamic play facilitated exercises that were unique and non-threatening, the responses they elicited were far from superficial. As noted, group process was a key component in the girls' group work, appropriate for their age and level of development, and there was significant collective effort by all group members in learning about conflict, cooperation, and negotiation. These techniques helped recreate a physical sense of safety in attachment and relationship, and facilitate immediate and accessible expression through the use of art and embodied improvised play.

Since the Family Dynamic Play approach implemented mutual activity for reconnecting safely negotiated relationships between Sylvie and her children, and because it was rooted using the considerations of attachment as affected by trauma (Harvey, 1983, 1994a, 1997, 2000), it was an appropriate and useful method for this group. Dramatic improvisation helped facilitate negotiation, communication, and recognition of internal states for participating family members in developmentally and emotionally accessible ways. Providing a playful and encouraging space, this creative arts approach allowed safety in exploration of desired ways of "being" without judgment. The structured, semi-directed activity using the body as a tool of expression and communication helped to nourish a bodily-felt trust inherent in recreating secure relationships (Bowlby, 1969; Harvey, 2000), and in reclaiming that the body can be used for security, protection, and ways of relating that are not intimidating and non-physically violent. One mother wrote in her evaluation, "*Ma fille a appris à quel point un papillon a besoin de sortir. Mais c'est le groupe qui lui a montré à quel point elle avait ses propres ailes/* My daughter learned to what degree a butterfly has to get out [from the cocoon]. But it was the group that showed her the degree to which she had her own set of wings."

References

Ainsworth, M. D. S., Blehar, M. C., Waters, E., & Wall, S. (1978). *Patterns of attachment: A psychological study of the Strange Situation.* Hillsdale, NJ: Erlbaum.

Andersen-Warren, M., & Grainger, R. (2000). *Practical approaches to dramatherapy: The shield of Perseus.* London: Jessica Kingsley Publishers.

Axline, V. (1964). *Dibs: In search of self.* New York: Ballantine.

Bair-Merrit, M. H., Blackstone, M., & Feudtner, C. (2006, February). Physical health outcomes of childhood exposure to intimate partner violence: A systematic review. *Pediatrics, 117*(2), 278-290.

Baker, L., & Cunningham, A. (2005). Apprendre à écouter, apprendre à aider : Comprendre la violence faite aux femmes et ses effets sur les enfants. London: Centre for Children and Families in the Justice System.

Baker, L. A., & Cunningham, A. J. (2004). *What about me! Seeking to understand the child's view of violence in the family.* London: Centre for Children and Families in the Justice System.

Bancroft, L., & Silverman, J. G. (2002). *The batterer as parent: Addressing the impact of domestic violence on family dynamics.* Thousand Oaks: Sage.

Berman, H., & Jiwini, Y. (2001). *Violence prevention and the girl child: Phase two report: In the best interests of the child.* Vancouver: FREDA Centre for Research on Violence Against Women & Children.

Bhola, S., & Nelson, T. (1990). *Cross-cultural training manual: Service providers training manual.* Calgary: Calgary Immigrant Woman's Centre.

Boal, A. (1995). *The rainbow of desire: The Boal method of theatre and therapy.* London: Routeledge.

Bowlby, J. (1969/1982). *Attachment and loss: Vol. 1: Attachment.* New York: Basic Books.

Brooke, S. L. (2006). *Creative arts therapies manual: A guide to the history, theoretical approaches, assessment, and work with special populations of art, play, dance, music, drama, and poetry therapies.* Springfield, IL: Charles C Thomas, Publisher, Ltd.

Boyd, K., & Klingbeil, K. S. (1984). Emergency room intervention: Detection, assessment, and treatment. In A. R. Roberts (Ed.), *Battered women and their families* (pp. 5-32). New York: Springer.

Carlson, B.E. (2000). Children exposed to intimate partner violence: Research findings and implications for intervention. *Trauma, Violence, and abuse, 1*(4), 321-342.

Canadian Centre for Justice Statistics / Centre canadien de la statistique juridique (2001). *La violence familale au Canada: un profil statistique.* Ottawa: Statistics Canada (Catalogue 0000085-224-XIF).

Cattanach, A. (1994). The developmental model of dramatherapy. In S. Jennings, A. Cattanach, S. Mitchell, A. Chesner, & B. Meldrum (Eds.), *The handbook of dramatherapy* (pp. 28-41). London: Routeledge,

Emunah, R. (1994). *Acting for real: Drama therapy: Process, technique, and performance.* New York: Brunner/Mazel.

Erikson, E. (1950). *Childhood and Society.* New York: Norton.

Federal-Provincial-Territorial Ministers Responsible for the Status of Women / Ministres fédéral, provinciaux et territoriaux responsables de la condition féminine (2002). *Évaluation de la violence contre les femmes: un profil statistique.* Ottawa: Status of women Canada.

Fondation pour l'enfance (Ed.). (2000). De la violence conjugale à la violence parentale: Femmes en détresse, enfants en souffrance. Ramonville Saint-Agne: Fondation Erès.

Fortin, A. (2005). *Le point de vue de l'enfant sur la violence conjugale à laquelle il est. exposé.* Publication du CRI-VIFF (Centre de recherche interdisciplinaire sur la violence familiale et la violence faite aux femmes), Collection Études et Analyses, no. 32, mars 2005.

Garvey, C. (1977; 1990). *Play.* Cambridge, MA: Harvard University Press.

Gauthier, L. (1998/1999, Fall/Winter). La formation en matière de violence faite aux femmes et aux enfants en Ontario français. In Ontario Institute for Studies in Education (Ed.), *Confronting violence in women's lives: Documentation sur la recherche féministe, 26*(3), 13-34. Toronto: University of Toronto Press.

Grainger, R. (1996). Artistic expression and the embodiment of social constructs. *The Arts in Psychotherapy, 23*(2), 137-140.

Harvey, S. (1983). Dynamic play therapy: Expressive play intervention with families. In K.J. O'Connor & C.E. Schaefer (Eds.), *Handbook of play therapy, volume Two: Advances and innovations* (pp 85-110). Toronto: Wiley.

Harvey, S.A. (1987). *Parent-infant relationships.* UK: John Wiley & Sons, Inc.

Harvey, S.A. (1990). Dynamic play therapy: An integrated expressive arts approach to the family therapy of young children. *The Arts in Psychotherapy, 17*(3), 239-246.

Harvey, S.A. (1994a). Dynamic play therapy: Creating attachments. In B. James, *Handbook for treatment of attachment-trauma problems in children.* New York: Lexington.

Harvey, S.A. (1994b). Dynamic play therapy: Expressive play intervention with families. In B. James, *Handbook for treatment of attachment-trauma problems in children.* New York: Lexington.

Harvey, S.A. (1997). Dynamic play therapy: A creative arts approach. In K. O'Connor & L. Braverman (Eds.), *Play therapy theory and practice: A comparative presentation.* New York: Norton.

Harvey, S.A. (2000). Family dynamic play. In P. Lewis & D. R. Johnson (Eds.), *Current approaches in drama therapy* (pp. 379-409). Springfield, IL: Charles C Thomas, Publisher, Ltd.

Health Canada (1991; rev.1996). Wife abuse - the impact on children. *Information from the National Clearinghouse on family violence* (Cat. H72-22/7-1996E). Ottawa: Health Canada Printing Office.

Irwin, E. (2000). Psychoanalytic approach to drama therapy: Defining and finding a therapeutic framework. In P. Lewis & D. R. Johnson, *Current approaches in drama therapy* (pp. 27-48). Springfield, IL: Charles C Thomas, Publisher, Ltd.

Jaffe, P. G., Wolfe, D. A., & Wilson, S. K. (1990). *Children of battered women.* London: Sage.

Jiwini, Y., Gorkoff, K., Berman, H., Taylor, G., Vardy-Dell, G., & Normandeau, S. (1999). *Violence prevention and the girl child: Phase one report.* Vancouver: FREDA Centre for Research on Violence Against Women & Children.

Johnstone, K. (1994). *Don't be prepared: Theatresports for teachers.* New York: Routeledge.

Johnstone, K. (1999). *Impro for storytellers.* New York: Routeledge.

Jones, P. (1996). *Drama as therapy: Theatre as living.* London: Routeledge.

Jones, P. (2005). *The arts therapies: A revolution in healthcare.* New York: Routeledge.

Jung, C. C. (1966). *Man and his symbols.* Garden City, NY: Doubleday.

Landy, R. (1990). Role theory and the role method of drama therapy. In P. Lewis & D. R. Johnson, *Current approaches in drama therapy* (pp. 50-69). Springfield, IL: Charles C Thomas, Publisher, Ltd.

Klein, M. (1955). The psychoanalytic play technique. *American Journal of Orthopsychiatry, XXV,* 223-237.

Moreno, J. L. (1985). *Psychodrama: First volume.* Ambler, PA: Random House, Inc.

Niagara Regional Police Service. (2005). *Annual Report, 2005.* Retrieved from http://www.nrps.com/report/default.asp (April 14, 2007).

Ontario Institute for Studies in Education. (1998-1999, Fall/Winter). Confronting violence in women's lives. *Resources for Feminist Research / Documentation sur la recherche féministe, 26*: 3-4. Toronto: University of Toronto Press.

Osofsky, J. (1998). Children as invisible victims of domestic and community violence. In G. Holden, R. Geffner, & E. Jouriles (Eds.), *Children exposed to marital violence: Theory, research, and applied issues* (pp. 95-117). Washington, DC: American Psychological Association.

Ouimette, J. (2005) *La force de s'affranchir.* Montréal : Les éditions de l'homme.

Piaget, J (1962). *Play, dreams, and imitation in childhood.* New York: Norton.

Schechter, S., & Gary, L. T. (1988). A framework for understanding and empowering battered women. In M. Straus (Ed.), *Abuse and victimization across the life span* (pp. 240-253). Baltimore: John Hopkins University Press.

Slade, P. (1954). *Child drama.* London: University Press.

Spolin, V. (1963). *Improvisation for the theatre.* Northwestern University Press.

Statistics Canada. (2005). *Family violence in Canada: A statistical profile 2005.* Canadian Centre for Justice Statistics: Ottawa, Catalogue no. 85-224-XIE.

Statistics Canada. (2006). *Measuring violence against women: Statistical trends 2006.* Minister of Industry: Ottawa, Catalogue no. 85-570-XIE.

Sutton-Smith, B. (1981). Sutton-Smith Lazier Scale of Dramatic Involvement. In G. Schattner & R. Courtney (Eds.), *Drama in therapy, Vol.1.* New York: Drama Book Specialists.

Ward, W. (1957). *Playmaking with children.* Englewood Cliffs, NJ: Prentice-Hall, Inc.

Ward, W. (1930). *Creative dramatics.* New York: Appleton, 1930.

Way, B. (1967). *Development through drama.* London: Longman.

Winnicott, D. W. (1971). *Playing and reality.* London: Pelican.

Winnicott, D. W. (1953). Transitional objects and transitional phenomena, A study of the first Not-me possession. *International Journal of Psychoanalysis, 34*, part 2.

BIOGRAPHY

Athena Madan (MA) received her MA in Creative Arts Therapies from Concordia University in Montréal. Her writing and publication research include: attachment and psychopathology; bereavement with survivors of suicide; symbolic play in child trauma due to domestic and organised violence; and creative arts in meaning-making with survivors of torture. Previous experience includes conduct disorder, youth at-risk, juvenile delinquents, drug and alcohol addiction, schizophrenia, and terminal illness (cancer, AIDS) populations. Having shared a private practise in Montréal before relocating to the Niagara region, Athena is currently working at the *Centre de santé communautaire Hamilton / Niagara* with trauma, abuse, and mental health cases. The Centre's website address is www.centredesantecommunautaire.com.

Chapter 16

TRANSFORMING THE HIDDEN TRAUMA OF ABUSE: INCORPORATING ART AND NARRATIVE THERAPY WITH CHILD SURVIVORS OF DOMESTIC VIOLENCE

ALEXIA ELECTRIS AND JANICE HNATH

Introduction

Growing up in a violent home is a terrifying and traumatic experience. Each child living in a violent home has his/her own story; some children witness verbal or physical abuse between family members and some children both witness the abuse as well as become direct victims of verbal, physical, and or sexual abuse. Regardless of the severity of the domestic violence that children witness or are subjected to, they have one element in common - they have all been traumatized in some way. The "essence of psychological trauma is the loss of faith that there is order and continuity in life. Trauma occurs when one loses the sense of having a safe place within or outside oneself to deal with frightening emotions and experiences" (van der Kolk, 1987, p. 31). As a result, traumatized children are left unable to understand and articulate their experiences. The extent to which a child suffers depends on the child's experience, chronicity, age, gender, temperament, and coping skills (Knapp, 1998; Schewe, n.d.).

The American Psychological Association (1996) reports 3.3 million children are exposed to domestic violence annually. Evans (1997) estimates as many as 90 percent of those children see and hear the violence. Domestic violence can affect every aspect of a child's life, growth, and development. Children who are exposed to violence in the home are more likely to exhibit long lasting psychological, developmental, behavioral, and physical health problems including Post Traumatic Stress Disorder (PTSD), depression, anxiety, and violence towards peers (Jaffe & Sudermann, 1995; Knapp, 1998).

According to Wolfe, Wekerle, Reitzel and Gough (1995), children lack the internal resources to understand and integrate their trauma. Therefore, they are more likely to engage in at-risk behaviors such as suicide, drug abuse, truancy, and sexual assault crimes. Many children traumatized by violence in the home experience a loss of control, low self-esteem, and pervasive fear characterizing their shattered sense of self. Nevertheless, when properly identified and addressed, the effects of domestic violence on children can be alleviated.

Treating the Trauma of Domestic Violence

Treating children affected by intrafamilial violence is often challenging due to the crucial role that secrecy holds within the family structure. Children are often forbidden to speak about the violence that occurs in the home by spoken or unspoken family rules, thus, leaving children without an outlet to voice and express their feelings about the violence. Children are commonly discouraged from reporting abuse and when they have the courage to voice their abuse, they are not always believed; therefore, the feelings of shame and anger that accompany domestic violence lie hidden beneath the surface, not to be shared with others (Stronach-Buschel, 1990).

The nature of Post-Traumatic Stress Disorder (PTSD) is such that it does not allow children to integrate the trauma experience into their understanding of themselves and their world. van der Kolk, van der Hart and Burbridge (1995) states:

> The goal of treatment is to find a way in which people can acknowledge the reality of what has happened without having to re-experience the trauma all over again. For this to occur, merely uncovering memories is not enough: they need to be modified and transformed, i.e., placed in their proper context and reconstructed into neutral or meaningful narratives. Thus, in therapy, memory paradoxically becomes an act of creation, rather than the static recording of events which is characteristic of trauma-based memories. (para. 8)

Telling the trauma story is essential to treatment of Post Traumatic Stress Disorder (PTSD). In order to feel empowered and create future positive intimate relationships, it is fundamental to the healing process that survivors of domestic violence find their voice through the telling of their stories (Peacock, 1991); however, children cannot start conversations about subjects that overwhelm them, or those that are hidden in their psyches. To help children recognize and incorporate the traumatizing events that they have experienced, James (1989) suggests that a direct dialogue about the trauma be combined with guided play.

Art Therapy and Trauma

Art therapy is commonly used with traumatized children to help them express their feelings in a medium that is familiar to them. Current trauma research suggests that imagery-specific techniques such as art therapy are among the most effective in reducing PTSD symptomology (Burch & Powell, 1980; Garrett & Ireland, 1979; Golub, 1985; Howard, 1990; Levin, Lazrove, & van der Kolk, 1999; Orr, 1997; Wollman, 1993). Trauma is initially embedded in the brain's memory as photographic images without any linguistic components. Intrusive and distressing memories often replay themselves in the mind of the survivor as flashbacks, nightmares, and phobic images. Trauma survivors describe traumatic memory as moving pictures that can be triggered and surface at unpredictable times (Herman, 1997; van der Kolk, van der Hart & Burbridge, 1995). Johnson (1987) suggests that art therapy can access and recall traumatic memories without causing one to relive the intense emotions associated with the memories.

For traumatized children who are left feeling helpless, art therapy offers a safe space to master their feelings, integrate their trauma, and change the outcome (Brooke, 2007). Creating art can tap into the unconscious and help children uncover details of the trauma memory that they may not be able to access on a verbal level. Through the process of externalizing one's trauma, art therapy provides individuals with a constructive method that heals and transforms traumatic imagery (Avidar, 1995; Peacock, 1991; Stronach-Buschel, 1990).

Storytelling

Stories are universal to all cultures and have traditionally been passed from one generation to the next. Although the exact origins of storytelling remain a mystery, historians, anthropologists, and psychologists have documented the use of storytelling since the beginning of human existence for the purpose of entertainment, education, and the preservation of cultural morals and values (Storytelling, n.d.).

Children frequently create stories in their everyday play. They intuitively understand the structure and elements of a story and are well adept at writing stories. The framework of a story allows children to easily access their trauma, change the outcome of the traumatic event, and actively create meaning out of their trauma. The structure of a story provides not only the necessary containment of the trauma story, but also the adequate distance and safe projections of feelings onto unrelated characters that allow children to begin owning and integrating their feelings (Avidar, 1995).

Therapeutic Applications of Storytelling

Bibliotherapy and narrative therapy are common therapy techniques that use storytelling to help children examine their lives (Burnes, 2005; Carlson, 1997; Montabalo-Phelps, 2003; Reichert 1998; Salans 2005). Bibliotherapy is based on the premise that individuals relate to characters in literature. The stages of bibliotherapy consist of identification, catharthis, and insight. In a typical bibliotherapy session, the therapist selects a piece of literature that closely parallels a child's real life problems. The therapist uses the metaphors from the story to help the child find solutions to his/her own problems (Bibliotherapy, n.d.a). Narrative therapy was established around the idea that an individual's life is shaped by the meaning he or she assigns to his or her life experiences. The goal of narrative therapy is to help people externalize their internalized stories in order to recognize that "the problem is the problem, the person is not the problem" (White & Epston, 1990, p. 39).

Although some theorists feel that children should not dwell on the trauma, in the safety of a therapeutic relationship, children are able to safely retell and/or reenact the traumatic event through the creation of individual or group stories (Groves, 1999; Peled & Edelson, 1995; Wilson, Cameron, Jaffe, & Wolfe, 1989). The use of drawings and storytelling has been extensively documented as an effective method of communication (Brooke, 2007; Reichert, 1998). In their witness and violence paper, Pynoos and Eth (1986) discuss a trauma interview technique that combines drawing and storytelling as a means to gain insight into the child's emotional response and areas where emotional support and coping skills are needed. According to Gardner, the child's documented story provides the child a sense of externalization, preventing the child from fixating on the trauma (as cited in Avidar, 1995).

Integrating Art Therapy and Narrative Therapy in Clinical Practice

This section will discuss the theoretical similarities between art therapy and narrative therapy and the clinical application of integrating the two therapies. Both art therapy and narrative therapy provide children with the opportunity to uncover hidden aspects of the self, explore role identity, and promote creativity and self-expression. In both art therapy and narrative therapy, the therapist has multiple roles and responsibilities as a guide, a non-judgmental witness, and a participant.

Narrative therapy is enhanced by the addition of art therapy. Art therapists often encourage children to create spontaneous stories based on their artwork. Narrative therapists guide children to reconstruct their trauma stories by means of fictional or actual characters and events. While narrative therapy provides a space for children to rewrite their trauma stories, art therapy provides an outlet for children to transform trauma images from their traumatic experiences. Together, art and narrative therapies have the capacity to transform trauma by helping children discover new insights and perspectives.

The combination of art and narrative therapies provides children with the opportunity to become creators, thus, changing their roles and self-perceptions from victims to survivors. Children are given full control of their stories by performing the roles of a writer, an artist, an editor, and a director. By actively choosing the words and images that construct their stories, children learn problem solving skills and regains a sense of control and empowerment over a terrifying experience (Avidar, 1995; Carlson, 1997).

When we applied art therapy to narrative therapy, the text of the story was accompanied by the child's artwork, illustrating the characters and setting of the story. We feel the advantage of incorporating art and narrative therapies is the end product – a book or video that contains proof of the child's perceived trauma. The resulting book or video tangibly documents and records the child's experience of the abuse. Under the guise of a story, the child can safely share the book or video with friends and family, alleviating the fear of betraying his/her family's secret.

Applying Art Therapy and Narrative Therapy in a Domestic Violence Shelter

Women residing in domestic violence shelters often escape to the shelter immediately following a violent episode or crisis in the family. In most cases, children have witnessed the abuse of their mothers or have been directly subjected to verbal, physical, and or sexual abuse. Upon entering a domestic violence shelter, children often appear visibly scared and anxious. In order to attain safety, they have had to leave their neighborhoods, their schools, their friends, and often times they leave their fathers or other loved ones.

Once admitted to the shelter, families are advised not to return to their neighborhoods and typically stay in the domestic violence shelter for an average of 3-6 months. Often times, children do not understand what happened and or why they are separated from their family and friends. A common fear of the children is the fear that their mothers will abandon them in their crisis as abruptly as they abandoned their batterers.

While residing in a domestic violence shelter, battered mothers routinely receive case management, advocacy, and counseling to assist with the primary goal of locating permanent safe housing for the entire family. While their mothers focus on finding a new residence and their own emotional needs, the children are left to manage their own emotions of anger, confusion, fear, guilt, shame, and helplessness. In an effort to alleviate tension and adapt to the climate of the shelter, some children withdraw while others become aggressive.

As it is not uncommon for children to know more about the abuse that occurred than their mothers acknowledge or recognize, children have historically been the neglected residents of the shelter; however, more recently, shelters have begun to emphasize the need for the intervention and treatment of the residing children. The major treatment goal for children residing in a shelter is to reduce anxiety, fear, anger, and feelings of helplessness associated with family violence. Due to the short term stay in a domestic violence shelter, the treatment goals have to be modest and should emphasize short term art therapy techniques in which a feeling of internal control is created. The sense of control is essential to the stabilization of children traumatized by family violence (Malchiodi, 1997).

While working in a domestic violence shelter, we encountered agitated and anxious children who preferred creating art with three-dimensional materials rather than two dimensional materials. Art materials such as clay, papier mâche_, and wood can be pounded, pinched, and pulled to create structural forms. The tactile quality of these materials allowed the children to sublimate harbored feelings of anger and anxiety. However, we began to notice that our offices were cluttered with art left behind by children and we recognized that most of the children had no connection to their artwork after the moment of creation. It seemed that the process of releasing emotions was more meaningful than the actual art piece. For those children that developed a connection to their art, it was usually too large to transport to their new home. Although we felt it was positive that the children began to self-regulate through creating art, it seemed that the act of creating art only captured a fragment of their domestic violence experience.

In the pursuit of a holistic therapeutic intervention that provided children with the opportunity to sublimate and externalize their trauma, we began combining art and narrative therapies. The art seemed to help children access their hidden trauma while the structure of a story seemed to help children verbally externalize their trauma. We noticed that when they introduced art and stories into therapy sessions, children created stories that closely paralleled their perception of the endured domestic violence, but changed the outcome by developing conflict resolutions that were empowering.

For example, many children created hero figures as a means to negotiate their feelings about their inability to protect themselves and their family from abuse. The hero allowed them to enact the fantasy of rescuing their families from harm. A story written by a ten-year-old girl titled, "The Transforming Girl," illustrates this point. She wrote, "If anybody is hurt or they are feeling sad, I can come talk to them and ask them, 'What's the matter?' Or if somebody is being beaten up, I can come and rescue them. I can change into anything! I can turn into a monster and scare the bad one away, and they will run like a chicken."

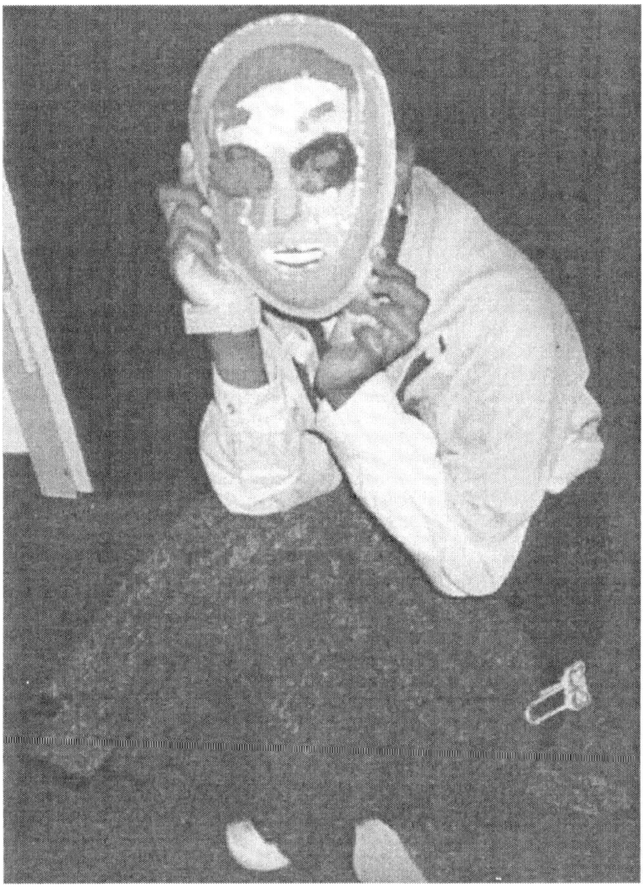

Figure 1. The Transforming Girl.

Figure 1 represents the persona of "the transforming girl." The mask in Figure 1 provided the girl with the opportunity to express her desire to feel powerful and protective of her mother. She created a costume and dressed up as this hero and posed for a photograph. Her picture and story were exhibited in an art show at the shelter. When she left the shelter, she took her matted picture, but chose to leave the mask in the therapist's room. Although wearing the mask helped her gain a new perspective of herself as a competent, autonomous individual, it was the portrait that became meaningful enough for her to take to her new home because it preserved the memory of feeling powerful and safe.

Story Development

Whether a story is in the form of a myth, a legend, a fairy tale, a fable, or an epic adventure, the structure of a story remains the same–there is a plot, a setting, and a protagonist and an antagonist character. The five basic elements of a plot consist of an introduction, a rising action, a climax, a falling action, and a dénouement (Short story elements, n.d.). A story is essentially determined by a character's actions. The character may be in conflict with himself, other characters, nature, and or society (Sanchez & Stewart, 2006).

We recognized that the children we met in the domestic violence shelter often spontaneously developed stories after they made characters out of art materials. Once the children connected a character to their artwork, we encouraged them to give life to the characters by considering a series of questions about the characters' physical attributes, thoughts, feelings, dreams, morals, and relationships with others. Once the characters were brought to life, the plot of the stories began to unfold. As the stories were developed, we supported and guided the children in structuring and organizing their trauma stories into a clear, coherent and sequential order. As the story progressed further, the children were engaged in a dual process of writing and creating artwork to symbolize other pieces of the story. Once the story and artwork were complete, the children were presented with the option to arrange their stories into a book or a video.

Storybook

If the children chose to translate their stories into books, we assisted them in staging and photographing the artwork that best depicted the parts of the trauma they wanted to present to others. Once we printed the photographs and the children selected the final pictures, the books were made. We provided children with various options for creating books. Some children chose to use materials such as cardboard, fabrics, sequins, feathers etc. to create elaborate books, while some simply chose to staple a stack of paper together. If age appropriate, we instructed children on how to use a computer to type the story and insert the digital photos into the text. Regardless of the method used to make the book, the book's function was to contain the trauma story and acted as a transitional holding environment (Robbins, 1987).

By allowing children to stage and create photographs for their trauma story, they decide which aspects of the memory to preserve and which to reject. Electris (2003) described photographs as a witness and a voice to the child's often secret pain and trauma experience. Pictures evoke memory in our lives but do not preserve meaning in the same way memory does. The sounds, smells, and movements associated with that memory can be evoked by the photograph, but not conveyed. When children look through the camera lens, they have control over the snapshot moment they choose to present. In conjunction with the text of the story, the photographs of artwork offer further distance from the trauma. Through this form of vicariously witnessing their trauma, children gain new insights and perspectives into their experience.

Video

If the children chose to make their story into a film, we assisted the children in narrating, directing, and filming the story. Filming a story gave children the opportunity to play and master different roles such as narrator, scene director, and cameraman. The video camera was used because it enabled children to recreate the traumatic memory as they saw and felt it. The children's perception of the traumatic event was brought to life in the video. Regardless of whether or not the story was believed or accepted by family and friends, the video offered a space free of judgment.

When we used a video camera in a group setting it enhanced the group process. We used two different methods when incorporating the video camera into a group session – either the group worked together to film their collaborative story or each group member filmed their own personal story and edited it together into one video. Both methods provided the group members with a safe environment to be a witness, either to each other's individual stories or to the collective story.

Videotaping children's trauma stories allows them to gain some control over the memories that haunt them. The video camera allows children to confront and control the environmental elements they were unable to in the past such as sounds, people or places. They now have control of the fear-based reactions and can transform them into sources of creativity. Unlike flashbacks and nightmares that are unpredictable, videos are made with conscious control and can be re-recorded and edited if necessary (O'Rourke, 2001).

Individual Applications

An important aspect of joining art and narrative therapy is the application of the technique during individual therapy. The following case example highlights Electris' use of art and narrative therapy in individual therapy. It also illustrates how the process of creating a story can produce a meaningful experience beyond the making of the art alone.

Jada

Jada, a nine-year-old girl entered the domestic violence shelter because her mother was escaping her abusive boyfriend for the fourth time. Jada presented as a parentified child who was extremely protective of her mother. As a result, she was adept at hiding her feelings in order to prevent upsetting her mother.

When I began meeting with Jada for individual therapy, she was reluctant to express her feelings of fear, anger, and sadness because it was an unfamiliar role. During one session, she chose to create a mask which she decorated over several sessions. As she added embellishments to her mask, she told me she was creating a superhero with magical powers. The superhero's powers were stored in the superhero's cape which we sewed together over the next few months. While Jada worked on the cape she spoke about her fears and particularly expressed feelings of terror at the thought of her mother's return to the batterer. It became clear that she restricted her emotions because it was the one thing she could control.

Throughout the therapy process, Jada eventually began to express her fears, but was still resistant about expressing anger towards her mother or her mother's batterer. To help Jada access and externalize her anger, I invited her to make a book about the superhero. Jada accepted enthusiastically. While writing the story, she decided to create a villain mask so her hero could protect the world from harm.

When Jada's story was finished, Jada asked me to photograph her playing the role of the hero. Figure 2 illustrates the superhero kicking the villain, who symbolizes her mother's batterer. By playing the superhero in the photograph, Jada was able to express her anger towards the batterer. After the photograph was taken, she crumbled the remains of the mask and discarded it in the garbage. Through destroying the mask, Jada was able to sublimate her revenge fantasy. The photograph of this scene empowered Jada to gain control over her feelings towards the batterer, gave her hope that her mother would not return, and provided her with a healthy and safe outlet to express her emotions attached with to trauma in a positive and constructive way.

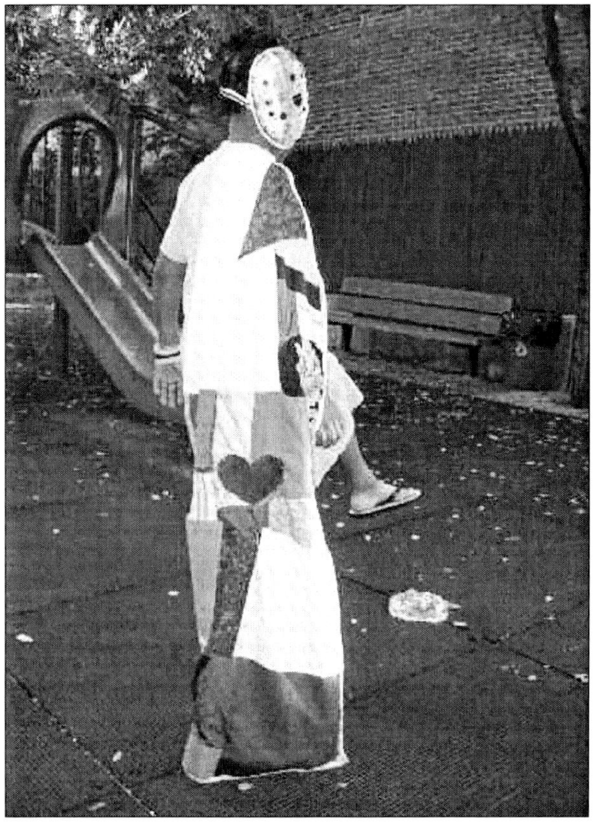

Figure 2. Jada's Superhero.

Jada glued the pictures alongside her written words into a store made book and invited her mother into the next session to read her story to her. Immediately after reading the story to her mother, Jada asked her if she would ever return to the batterer. The book provided Jada with an opportunity to begin to share her repressed feelings with her mother. In turn, Jada's mother learned how strongly Jada was affected by repeated returns to the batterer.

Group Applications in a Domestic Violence Shelter

We found the combination of art and narrative therapies to be incredibly powerful and beneficial when utilized with children's groups. Children typically entered the domestic violence shelter knowing that what happened in the home must be kept a secret. This message caused them to feel isolated and assume that only their family was troubled by abuse and violence.

Writing a collaborative story provided them with a place to feel accepted and understood. Sharing their story with one another lessened the loneliness and shame of their victimization. Additionally as they began to understand that they were not alone in their experience, they started to develop positive, meaningful connections with each other. As the positive interactions between one another increased they began to learn non-violent ways to manage conflicts that arose in the group. The following case examples document our application of therapeutic storytelling with groups of children residing in the shelter.

The Sea Monster

In a domestic violence shelter, Hnath and an art therapy intern co-lead a group consisting of 6 children between the ages of 9 and 12 years old. The group met over a period of three months. After setting up the group expectations in the initial group, the group members were engaged in an art directive that provided them with the opportunity to introduce themselves to one another. While working on this initial directive, the members had difficulty following the group expectations and required a lot of redirection. It was clear that their behavior and inability to regulate their emotions stemmed from growing up in violent homes.

In the following session, we directed each member to make a three-dimensional container using clay. The clay container was meant to serve as a holding environment for their emotions to help them learn affect modulation. Although the creation of the container seemed to ground the members and decreased the need for redirection, they seemed disconnected from their art and dissociated from their trauma. It was clear that the group members required an intervention that would not only allow them to sublimate their feelings, but also allow them to safely reconstruct traumatic memories.

Consequently, in the next session we directed the members to transform their containers into characters and introduced the idea of writing a story together that would include all of the group's characters. The members in the group immediately accepted the idea and began exploring plots that would involve all of their characters. Once a plot was agreed upon, they took turns developing sentences and recording the story onto paper. The text of the story was completely written by the group members. We remained neutral throughout the process and intervened only when the group needed help remaining on task or assistance with problem-solving.

As the members wrote the story, they also worked together to create additional objects and scenery to enhance the story. Once the members finished writing and illustrating the story, they chose to develop their story into a book and took turns using the digital camera to photograph scenes from the story. After the group agreed on what photographs they wanted to accompany each part of their story, we helped the children use a computer to compile their words and photographs into a text which was later bound with a book binding machine. Each member received their own copy of the book in the final group session. The members expressed deep feelings of satisfaction and pride in the finished product and chose to show it to their families and friends. Their story titled, "The Sea Monster" is as follows:

> Once upon a time on a planet called Salest, lived many sea monsters. The sea monsters lived underwater. Salest was a planet full of water, except one part called Mystery Island. Mystery Island was 200 acres long. There were only eight people remaining who lived on Mystery Island. Four boys, two girls, and two women lived on this island. The boy's names were Rashawn, Jonathon, Joseph and Malik. The girl's names were Jessy and Yolanda. The women's names were Jennifer and Christina.

The most dangerous creature was Infoury. Infoury killed anything in his way. Infoury's weakness was a weed on his back. Long ago there were more than one of the Infoury's. All of them killed hundreds of people because they wanted land and the people were food to them.

The people wanted to kill Infoury with the most powerful device on the planet. It was found in the black water deep in the sea. It was dangerous for the people to dig for the device because Infoury may attack. Rashawn, Jonathon and Malik went to dig for the device underwater. They were armed for protection just in case Infoury attacks. They start digging and the device pops up. They took the device to the island to build the bomb. The bomb is ready to kill Infoury. They went out to look for Infoury. Whey they found Infoury, they threw the bomb on Infoury and went back to the island. They pushed the button and Infoury blew up. "Booooommmmm!" They lived happily ever after.

As the members worked together to create "The Sea Monster," they began to develop a strong bond with one another that enabled them to process their feelings of anger and hatred toward their batterers, rather than acting out aggressively toward one another. The strong attachment bond that they developed with one another is illustrated in a photograph from their book (see Figure 3).

As seen in their story, the group members identified Infoury as the abuser. Stronach-Buschel (1990) wrote about children identifying with the aggressor and or having revenge fantasies that stem from feelings of helplessness and guilt at their inability to intervene in episodes of violence that occur in the

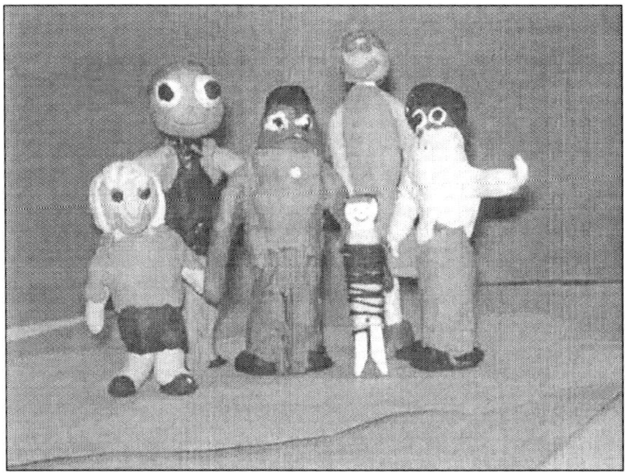

Figure 3. The people living on Mystery Island.

home. The feelings of powerlessness and helplessness that the group members experienced when living in a violent home were transformed through their choice to kill Infoury. Infoury was a threat to the characters' existence. Rather than becoming a victim to Infoury's wrath, the group decided to take control of the situation by protecting themselves from impending harm. Killing Infoury provided the members with an opportunity to vicariously feel powerful and safely express their revenge fantasy towards their own abuser.

At the end of the story, the members debated about saving a bomb in case of future attacks from other harmful creatures. They eventually decided that future protection was not necessary because Infoury's death brought them safety. Their decision suggested that they now felt a sense of control over their situation and their future.

The Happy and Helpful Town

Another group at the shelter co-led by Electris and an art therapy intern was comprised of six girls between the ages of 9 and 11. The group met weekly for approximately four months. From the start of the group, the girls were extremely energetic and easily over-stimulated. It was difficult for them to connect with each other, as they often appeared guarded and un-empathic towards one another. They were not respectful of each other's boundaries or feelings because they were each struggling to be the one in control.

When they created art, they appeared to have an insatiable hunger for materials, and frequently took materials from each other. Living in the shelter, they had little belongings, as they had left most of their possessions behind, and they tried to meet their needs for material items through the group. The girls brought a feeling of disorganized chaos to the group that made it difficult for them to connect to each other in a meaningful way. In an effort to contain and focus the girls, we introduced structured directives with pre-selected materials. Although the girls enjoyed the art projects and the structured directives provided some containment for their emotions, they still did not appear to be connecting or relating to each other positively.

Two months into the group, we decided that the group members would benefit more from the sessions if they were to feel in control of their treatment. This treatment goal was accomplished by allowing the children to select a theme and their own directive, using any materials they chose. At the beginning the next group, we started the session by opening up the art supply closet and asking the group members to agree upon an art directive. The group members came up with two main ideas: to build a house and to create art about a friend. We suggested that they combine the two ideas by each building a house and deciding who would live in the home, which could include friends. The girls agreed and spent several weeks building and decorating their individual homes. As they became invested in their individual projects the conflicts between one another decreased.

As they shared ideas and materials, they began to develop positive relationships with one another and decided to join their homes together. While sitting around the table filled with large houses, they remarked that they had created their own town and named it, "The happy and helpful town." In an attempt to provide the group with a sense of structure and containment, we encouraged the members to write a story together about their town that could be made into a book or a video.

The members loved the idea of creating a video that would capture their collaborative story. We assisted the girls in the process of videotaping by creating a structure in which each girl had an opportunity to direct and film a part of the story. Each girl had a turn directing, filming, and using art props to act out the story. We narrated the story by reading the group's script as the girls filmed in order to provide a single, consistent voice to the story. In the final group session, the members watched the video together and received their own copy of the edited video. The story they wrote is written below:

> Once upon a time, there was a little town called *Happy and Helpful*. In the town of *Happy and Helpful*, everyone knows each other, and when someone new comes to town, the people throw a party to welcome strangers. In our town, people protect each other. They have rules: No bad words, no fighting, no smoking, and no riding bikes on hills.
>
> One day there was a big fire. The people of the town were not sure what to do, because they're not used to danger. One day, an evil stranger comes to town named Dr. Evil. He was a big, fat man with a big mustache and

long eyebrows. He lived on the hill across the street and underground. He hated being happy and helpful. And he walked through the town pushing down old ladies. An old lady, Ms. Medea, who was good friends with everyone called the police. She was angry because she was pushed down. Dr. Evil ran away back to his hideout. Ms. Medea told the police what happened.

The next day, Dr. Evil changed the weather so the townspeople wouldn't be so happy. He created a tornado with his weather machine. The village people became very angry with one another, after they saw the damage. The townspeople thought someone in the village changed the weather, until they realized that Dr. Evil had done it after reviewing the security cameras.

The village people found out where Dr. Evil's hideout was. They went there and tortured him with niceness and tried to be his friend. "I love you Dr. Evil. You're the best. Oh, man. Can we stay over? I want to help you do your homework, awwh! You're so kind!" they said.

"Please stop! This gives me a headache!" he yelled. "My head hurts!" The village people told him that they would stop if he started to be nice. He agreed. However, he was only nice for three days. After that, he started to steal people's jewelry and their animals from the farm. They yelled, "Give us back our animals." The president and the mayor, along with the village people, were furious! "This is the last straw! Dr. Evil, you have to go! This is the town of *happy and helpful*, and we do not have mean people here," said the villagers.

Looking at all the damage, Dr. Evil realized that what he did was really bad. He told the village people that he didn't mean to hurt anyone and apologized, before leaving the town forever. After Dr. Evil left, the villagers were sad because they were going to miss him. But they were also happy he was gone. So now, the town of happy and helpful was back to being happy and helpful.

As the girls wrote the story of "Happy and Helpful," it became clear that they were all telling the same story, the story about being a victim of domestic violence. The group members created Dr. Evil as an antagonist character representing their batterers. The physical and emotional pain that they suffered living in a violent home was symbolically portrayed through the physical destruction of the town. Dr. Evil's destructive effect on the fictional town provided the group members with enough distance and safety to express their conflicted feelings about their own estranged family.

The process of filming eventually became a canvas for the group members to paint out their painful feelings about this disruption in their own personal lives. The girls were highly anxious on the day of filming and as they began to film Dr. Evil invading the town, conflicts arose and they started to argue with one another. With our redirection and support, the group members were able to continue filming. However, when we began to film the eviction of Dr. Evil, the members of the group began to regress. The filming was halted until we recognized and acknowledged that saying goodbye to Dr. Evil created conflicted feelings, similarly to their feelings about leaving home and entering the shelter. The group members shared that leaving the batterer provided them with a sense of relief and safety, but that they also felt sad leaving the batterer and other family and friends behind. We encouraged the members to incorporate their conflicted feelings into the end of the story. As a result, the filming was successfully completed.

It was evident that by not setting limits on the materials or ideas available, the children were able to let go of their preoccupation of feeding themselves and "getting enough." By allowing creative freedom as well as providing the children with a sense of autonomy, the children became more involved in the creative therapeutic process and interacted positively in the group setting.

This therapeutic intervention provided a safe and constructive setting for the children to gain control over the negative feelings associated with the trauma and alleviated some of the anxieties of the abuse. It also provided the children with various forms of social skills training, which included appropriate group and social interaction and respect for others' ideas. Additionally, the experience of creating a group video story helped the children become more empathic towards each other, and allowed them to become more reflective and insightful on what they had each experienced.

Conclusion

The awareness that domestic violence is widespread has been known for years: "25% to 30% of American women are physically harmed by an intimate partner at least once in their lifetimes, and that 12% of husbands assault their wives each year" (Schewe, n.d.). More recently attention has been focused on the 3.3 million children exposed to domestic violence annually (American Psychological Association, 1996).

Trauma associated with domestic violence often overwhelms children and can cause long lasting scars if left untreated. van der Kolk stated that "the imprint of trauma doesn't sit in the verbal, understanding, part of the brain, but in much deeper regions [sub-cortical brain, nervous system, body] . . . then to do effective therapy, we need to do things that change the way people regulate their core functions, which probably can't be done by words and language alone" (Trauma therapy, n.d.). The alarming statistics above and van der Kolk's statement suggest the need for an effective treatment for children victims of domestic violence.

We found that combining the techniques of art and narrative therapies was a powerful, holistic intervention that broke the silence of domestic violence by giving a voice to the silent victims. When children simply retell their trauma stories, it seems to reinforce the damaging psychological effects on the children. However, we discovered that creating these stories, either with actual or fictional characters and circumstances allowed children to reshape the trauma and create a new outcome. A different outcome can create a long term personal change. The words and images created equipped children with a new knowledge and perspective of themselves that allowed them to rediscover a sense of who they were and regained a sense of security. The book or video developed in this treatment method was a tangible product that provided containment and validated the child's feelings and perceptions of the traumatic event.

When we incorporated art and narrative therapies into the treatment of children at the domestic violence shelter, we found it created a safe environment and structure for children to voice their fears, longings, revenge, and concerns in a symbolic form. Narrative therapy helped the children re-author their trauma in their own terms and art therapy helped children transform the trauma images that haunted them. Writing a story and creating art about the trauma seemed to create a healthy detachment that allowed the children to embody the characters and events in their story, thus re-integrating their trauma. Although the case examples highlighted were limited to children residing in a domestic violence shelter, we believe that this technique would also be effective in treating all types of trauma and can be applied to adults and families.

Terms

Art Therapy: A form of psychotherapy which uses art and the creative process as a means of expression, where the interpretation of the inner meaning is used for therapy. The therapeutic technique uses creative expression that may assist in exploring personal problems and in healing emotional traumas through non-verbal expressions. Art therapy integrates the fields of visual art, with psychology and therapy (Olivera, Toler & Trevithick, 2001).
Bibliotherapy: Having originated as a form of play therapy, this expressive therapy consists of selecting reading material that a child or teenager will be able to identify with and reading it to them. This technique can consist solely of reading, or can be followed with discussion or a play activity (Bibliotherapy, n.d.a.).
Narrative Therapy: A form of psychotherapy using narrative to capture a client's history. The importance is placed upon a client telling and retelling their story so that the therapist may understand the client better (Narrative therapy, n.d.b).

Parentified child: Children under the age of 18 who provide care to a family member. This occurs when children are not allowed to act like children and must assume grown-up responsibilities (Kass, n.d.).

Post Traumatic Stress Disorder (PTSD): An anxiety disorder that can develop after exposure to a terrifying event or ordeal where physical harm occurred or was threatened to one's own or another's life. PTSD symptoms in children include intense fear, helplessness, or horror. Additionally, children often re-enact the traumatic event (in play, dreams, or behaviors), withdraw or avoid cues associated with the event, and present with physiological hyper-reactivity (hypervigilance, sleep problems or anxiety) (Hamblen, n.d.).

References

American Psychological Association. (1996). *Violence and the family: Report of the American Psychological Association Presidential Task Force on Violence and the Family.* Retrieved December 21, 2006, from http://www.acadv.org/children.html

Avidar, A. (1995). Art therapy and pervasive trauma: Working with children in violent communities. *Pratt Institute Creative Arts Therapy Review, 16,* 10-16.

Bibliotherapy. (n.d.a). Retrieved February 21, 2007, from http://maxweber.hunter.cuny.edu/pub/eres/EDSPC715_MCINTYRE/Biblio.html

Bibliotherapy, (n.d.b). Retrieved March 5, 2007, from http://en.wikipedia.org/wiki/Bibliotherapy

Brooke, S. L. (2007). *The use of the creative therapies with sexual abuse survivors.* Springfield, IL: Charles C Thomas, Publisher, Ltd.

Burch, E. A., & Powell, C. H. (1980). The psychiatric assessment of a Vietnamese refugee through art. *American Journal of Psychiatry, 137,* 236-237.

Burnes, G. W. (2005). *101 Healing stories for kids and teens: Using metaphors in therapy.* Hoboken, NJ: John Wiley & Sons, Inc.

Carlson, T. D. (1997). Using art in narrative therapy: Enhancing therapeutic possibilities. *The American Journal of Family Therapy, 25*(3), 271-283.

Electris, A. (2003). *Video storytelling with art and text: Working through trauma body image disturbance.* Unpublished master's thesis, Pratt Institute, Brooklyn.

Evans, K.G. (1997, July-August). If mom's battered, kids suffer. *Children's Advocate.* Retrieved October 21, 2006, from http://www.4children.org/news/7-97mbat.htm

Garrett, C. A., & Ireland, M. S. (1979). A therapeutic art session with rape victims. *American Journal of Art Therapy, 18,* 103-106.

Golub, D. (1985). Symbolic expression in post traumatic stress disorder: Vietnam combat veterans in art therapy. *The Arts in Psychotherapy, 12,* 285-296.

Groves, B. M. (1999). Mental health service for children who witness domestic violence. *The Future of Children, 9*(3), 122-132.

Hamblen, J. (n.d.). PTSD in children and adolescents. *National Center for PTSD Factsheet.* Retrieved March 4, 2007, from http://www.ncptsd.va.gov/ncmain/ncdocs/fact_shts/fs_children.html

Herman, J. (1997). *Trauma and recovery: The aftermath of violence - from domestic abuse to political terror.* New York: Basic Books.

Howard, R. (1990). Art therapy as an isomorphic intervention in the treatment of a client with Post Traumatic Stress Disorder. *American Journal of Art Therapy, 28,* 79-86.

Jaffe, P., & Sudermann, M. (1995). Child witness of women abuse: Research and community responses. In S. Stith & M. Straus. *Understanding partner violence: Prevalence, causes, consequences, and solutions. Families in Focus Services: Vol. 2.* Minneapolis, MN: National Council on Family Relations.

James, B. (1989). *Treating traumatized children: New insights and creative interventions.* New York: The Free Press.

Johnson, D. (1987). The role of the creative arts therapies in the diagnosis and treatment of psychological trauma. *Arts in Psychotherapy, 14,* 7-13.

Kass, A. (n.d.). Robbing our children of childhood: Parentified children suffer later. Retrieved March 20, 2007, in http://www.divorcerecovery101.com/kass18.html

Knapp, J. F. (1998). The impact of children witnessing domestic violence. *Pediatric Clinics of North America, 45*(2), 355-364.

Levin, P., Lazrove, S., & van der Kolk, B. (1999). What psychological testing and neuroimaging tell us about the treatment of post traumatic stress disorder and eye movement desensitization and reprocessing. *Journal of Anxiety Disorders, 13*(1-2), 159-172.

Malchiodi, C. (1997). *Breaking the silence: Art therapy with children from violent homes.* Bristol, PA: Brunner/Mazel.

Montabalo-Phelps, L. L. (2003). Discourse of survival: Building families free of unhealthy relationships. *The Journal of Family Communication, 3*(3), 149-177.

Narrative Therapy (n.d.). Retrieved March 4, 2007, fromhttp://en.wikipedia.org/wiki/Narrative_therapy

Olivera, B., Toler, R., & Trevithick, C. (2001). Appendix. In M. Farrelly-Hansen (Ed.), *Spirituality and art therapy: Living the connection.* London: Jessica Kingsley Publishers.

O'Rourke, R. (1997). Anya's movies. In B. Chalfour (Ed.), *Afterimage* (Vol. 29, No. 3, p. 5). Rochester, NY: Visual Studies Workshop.

Orr, S. P. (1997). Psychophysiologic reactivity to trauma-related imagery in PTSD: Diagnostic and theoretical implications of recent findings. *Annals of the New York Academy of Science, 821,* 141-124.

Peacock, M. E. (1991). A personal construct approach to art therapy in the treatment of post sexual abuse trauma. *American Journal of Art Therapy, 29*(4), 1-11. Retrieved November 19, 2006, from the EBSCOhost database.

Peled, E., & Edelson, J. (1995). Process and outcome in small groups for children of battered women. In E. Peled, G. Jaffe & J. L. Edleson (Eds.), *Ending the cycle of violence: Community responses to children of battered women.* Thousand Oaks, CA: Sage Publications.

Pynoos, R. S., & Eth, S. (1986). Witness to violence: The child interview. *Journal of the American Academy of Child Psychiatry, 25,* 306–319.

Robbins, A. (1987). *The artist as therapist.* New York: Human Sciences Press, Inc.

Reichert, E. (1998). Individual counseling for sexually abused children: A role for animals and storytelling. *Child and Adolescent Social Work Journal, 15*(3), 177-185.

Salans, M. (2003). *Storytelling with children in crisis: Take just one star - how impoverished children heal through stories.* London: Jessica Kingsley Publishers.

Sanchez, T. R., & Stewart, V. (2006). The remarkable abigail: Storytelling for character education. *High School Journal, 89*(4), 14-21.

Schewe, P. A. (n.d.). *Interventions for children exposed to domestic violence.* Paper presented to the Illinois Department of Human Services. Retrieved January 19, 2007, from http://www.uic.edu/depts/psch/idhs/Childwitnesses.htm

Short story elements. (n.d.). Retrieved January 21, 2007, from http://hrsbstaff.ednet.ns.ca/engramja/elements.html

Stronach-Buschel, B. (1990). Trauma, children and art. *The American Journal of Art Therapy, 29,* 48-52.

Storytelling. (n.d.). Retrieved January 21, 2007, from http://en.wikipedia.org/wiki/Storytelling

Trauma therapy. (n.d.). Retrieved February 25, 2007, from http://www.erikahilliard.com/trauma_therapy.html

van der Kolk, B. A. (1987). *Psychological trauma.* Washington D.C.: American Psychological Press.

van der Kolk, B. A., van der Hart, O., & Burbridge, J. (1995). *Approaches to the treatment of PTSD.* Retrieved August 10, 2006, from David Baldwin's Trauma Information Pages Web site: www.trauma-pages.com/a/vanderk.php

White, M., & Epston, D. (1990). *Narrative means to therapeutic ends.* New York: Norton.

Wilson, S. K., Cameron, S., Jaffe, P., & Wolfe, D. (1989). Children exposed to wife abuse: An intervention model. *Social Casework: The Journal of Contemporary Social Work, March,* 180-184.

Wolfe, D. A., Wekerle, C., Reitzel, D., & Gough, R. (1995). Strategies to address violence in the lives of high risk youth. In E. Peled, P. G. Jaffe, & J. L. Edleson (Eds.), *Ending the cycle of violence: Community responses to children of battered women.* New York: Sage Publications.

Wollman, D. (1993). Critical incident stress debriefing and crisis groups: A review of literature, *Group, 17*(2), 70-83.

Biographies

Alexia Electris, MPS, ATR, L-CAT is a New York State licensed art therapist. Ms. Electris is currently enrolled in a doctoral program for clinical psychology at Long Island University and is working at Brooklyn Center for Psychotherapy and New Directions substance abuse outpatient treatment center. Previously, Ms. Electris worked with traumatized children and families in a domestic violence shelter. Ms. Electris has extensive training in the treatment of trauma, including Eye Movement Desensitization and Reprocessing (EMDR) trainings. Ms. Electris is also a certified instructor for Non-Violence Crisis Intervention (CPI). In addition, Ms. Electris has conducted trainings on trauma and domestic violence at various shelters and is also part of Garrison Institute's faculty for their domestic violence wellness program for shelter workers.

Janice Hnath, MPS, BCSCR, ATR-BC, L-CAT is a New York State licensed art therapist and board certified in school crisis response. She currently works at Safe Horizon as a manager of their school programs, which educates youth about domestic violence and teen dating abuse. Ms. Hnath also provides part-time art therapy services to at-risk youth as an alternative to detention program in conjunction with the Office of the Kings County District Attorney and the Youth in Congregations Partnership (YCP). She also maintains a small private practice in Queens, NY. Ms. Hnath previously worked in a domestic violence shelter providing individual, group, and family art therapy. Ms. Hnath has conducted numerous trainings on trauma and domestic violence. Additionally, she is on the faculty of Garrison Institute's domestic violence wellness program for shelter workers. She is currently in the process of becoming a trained EMDR practitioner. Ms. Hnath is a member of the American Art Therapy Association and the American Academy of Experts in Traumatic Stress.

Chapter 17

SUPERVISION ISSUES IN FAMILY VIOLENCE CASES

DAWN LORRAINE MCBRIDE

Introduction

> A counselor, somewhat new to the field of family violence work, debriefs her frustration to you, the agency supervisor, at her client's decision to return to an abusive partner. You sense the counselor is feeling disheartened the client did not listen to her advice to remain at the shelter for another week. You wonder if the counselor is personalizing the client's decision as a counter transference reaction given her unusual amount of frustration. Further, you wonder if a risk assessment was done before the client left the session to ensure the client's safety. All these thoughts, and more, are running through your mind as the counselor stands before you. You question the best way to approach this counselor as there are a host of options and each option is dependent on many variables such as the counselor's developmental competency stage, her personal background, and her personality style.

This is just one of the many scenarios supervisors have to contend with when supervising therapists who carry a caseload of clients with a family violence background. Supervisors need to adopt a new way of thinking when they become a supervisor (Pearson, 2006). They need to think and act like an educator/trainer, consultant, and counselor (Bernard, 1997; Stoltenberg & Delworth, 1987) with the mandate to always look after the best interests of the client but at the same time ensure the counselor is gaining therapeutic competence. It is a juggling act that can be taxing, particular if the supervisor has not received training in the art and science of supervision. The lack of training of supervisors is a significant concern, particularly since many universities still fail to offer graduate counselor courses in supervision (Nelson, Johnson, & Thorngren, 2000). Furthermore, it is not uncommon for therapists (often those working for non-profit agencies such as shelters) to be promoted to the role of supervisor without receiving training in the understanding and application of the theoretical underpinnings associated with supervision (Lindblad-Goldberg, 1996; Nelson et al., 2000), especially as it relates to supervising family violence cases. Thus, this chapter is timely.

The context of this chapter is specific to supervising counselors with clients who were/are in a domestic relationship (e.g., dating, common-law, marriage) characterized by abuse. The guiding assumption is that both males and females can be perpetuators and/or victims of abuse and that abuse occurs in both same-sex and heterosexual relationships. Perhaps not surprisingly, the body of academic literature on supervision practices is limited as noted by Bradshaw, Butterworth, and Mairs (2007) and Edwards and associates (2005). Furthermore, the literature is even scarcer when it pertains to family violence and supervision issues. Consequently, much of the material in this chapter is drawn from my experiences as a clinical supervisor and educator on family violence.

To explore issues in family violence supervision, this chapter begins with an overview of the developmental stages of counselors. If the supervisor does not align with the needs of the supervisee, significant conflicts will likely occur. The next major section explores the value of knowing the supervisor's and supervisee's personality profiles as it relates to maximizing communication and learning practices. The last section in this chapter discusses the inherent risk of family violence therapists experiencing vicarious traumatic reactions and the role of the supervisor in helping the supervisee overcome the effects of listening to stories of trauma. The chapter concludes with an experiential activity family violence supervisors can use to promote discussion of self-care in their supervisees.

Developmental Stages of Supervisees

Intuitively, supervisees are in different stages of developing professional competence. As noted by Pearson (2001), knowledge of these stages allows supervisors to decide on the amount of structure needed in the supervision sessions including the balance between teaching, consulting, practicing the skills, and exploring supervisee's personal reactions and beliefs. Many writers have written about these developmental stages, notably Loganbill, Hardy, and Delworth (1982, a very comprehensive review) and Worthington (1987, an excellent review). Since these stages are described at length elsewhere, I will present three integrative stages, based on the work of Stoltenberg and Delworth (1987), using the same descriptive headings (levels) as Hawkins and Shohet (1989, p. 52) to reflect the main focus of the supervisee.

Level I: Self centered–Can I make it in this work?

If you are helping newcomers to the field of counseling and/or to the field of intervening in family violence cases, it is likely the counselors are grappling with anxiety, uncertainty, self-doubt, and confusion. These counselors (known forth as supervisees) will be dependent on the supervisor for guidance, reassurance, and support (Stoltenberg & Delworth, 1987). As noted by Costa (1994), supervisee anxiety needs to be addressed, for if it continues, supervisees may rely on unhealthy defense mechanisms to cope with the anxiety (e.g., submissive, blaming, projection, displacement, intellectualization). This reaction could interfere with the supervisees learning process and could put them at risk of developing poor working alliances with their clients (Ackerman & Hilsenroth, 2001). One strategy (among seven described by Costa) to reduce anxiety is to have the supervisees list their irrational fears and beliefs about supervision (and working with family violence clients). I would then follow this exercise with cognitive behavioral exercises to challenge their irrational beliefs. Throughout this normalizing and instructional phase, it is of crucial importance to create a trusting, caring, and nonjudgmental relationship with the supervisees. A strong working alliance between a supervisee and supervisor will promote safety for exploration and will act as a buffer when negative events occur in counseling (Ramos-Sanchez et al., 2002, a good empirical study on the value of good working in supervisory relationships; Worthington & Roehlke, 1979, a classic article on what supervisees find helpful from their supervisors).

Structured supervision sessions are highly valuable when working with supervisees at level I. The work of Bradley and Whiting (2001) and Powell (2004) provide ample resource material that can be used during structured supervision sessions (e.g., supervisee goal sheets, pre-post evaluations, case review forms, live observation forms, supervisory record, etc.). In addition, see Appendix A for an interview schedule to help build the relationship between the supervisee and supervisor as well as outline the expectations for supervision (McBride, 2007).

Supervisees in this stage need to learn about the dynamics of family violence and how counselors manage the intensity in these sessions. To meet this learning need, two required readings I assign family violence supervisees are Herman's (1997) book on the impact of trauma and the recovery from it and Dutton's (1995) narrative account of a group program for men who have abusive histories. I also encourage supervisees, before they start work with family violence clients, to observe a diverse range of family violence sessions (e.g., intake, group and individual sessions, crisis sessions, etc.) being facilitated by a number of different counselors. This exposure hopefully demonstrates there is more than one way to counsel family violence clients and that there is "no perfect session," which can have the effect of reducing supervisee performance and evaluation anxiety. In debriefing their observations, I ensure there are no judgments or criticisms of fellow counselors as it preserves the cohesiveness of the agency and promotes a safe atmosphere for learning. This is an important piece to note, as it is a precaution against vicarious traumatization, which will be explained later in the chapter.

Once level I supervisees start to counsel family violence clients, it is critical the supervisor observes the sessions of the supervisees and/or reviews the content of the session (e.g., reviews the counseling tapes and/or written transcripts). This is because supervisees at this particular stage tend "to focus on specific aspects of the client's history, current situation, or personality assessment data to the exclusion of other relevant information. Grand conclusions may be based on rather discreet pieces of information" (Stoltenberg & Delworth, 1987, p. 56). I find this is a very common reaction when a therapist (at any skill level) feels overwhelmed with the volume and intensity of the multiple issues often associated with working with family violence cases (i.e., a common family violence client scenario: The client has numerous systems involved in the case, has active PTSD symptoms such as flashbacks, has an unending list of resolved family of origin issues, and is at risk for suicide). Guiding level I supervisees on how to prioritize clients concerns and manage the long list of issues is a process that requires active involvement from the supervisor. In fact, co-therapy or direct observations behind a mirror using a telephone are my preferred strategies when working with counselors new to family violence work. This format of supervision allows me to guide the counseling session if the supervisee(s) is uncertain what to say or do next or focuses on issues that do not require immediate attention. An excellent book on co-therapy by Roller and Nelson (1991) and the chapter by Goodyear and Nelson (1997) provides an informative review of the major supervision methods (e.g., bug in the ear, group supervision, reflecting teams, case presentations).

In addition to the narrow perspective level I supervisees are prone to have when processing client information, I find counselors new to trauma work tend to either block (or deny) their emotional and physical reactions during session work or become very overwhelmed with these sensations. Teaching counselors how to ground themselves when hearing stories of violence and despair is critical to prevent emotional burnout and vicarious traumatization. To this end, I assign Pearlman and Saakvitne's (1995) excellent chapter on specific strategies to manage the content when listening to client's stories of experiencing or inflicting abuse. I also actively invite supervisees to process with me what they felt in their body while working with a family violence client. For example, I might ask a supervisee: "what was happening in your body as you heard the husband describe? . . . , "I notice you grimaced at the disclosure of . . . put words to your grimace," "were you aware of making this grimace?" and/or "what sensations or thoughts are you aware of that might give you a clue of a grimace starting to form?"

Overall, supervisees new to the field of counseling and/or working with family violence cases may be highly anxious but are often highly motivated to learn (level I; Stoltenberg & Delworth, 1987). Navigating through this level requires the supervisor to assume a nurturing role, combined with sharing family violence literature and indirectly exposing the supervisee to family violence cases to prepare them to move to level II. This is one of the most taxing levels for the supervisor because of the steady demand for assistance and the need for the supervisor to constantly monitor how much information and processing the supervisee can handle to avoid overwhelming the already insecure, anxious supervisee.

Level II: Client centered–Can I help this client?

By this point, supervisees have gained some confidence in working with family violence cases. There is also an overall reduction in expecting the supervisor to offer "cookbook" solutions (Powell, 2004). Likewise, experienced therapists new to family violence work, and who are in level II, will come to realize many of their counseling skills can be integrated to help clients with an abuse/abusive history. To the relief of their supervisors, supervisees at this stage are often able to remain somewhat grounded before, during and after a trauma session. As a result of their anxieties decreasing and their confidence building, they become more client focused (Stoltenberg & Delworth, 1987). However, there is more of a risk at this stage for supervisees to over identify, become enmeshed, or emotionally distant from their clients (Powell). This may be demonstrated by the supervisee accepting calls at home from clients who are wanting to leave their partners, if the counselor has a vested interest in making sure clients do leave their abusive spouses. Or, in facilitating groups for those who abuse, the supervisee may act reserved and decline to socialize with the group members during the coffee breaks.

Supervisees in level II are described by Haber (1996) as being like adolescents undergoing a rapid and turbulent growth process characterized by wanting to become autonomous but at the same time recognizing (hopefully) that they still need guidance and support. It is also common for level II supervisees to experience fluctuations in their confidence and motivation as they realize therapy is not easily learned or powerful enough as they start to encounter therapeutic failures (Stoltenberg & Delworth, 1987). Consequently, Hawkins and Shohet (1989) warn supervisees, at this point, may become disillusioned with the supervision process and become frustrated with the supervisor. They wisely recommend these supervisee feelings need to be monitored, processed and/or contained as these feelings could leak into their counseling sessions, which may be one of the explanations why the therapist in the opening case was so frustrated at her client for returning to her abusive partner.

The supervisor's role, in this level, is to provide "a transparent safety net, giving counselors the courage to venture out with the knowledge that someone is there to catch them should they fall" (Powell, 2004, p. 89). This can be a very challenging stage to navigate as the supervisor is now seen as fallible so there is often more challenging of the supervisor's feedback (Hawkins & Shohet, 1998). In addition, even though there is significant value in allowing the supervisees to learn from their mistakes (much like parenting an adolescent; Hawkins & Shohet) supervisors still need to ensure the supervisee's clients are safe and receiving appropriate care.

One of the ways I manage this balance between respecting autonomy and ensuring client care is to outline clear, non-negotiable expectations as to when I must be consulted, particularly with family violence cases (see Appendix B, McBride 2006). I find this list serves as a face saving mechanism as the supervisee can start off the supervision session by saying "you told me I have to consult with you when. . . ." This encourages the supervisee to come forth with therapeutic problems rather than get caught in the shameful circle of "I should know what to do." An excellent article on the experience and behavior of shame in supervision sessions is by Hahn (2001). I highly recommend supervisees read this article and process it with their supervisors as a way to prevent shame from flourishing as the supervisee works through the "dependency-autonomy" conflicts.

Level III: Process oriented–How are we relating together?

Level III supervisees have a "mature awareness of their own strengths and limitations . . . they can empathize with a client while maintaining sufficient objectivity. . . . As a result, they can make therapeutic use of their own and client's reactions. . . . [Their] motivation is steady, consistent, realistic, and balanced" (Powell, 2004, pp. 92-93). This awareness and objectivity allows theme to refine what Hawkins and Shohet (1989) refer to as, "helicopter skills" (p. 51) where they have the skill to gain a holistic view of the situation. Consequently, their assessment and case conceptualization skills are sharp and thus, they can be trusted to seek supervision when needed as they will know when they are at an impasse (Stoltenberg & Delworth, 1987). Pearson (2001) notes supervision sessions "come alive . . . primarily in the form of self-challenge, and a deeper exploration of personal reactions and relationship processes. At this level, the supervisor essentially follows the counselor's lead in determining the content of supervision" (p. 176). In other words, as the supervisee becomes more effective, Worthington (1987) advocates the supervisor can become more reactive.

There are two inherent dangers I have witnessed with level III supervisees, particularly those based in rural communities or in non-profit agencies. First, supervision sessions are not as regular and are frequently rescheduled or canceled as the supervisor may not see the value in regular supervision with a skilled clinician, particularly if the supervisor has a heavy case load of level I and II supervisees. In my opinion, this puts the counselor at great risk for burnout, vicarious traumatization, and/or counter transference issues. Second, I find level III supervisees are often promoted to supervisor status with little to no support or guidance, as it is assumed that if they can counsel family violence clients, they can supervise. This is most unfortunate as supervisors-in-training also navigate a very similar developmental process paralleling supervisees, indicating new supervisors would also need a considerable amount of support and guidance (see Stoltenberg & Delworth, 1987). Of relevance, the ethical guidelines of the Association for Counselor Education and Supervision clearly stipulate counselors should receive training in supervision before becoming supervisors (Nelson, Johnson, & Thorngren, 2000).

Regardless of the developmental level of the trainee (supervisee or the supervisor in training), there is an inherent need to "think and talk freely, reflectively, without censorship" in their supervision sessions (Mollon cited in Hahn, 2001, p. 281). The use of measures, such as the Manchester Clinical Supervision Scale (Edwards et al., 2005) can provide feedback on the success of creating this type of safe environment. Another measure I rely on to increase the quality of positive interactions with my family violence supervisees is the Myers Briggs Type Indicator personality test, which will be discussed next.

Using Personality Profiles in Supervision

In many cases, when I am asked to be a consultant for a problematic therapist-client relationship or supervisee-supervisor relationship, I usually find the problem originates in one or two areas: (i) lack of clarity and/or agreement on the goals for change as defined by the client, counselor, and/or supervisor, or (ii) personality differences in interpersonal communication, where one or more individuals do not feel understood or supported. Revisiting and re-writing the goals from all stakeholders' perspectives, and achieving consensus of these goals, address the former problem. The work of Cormier and Nurius (2002) is a good resource on this topic. In terms of addressing the latter problem of interpersonal difficulties, I often rely on the Myers Briggs Type Indicator (MBTI: Myers, McCauley, Quenk, & Hammer, 1998).

The MBTI personality assessment tool, based on Jungian theory, has the potential to help uncover personality preferences as it relates how one prefers to structure interactions and learn new information and/or make decisions (Myers et al., 1998). This can be critical information for a supervisor to know about their supervisees. A good resource is the book "What type am I?" by Baron (1998). Hogan and Champagne (Personal Style Inventory, n.d.) have a non-copyrighted Inventory and follows the same theory and presentation style as the MBTI (a free copy is available at http://home.ica.net/~oyar/perstype.pdf)

Briefly, MBTI (which also applies to the Personal Style Inventory, n.d.) are composed of four sets of preferences, which forms a four-letter preference code. Each preference will be briefly explained, amplified with the use of supervisee-supervisor examples drawn from my family violence experiences.

Introversion (I) or Extroversion (E): How do you get energized?

Supervisees with strong preferences towards Introversion (I) type interactions tend to rejuvenate when they are by themselves, whereas supervisees with a strong orientation to Extroversion (E) are likely to be quite open and interactive with others as well as driven to connect with people to feel re-energized (Baron, 1998). Thus, it is common for those with a strong E preference to seek out the supervisor to debrief after intense family violence counseling sessions. A supervisee with strong Introversion preferences may be more inclined to spend time alone before debriefing with a supervisor or colleagues.

Both behavior preferences can be judged negatively: Supervisees with introversion tendencies are often being judged for not being more social with one's peers and/or for not seeking support earlier. And, those with a strong E preference for being needy, as they may want considerable connection time from their supervisor. To prevent this negative characterization, I find it useful to introduce the strengths and potential weaknesses of each preference to the supervisees, and how this information can enhance and distract the quality supervision. I also recognize that supervisees with a strong E preference may need to learn how to contain their need to debrief until the next scheduled supervision sessions and/or learn other ways to appropriately debrief when the supervisor is not available. Further, both preference styles, but perhaps more so with I's, benefit from clear expectations as to when they must consult with their supervisor. This will minimize the I's tendency to be too reflective and independent when needing to make clinical decisions (see Appendix B for my expectations when supervisees need to seek consultation).

Sensing (S) or Intuition(N): How do you receive information?

Those with a strong preference for Sensing (S) tend to be very detail orientated, careful, practical, and are driven to learn the facts (Personal Style Inventory, n.d.). This is in sharp contrast to the preference of Intuition (N) individuals who are known for exploring possibilities and patterns, particularly with novel problems (Baron, 1998). Such people are typically drawn to supervisors who ask constructive based questions. When working with supervisees with a strong N preference, it is important to ensure they are explaining key concepts and techniques to clients in the amount of detail required (e.g., safety precautions, time out procedure, what to say to a lawyer when advocating for child visitation rights). It has been my experience that supervisees with a strong N profile tend to regard communicating details as rather tedious. On the other hand, supervisors could maximize the learning for supervisees with a strong preference for S by catering to their need to have extensive detailed explanations. Supervisors would be wise to observe the amount of detail S type supervisees share with their clients, as they may have a tendency to be overly specific and not leave enough time for the client to engage in self-discovery such as processing what the counselor is suggesting or practicing by using role plays.

Thinking (T) or Feeling (F): How do you make decisions?

Those with a strong Thinking (T) preference are often driven by principles of fairness and logic where as those with strong Feeling (F) preferences tend to place emphasis on the relationship factors as the main priority when making decisions (Baron, 1998). A supervisee (or supervisor) with a high T preference might argue that child welfare should remove the children from the home because the parents are physically abusive to each other and it is the law to protect children from witnessing such abuse, despite the parents clearly loving their children. In the same situation, a supervisee (or supervisor) coming from a strong F orientation may be more inclined to advocate the family needs to stay together, to keep the parents motivated to change their abusive ways. Neither approach is wrong in itself; however, both supervisors and supervisees need to be aware of how their preferences in making decisions can color their ability to explore the relevant options.

Judging (J) or Perceiving (P): How do you interact with others?

Those with a strong Judging (J) preference are likely to be well organized, active note takers, not easily distracted, and seem prepared well in advance (Personal Style Inventory, n.d.). They indicate a strong preference for supervision sessions to be structured and to start/end on time. However, those supervisees (and supervisors) who have more of a Perceiving (P) preference are typically drawn to supervision styles that have more of a "go with the flow" style. They seem to prefer supervision sessions that are open-ended and process material in the moment, and may resist doing ample preparation work before supervisory sessions. They are often seen as being more flexible and open to change than those with a strong J preference (Baron, 1998). Both preferences have merit but at the same time can contribute to significant interpersonal clashes when they go unrecognized.

Of interest, Hammer (1993) reported counselors typically hold preferences toward INFJ, INFP or ENFP profiles. Thus, an INFJ type supervisee (or supervisor), for example, would be decisive in how things should be done, hold very firm values, drawn to seek connections, and be curious about why people do what they do. Supervisors would need to help INFJ supervisees do a thorough assessment before creating hypotheses. In addition, since an INFJ supervisee (or supervisor) may be inclined to lead very structured sessions, they also need to learn to allow the client open-ended time to process and raise whatever issues they want. On a similar note, pairing an INFJ with an ESFJ could be quite taxing, as both will see the need and format of supervision quite differently. To prevent an interpersonal clash, both would need to understand each other's personality profiles and then reach agreement in advance of their expectations for supervision (hence the need for the form found in Appendix A).

The connecting theme between the first two supervision issues (i.e., developmental stages of competency and personality profiles) is the need to have open communication where supervisors and supervisees can speak openly and directly about what they need from each other. There is often a perceived risk in asking for what you need and it is this fear of consequences that contributes to the profession's dark secret. This topic will be addressed next.

Addressing Vicarious Traumatization

Most people in the counseling field are aware of the profession's dark secret–vicarious traumatization (VT). McCann and Pearlman (1990), who were influential in naming the secret, describe VT as a serious internal reaction in response to listening empathetically to descriptions of client's traumatic experiences. With repeated exposure, helping professionals may experience VT, which results in cognitive shifts in their core beliefs about safety, trust, esteem, intimacy, and control as it relates to themselves and others, regardless of the amount of clinical experience they have. Counselors may further be haunted by flashbacks, intrusive thoughts, and somatic responses after listening to a client's traumatic material. For a brief yet informative account of a supervisee experiencing VT and how the supervisor intervened, read Rothschild (2002).

Saakvitne, Gamble, Pearlman, and Lev (2000) believe that VT is no one's fault as it "is the natural consequence of being human, connecting to and caring about our clients as we hear about, and see, the effects of trauma on their lives" (p. 157). I sense there is still a considerable amount of shame in the counseling profession, particularly among family violence workers, of disclosing vicarious trauma. As Hahn (2001) notes, "supervisees experience a strong desire to be competent and autonomous along with fears of being found wanting in some respect . . . and supervisors also struggle identifying their own shame and may inadvertently allow their supervisee to carry a disproportionate burden of shame" (p. 272). There is a cultural norm, along with personal drivers (beliefs) of "be strong," "keep trying," "be perfect" (Toth, 2004) that provide extensive reinforcement to cover feelings of inadequacy.

When these norms and beliefs are not overtly challenged, it promotes "projecting an illusion of self-sufficiency" (Hahn, 2001, p. 277). This internal and external pressure to be perceived as competent makes it very difficult to admit to having a client's traumatic material surface in one's dreams, thoughts, or in the form of flashbacks (McCann & Pearlman, 1990) or experiencing cognitive shifts (e.g., becoming more pessimistic, losing hope that the world is a safe place, having intimacy difficulties, etc.). These haunting experiences deepen the risk for anyone in the counseling profession to develop emotional exhaustion, compassion fatigue, and/or VT. It is my firm belief, supported by Hahn, that supervisors need to take a preventive role in addressing the role of shame in their sessions. Likewise, supervisors must provide a climate where it is acceptable (and encouraged) to pursue personal therapy to gain control and inner peace. The remaining section of this chapter will highlight three main strategies which supervisors can utilize to create a place where being impacted by trauma work is contained in support, not shame.

Supervisees' Actions in the Counseling Room

Those who work with trauma material need to take extra precaution in how they privately process client disclosures to foster an empathetic connection with their client (Rothschild, 2002). Many counselors are taught to "step into the client's shoes" to deepen the understanding what the client may be thinking, feeling, and behaving. In most cases, this is an effective strategy. However, when listening to traumatic material, a firmer boundary is needed so the horrors are contained externally and not within the counselor's body or mind. If the horrors do surface in the supervisee's private domain, then this needs to be processed immediately. To this end, the supervisor must alert the supervisee of the need to set boundaries with the material heard in the session and to develop effective tools to develop and maintain this boundary.

Ample VT prevention resources are available including Saakvitne, Gamble, Pearlman, and Lev's (2000) excellent training curriculum manual for working with survivors. A host of ideas are also listed in Pearlman and Saakvitne (1995) such as reminding oneself that the client has survived the trauma–the trauma is over. Or, lighting a candle at the start of the session and blowing it out after the session along with saying a small affirmation that the client's story is to be put at rest until the next session. Some counselors put a picture of something that connects them to the present (e.g., family, a recent holiday) that they can glance at while listening to a heavy disclosure. The overall message is to give permission, followed by support, for supervisees to take action to protect themselves.

It is important to stress to supervisees that in very few cases does a counselor need to listen to the minute details of the trauma being disclosed. Rather, teach them to listen for connecting themes such as limiting beliefs (e.g., She deserved it! I am not allowed to show anger! It IS my fault!) that can be therapeutically challenged to foster a discharge of held emotions. For example, I will invite a supervisee to play a section of her counseling tape where her client describes the violence he inflicted on his partner. After listening to the tape, I will ask the supervisee what were the key pieces to listen to and validate for the client. I also share with the supervisee how I might process the material I was listening to, as a way to role model. This demonstration shows it is not only inexperienced therapists who have to make the effort to set boundaries in regard to the clients' stories and the extent to which they are heard.

Supervisor's Actions in Supervision Sessions

The supervisor offers the supervisee coaching on how to meet therapeutic goals, assisting with case conceptualization, and providing feedback on their skill delivery. But, the work of trauma also requires the supervisor to be a container for the pain and despair the supervisee may be processing. This pain often stems from listening to client disclosures of how they were victimized or how they victimized others (Pearlman & Saakvitne, 1995). The supervisor needs to invite this level of processing and ensure it is held with utmost respect (e.g., supervisee is not later criticized on an evaluation form for not being able to stay grounded after a session). Family violence counselors need to know they have the freedom to turn to their supervisor who will offer them a safe place to have their own pain of helping others, witnessed, and validated (Pearlman & Saakvitne). This is an important role of a family violence supervisor because the supervisee will be violating confidentiality and/or not maintaining healthy boundaries if the supervisee turns to their family/friends for this level of emotional support.

Supervisees' Protective Behaviors

A comprehensive approach to protect and/or recover from VT involves three groups of activities, as described by Saakvitne and associates (2000). The first group involves engaging in activities that promote self-care, self-nurturing, and offer an escape from trauma exposure. Next are the activities that allow the negative elements of trauma work to be transformed into value and purpose, by finding meaning in the work we do and not losing hope. The last set of activities requires an acceptance of the reality of VT occurring in the helping profession. This entails a responsibility to address it by regularly monitoring and handling VT like reactions (e.g., periodically complete assessment tools on emotional fatigue, VT, etc.) and to address one's own unfinished issues in personal therapy.

To process many of these strategies with supervisees, I like to facilitate a modified version of the "Draw-a-Tree" task described in a workbook on VT (Saakvitne & Pearlman, 1996). I prefer to do this activity in a group setting to increase the range of ideas and to also normalize that reactions to client material is not something to be ashamed about but it does require taking action to minimize the impact this type of work has on one's private and professional life. The required supplies include blank paper and felts.

- Image what a healthy, well-grounded tree looks like. Draw this tree. This tree will be called your healthy tree.
- Recall how you feel after a very difficult session that didn't go very well for whatever reason. Draw another tree to represent how you are feeling after this type of session. What would your tree look like?

The group debriefing questions I use include:

1. What feelings and thoughts describe your two trees?
2. What are some differences between your two trees?
3. What type of protection does your healthy tree need to remain strong and in this state even if it exists in a taxing environment? (e.g., have extra water buckets, install a fence, add birds)
4. What does the second tree (i.e., the tree after a difficult session) need so it can return to a healthy state?
5. Transform your answers from question #3 and/or #4 into some concrete ideas as to what you can do (i.e., self care) to help the tree (you) stay strong.

Your answers	Transform	*A Concrete Self-Care Strategy*
EXAMPLE: Store more water	⟶	I need to make sure I drink enough fluids during my workday.

The message in this tree exercise is the responsibility we have to look after our inner healthy tree and to make it stronger and more resilient as time goes on. To do this, we need to acquire the skills and activities to keep our tree in good shape. When our trees become exhausted, we also need to have strategies in place to rejuvenate our tree. If you encounter difficulties in nursing your tree, then you need to have a plan in place to seek more support.

Conclusion

Saakvitne and associates (2000) captured the essence of this chapter when they wrote, "the most important factor in the success or failure of trauma work is the attention paid to the experience and needs of the helper" (p. 157). This chapter has provided over a dozen strategies on how to tune in to the needs of the supervisee working with family violence cases. These needs are critical issues in supervision and may often be overlooked if the supervisor is driven to put the client needs ahead of the supervisee. It was the premise of this chapter that the role of the supervisor is to address the supervisee's needs so the supervisee has the passion, energy, resources, and skill to help family violence clients.

APPENDIX A–SUPERVISION WITH DAWN MCBRIDE: GETTING TO KNOW EACH OTHER & OUTLINING SUPERVISION EXPECTATIONS (MCBRIDE, 2007)

This handout is a modified version of the Initial Supervision Session Checklist (ISSC) developed by Prest, Schindleer-Zimmerman, and Sporakowski (1992, pp. 130-133). The authors designed this handout to facilitate discussion between the supervisee and supervisor to help establish a clear contract for supervision, maximize the fit between supervisee and supervisor, and ensure the supervision sessions are purposeful.

Working through this handout will take approximately one or two hours as both supervisor and supervisee will share their answers to the questions. The use of prompts, paraphrasing, and seeking clarification, and/or examples will further enhance the relationship-building phase between the supervisee and supervisor. After the discussion, written copies of the relevant sections should be exchanged to allow for reflection and future reference. Relevant sections of this handout should be reviewed on a regular basis since expectations and counselor skill level will change overtime.

I. Interest in Counseling, Education, Training and Clinical Experiences

A. What factors lead to your decision to become a therapist?
B. What do you look forward to about your work (or future work) at this counseling centre?
C. Inquire about the following background characteristics of each other:

- Educational background (degrees, relevant courses, conferences attended, etc.)
- Training experiences.
- Work experience(s) and relevant volunteer experiences.
- Sense of mission/purpose/desire to work in the field of counseling.
- Educational plans as well as professional developmental plans and goals.

II. Theoretical Orientation

A. What models and specific schools of thought (e.g., feminist, systems, behavioral) have you trained in and also use on a regular basis? How do these models influence your beliefs on the nature of humans, problem development and maintenance, and personal growth?
B. What level of interest do you have in learning other new models, theories and styles?

C. In your opinion, what are some characteristics of a good therapist and a not so good therapist? Why might a poor functioning therapist be under-performing?

III. Philosophy of Supervision

A. Explore each other's perspectives and value of the supervision process, including the developmental competency stages of supervision and the experience of shame in supervision.

IV. Previous Supervision Experiences (Supervisee)

A. Describe your previous supervision experiences (e.g., which supervisor influenced you the most, liked/disliked about past supervision experiences, etc.).
B. What do you see as your strengths and areas of needed growth in terms of counseling (may be useful to assess developmental level)?
C. How would you rate your competence with:

- Facilitating the stages of therapy? The stages of change?
- Assessing for risk?
- Managing crisis sessions?
- Identifying & solving ethical dilemmas?
- Conducting assessment, informal & formal?
- Case planning, and preparing for case reviews?
- Advocating in the justice and child welfare systems?
- Working with trauma?
- Addictions and other DSM issues?
- Knowing community resources for basic needs and other social support services?
- Working with various age groups?
- Handling anger and other intense emotions in counseling sessions?
- Preventing emotional exhaustion and minimizing vicarious traumatization?

V. Supervision Goals

A. In order to establish and evaluate goals of supervision, the following topics need to be addressed:

- What are supervisee's goals that meet the definition of goal criteria (e.g., specific, measurable, observable, incremental, and realistic)?

- When will the goals be measured and how often?
- How does the supervisee plan to meet these goals (emphasize personal responsibility to ensure these goals are met)?

VI. Supervision Style and Techniques

A. In order to facilitate an optimum fit in terms of supervisory style, the following need to be addressed:

- A review of the various types/styles of supervision to facilitate clinical growth of the supervisee. Followed by a discussion on each other's preferred style & modality of supervision.

VII. Ethical and Legal Considerations

The legal and ethical parameters for the supervision process should be defined, discussed, and documented. At minimum, the topics should include:

A. The need to participate in an agency orientation. Furthermore, the supervisee is to take the initiative to be familiar with the organization's policies and procedures (e.g., refer to operating and policy manuals).
B. Emergency and back-up procedures available 24 hours a day. Furthermore, the supervisor's accessibility and who to consult with on the staff when the supervisor is not available.
C. Expectations of when the supervisee is to contact the supervisor for clinical consult.
D. Awareness and adherence to the organization's and professional codes of practice.
E. Confidentiality regarding the nature of ALL information pertaining to client data (e.g., client records, discussing client cases with non-staff or with inappropriate staff, not allowed to take any client material off site, etc.).
F. Specific issues to be dealt with in situations where dual roles exist (e.g., one is both a supervisee and staff member of supervisor).
G. Utilization of sense of self in supervision (e.g., genogram, life history, etc.) and differentiation between supervision vs. therapy. Majority of code of ethics states clearly that personal counseling is not to be part of the supervision process.
H. Process for dealing with issues that relate to supervisee's personal issues which may/are interfering with delivery of service to clients (e.g., family of origin issues, burn-out, transference issues with supervisor, and counter-transference issues with clients).

VIII. Practical Issues

Discuss and document the following:

A. Supervision schedule, location and duration of meetings.
B. Duration of supervision (e.g., first and last day of supervision).
C. Role of other supervisors and supervisees in the supervision sessions (e.g., spectator, co-supervisor, reflecting teams).
D. Process for handling conflictual issues between supervisee-supervisor.
E. Statistical record keeping for agency purposes.
F. File management and storage.
G. How to job shadow, observe other sessions, etc.
H. Number of cases for which the supervisee will be responsible for and clients are obtained.
I. Responsibility of the supervisee to maintain an accurate journal of supervision hours she/he has received, the supervisor's written comments (formal) and a brief summary of each formal supervision session including observation/job shadow experiences.
J. Consent forms to be signed by each client to discuss the case in supervision.
K. The responsibility of the supervisee to ensure **prior** to supervision meetings that:

- Proper forms (e.g., consent forms for supervision, case review worksheets) are completed ahead of time.
- For each case, a list of questions to ask supervisor, and/or identified areas of needed support has been prepared
- A supervisor room has been booked and is set up (e.g., chairs arranged, do not disturb sign posted).
- All necessary equipment is set up and in working order (e.g., TV/VCR and/or cassette player is ready to play).
- The tapes have been viewed by the supervisee and are cued in advance.
- All necessary materials (e.g., case review forms, video-tapes) are present.
- If live observation: Supervisee has confirmed his/her attendance and the supervisee has back-up plans for supervision if the client does not appear for live supervision (e.g., tape of a previous session, case presentation, audio clips, etc.).

Winding Down:

- What do we need to know about each other that we have not already discussed?

- What, if any, questions do you have?
- What was it like for you completing this form? What things would you want to keep in mind when having to ask clients a series of questions, much like the format on this form?
- When should selected questions from this form be reviewed to assess compliance and/or update information?

Appendix B–Indications When to Alert Your Supervisor for Therapeutic Support, Feedback and/or Direction (McBride, 2006)[1, 2]

1. Any sudden or unexpected change for the worse in the client's psychological or physical status.
2. Client's overt expression of suicidal ideation and/or threats of harm (real or perceived).
3. Children who appear to be suffering significant neglect and/or are in danger of being abused physically or sexually.
4. When there is a threat of/or actual removal of the children from the home.
5. Behavior change in the client that may suggest potentially destructive behavior toward others (e.g., collecting pills, buying a gun, etc.) even when intent is denied.
6. Significant deterioration in the client's mood with increased depression and/or anxiety.
7. Stagnation in the therapeutic process, i.e., after a series of two to three sessions at reasonable intervals. And/or, the therapist and/or client are at an irresolvable impasse.
8. The therapist is uncertain as to the treatment plan and/or the agenda for the next session.
9. The therapist feels a need to debrief the case after a heavy session.
10. Suspect psychotic symptomatology in client (i.e., delusions, hallucinations, bizarre actions).
11. Suspicion of organicity (i.e., persistent change in personality, alertness, and/or mood).
12. The client requests to see another agency counselor or speak to a supervisor.

---

1. This list was created by initially drawing on the work of Wright, L., & Leahey, M. (1984). *Nurses and families: A guide to family assessment and intervention* (pp. 225-226). Philadelphia: F.A. Davis.

2. The events are not presented in any particular order. This list is not exhaustive. If you have encountered an event not listed on this handout that you believe justifies consulting a supervisor, then please contact your supervisor.

13. The client conveys dissatisfaction with the therapist or with the treatment offered.
14. The client refuses to continue attending sessions when further treatment appears desirable.
15. The client shows noticeable discomfort or expresses concern about videotaping and/or observation and as a result refuses to attend further sessions.
16. The client refuses to sign a release of information form and/or consent form for supervision.
17. When there appears a possibility of conflict within or outside the agency with regard to the client, personally, or with any political, medical, or social agency.
18. When there is a possibility of some legal encounter or you a request/order to participate in legal proceedings.
19. When the client is in therapy elsewhere and/or is accessing numerous therapists.
20. A case conference needs to be called and/or you have been invited to a case conference.
21. The client misses two consecutive individual sessions with or without notifying the therapist of the cancellations.
22. When the therapist anticipates and/or is in an ethical dilemma or conflict with the feedback received from another supervisor other than your own.
23. When you have received feedback from another supervisor that seems to be in conflict with that received from your own supervisor.
24. The file is ready to be closed (only about 2-3 sessions remaining)
25. The client requests to review their file and/or wants a copy of their file.
26. The file is ready to be closed.

References

Ackerman, S., & Hilsenroth, M. (2001). A review of therapist characteristics and techniques negatively impacting the therapeutic alliance. *Psychotherapy: Theory, Research, Practice, Training, 38*(2), 171-185.

Baron, R. (1998). *What type am I? Discover who you really are.* New York: Penguin Group.

Bernard, J. (1997). The discrimination model. In C. E. Watkins, Jr. (Ed.), *Handbook of psychotherapy supervision* (pp. 310-327). New York: Wiley.

Bradley, L., & Whiting, P. (2001). Supervision and training: A model. In L. J. Bradley & N. Ladany (Eds.), *Counselor supervision: Principles, process and practice* (3rd ed.), (pp. 361-387). Philadelphia: Brunner-Routledge.

Bradshaw, T., Butterworth, A., & Mairs, H. (2007). Does structured clinical supervision during psychosocial intervention education enhance outcome for mental health nurses and the service users they work with? *Journal of Psychiatric and Mental Health, 14*, 4-12.

Cormier, S., & Nurius, P. (2002). *Interviewing and change strategies for helpers: Fundamental skills and cognitive behavioral interventions* (5th ed.). Pacific Grove, CA: Brooks/Cole.
Costa, L. (1994). Reducing anxiety in supervision. *Counselor Education and Supervisor, 34*, 30-40.
Dutton, D. (1995). *The batterer: A psychological profile.* New York: Basic Books.
Edwards, D., Cooper, L., Burnard, P., Hanningan, B., Adams, J., Fothergill, A., & Coyle, D. (2005). Factors influencing the effectiveness of clinical supervision. *Journal of Psychiatric and Mental Health Nursing, 12*, 405-414.
Goodyear, R., & Nelson, M. (1997). The major formats of psychotherapy supervision. In C. Watkins (Ed.), *Handbook of psychotherapy supervision* (pp. 328-344). New York: John Wiley & Sons, Inc.
Haber, R. (1996). *Dimensions of psychotherapy supervision.* New York: W.W. Norton & Company.
Hahn, W. (2001). The experience of shame in psychotherapy supervision. *Psychotherapy: Theory, Research, Practice, Training, 38*(3), 272-282.
Hammer, A. (1993). *Introduction to type and careers.* Palo Alto, CA: Consulting Psychologists.
Hawkins, P., & Shohet, R. (1989). *Supervision in the helping professions.* Philadelphia: Open University Press.
Herman, J. (1997). *Trauma and recovery.* New York: Basic Books.
Lindblad-Goldberg, M. (1996). Forward. In R. Haber, *Dimensions of psychotherapy supervision: Maps and means* (pp. vii-viii). New York: W.W. Norton & Company.
Loganbill, C., Hardy, E., & Delworth, U. (1982). Supervision: A conceptual model. *The Counseling Psychologist, 10*(1), 3-42.
McCann, I., & Pearlman, L. (1990). Vicarious traumatization: A framework for understanding the psychological effects of working with victims. *Journal of Traumatic Stress, 3*, 131-149.
Myers, I., McCauley, M., Quenk, N., & Hammer, A. (1998). *MBTI manual: A guide to the development and the use of the Myers-Briggs Type Indicator* (3rd ed.). Palo Alto, CA: Consulting Psychologists.
McBride, D. (2006). *Indications when to alert your supervisor for therapeutic support, feedback and/or direction.* Unpublished paper, Zayed University, United Arab Emirates.
McBride, D. (2007). *Education 719: Counselling practicum 1998 guidebook, revisions 2007.* Terrace, Canada: University of Northern British Columbia, Department of Education.
Nelson, M., Johnson, P., & Thorngren, J. (2000). An integrated approach for supervising mental health counseling interns. *Journal of Mental Health Counseling, 22*(1), 1-9. Retrieved February 2, 2007, from the PsycINFO database.
Pearlman, L., & Saakvitne, K. (1995). *Trauma and the therapist.* New York: W.W. Norton & Company.
Pearson, Q. (2006). Psychotherapy-driven supervision: Integrating counseling theories into role-based supervision. *Journal of Mental Health Counseling, 28*(3), 241-252. Retrieved January 22, 2007, from the PsycINFO database.
Pearson, Q. (2001). A case in clinical supervision: A framework for putting theory into practice. *Journal of Mental Health Counseling, 23*(2), 174-183. Retrieved February 6, 2007, from the PsycINFO database.
Personal Style Inventory. (n.d.). Retrieved January 22, 2007 from http://home.ica.net/~oyar/perstype.pdf
Powell, D. (2004). *Clinical supervision in alcohol and drug abuse counseling: Principles, models, methods.* San Francisco, CA: Jossey-Bass.
Prest, L., Schindleer-Zimmerman, T., & Sporakowski, M. (1992). The initial supervision session checklist (ISSC): A guide for the MFT supervision process. *The Clinical Supervisor, 10*(2), 117-133.

Roller, B., & Nelson, V. (1991). *The art of co-therapy: How therapists work together.* New York: Guilford Press.

Ramos-Sanchez, L., Esnil, E., Goodwin, A., Riggs, S., Touster, L.O., Wright, L.K., Ratanasiripong, P., & Rodolfa, E. (2002). Negative supervisory events: Effects on supervision satisfaction, and supervisory alliance. *Professional Psychology: Research and Practice, 33,* 197-202.

Rothschild, B. (2002). The dangers of empathy: Understanding the keys to vicarious traumatization. *Psychotherapy Networker, July/August,* 61-65.

Saakvitne, K., Gamble, S., Pearlman, L., & Lev, B. T. (2000). *Risking connection: A training curriculum for working with survivors of childhood abuse.* Lutherville, MD: Sidran Foundation.

Saakvitne, K., & Pearlman, L. (1996). *Transforming the pain: A workbook on vicarious traumatization.* New York: W.W. Norton.

Stoltenberg, C., & Delworth, U. (1987). *Supervising counselors and therapists: A developmental approach.* San Francisco: Jossey-Bass.

Toth, M. (2004). Dealing with fear of failure: Working with script concepts in the classroom. *Transactional Analysis Journal, 34*(3), 209-215.

Worthington, E. (1987). Changes in supervision as counselors and supervisors gain experience: A review. *Professional Psychology: Research and Review, 18*(3), 189-208.

Worthington, E., & Roehlke, H. (1979). Effective supervision as perceived by beginning counselors-in-training. *Journal of Counseling Psychology, 26*(1), 64-73.

Biography

Dawn Lorraine McBride, is a registered psychologist and an assistant professor in graduate counselor education at the University of Lethbridge, Canada. The prevention, assessment, and treatment of family violence is one of her main areas of research and clinical interest. For nearly ten years, Dawn worked at a large family violence treatment centre/emergency shelter that provided counseling to men, women, adolescents, and children who were the perpetrators, victims, or witnesses to abuse. At this centre, she held various positions including outreach coordinator, specialist therapist for difficult cases, clinical supervisor, and program manager. She designed and taught one of the first undergraduate and graduate level family violence assessment and treatment courses in Canada. Dawn has held teaching positions in the Middle East (Gulf Region) as well as presented at numerous international conferences. She has recently finished co-editing a book on learning and teaching across cultures in higher education. She also has a private practice specializing in mental health issues. You are welcome to contact the author at dawnm@apmcomp.com

NAME INDEX

C

D

E

F

G

J

K

L

M

N

O

P

SUBJECT INDEX